Atlas of
NORMAL *and* VARIANT
ANGIOGRAPHIC ANATOMY

Atlas of NORMAL and VARIANT ANGIOGRAPHIC ANATOMY

SAADOON KADIR, M.D.

Professor of Radiology,
Duke University School of Medicine;
Chief, Section of Interventional and Vascular Radiology,
Duke University Medical Center,
Durham, North Carolina

1991

W.B. SAUNDERS COMPANY *Philadelphia, London, Toronto, Montreal, Sydney, Tokyo*

Harcourt Brace Jovanovich, Inc.

W. B. SAUNDERS COMPANY
Harcourt Brace Jovanovich, Inc.

The Curtis Center
Independence Square West
Philadelphia, PA 19106

Library of Congress Cataloging-in-Publication Data

Kadir, Saadoon.

Atlas of normal and variant angiographic anatomy /
Saadoon Kadir.
    p.   cm.
ISBN 0–7216–2894–X
1. Angiography—Atlases.   2. Blood vessels—Atlases.
    I. Title.   [DNLM: 1. Angiography—atlases.
    WG 17 K113a]
RC691.6.A53K3 1991   611′.13′0222—dc20
DNLM/DLC   90–8144

Sponsoring Editor: Lisette Bralow
Manuscript Editor: Donna Walker
Production Manager: Frank Polizzano
Illustration Coordinator and Page Layout Artist: Joan Sinclair
Indexer: Julie Figures

Atlas of Normal and Variant Angiographic Anatomy   ISBN 0–7216–2894–X

Printed in the United States of America.

Last digit is the print number: 9   8   7   6   5   4   3   2   1

CONTRIBUTORS

MICHAEL F. BROTHERS, M.D., F.R.C.P.(C)

Assistant Professor of Radiology, Duke University School of Medicine; Staff Neuro-radiologist, Duke University Medical Center, Durham, North Carolina

Neurovascular Anatomy

CHRISTIAN DELCOUR, M.D.

Associate Professor of Radiology, Université Libre de Bruxelles; Department of Radiology, Hôpital Erasme, Université de Bruxelles, Brussels, Belgium

The Penile and Uterine Vessels

SAADOON KADIR, M.D.

Professor of Radiology, Duke University School of Medicine; Chief, Section of Interventional and Vascular Radiology, Duke University Medical Center, Durham, North Carolina

Regional Anatomy of the Thoracic Aorta; Arterial Anatomy of the Upper Exremities; Abdominal Aorta and Pelvis; Arterial Anatomy of the Lower Extremities; Superior Vena Cava and Thoracic Veins; Upper Extremity Veins; Inferior Vena Cava and Spinal Veins; Lower Extremities and Pelvis; Pulmonary Artery and Venous Anatomy; Gonadal Vessels; The Penile and Uterine Vessels; Celiac, Superior, and Inferior Mesenteric Arteries; The Portal Venous System and Hepatic Veins; Kidneys; Lymph Vessels and Nodes

CAROLINE LUNDELL, M.D.

Clinical Assistant Professor of Radiology, University of Southern California; Staff Radiologist, City of Hope National Medical Center, Duarte, California

Superior Vena Cava and Thoracic Veins; Upper Extremity Veins; Inferior Vena Cava and Spinal Veins; Lower Extremities and Pelvis; Celiac, Superior, and Inferior Mesenteric Arteries; The Portal Venous System and Hepatic Veins; Lymph Vessels and Nodes

BENT MADSEN, M.D.

Docent, University of Aarhus; Chairman, Department of Diagnostic Radiology, Kommune Hospitalet, Aarhus, Denmark

Adrenals

STEPHEN W. MILLER, M.D.

Associate Professor of Radiology, Harvard Medical School; Staff Radiologist, Massachusetts General Hospital, Boston, Massachusetts

Angiographic Anatomy of the Heart

WILLIAM PROTZER, M.D.

Associate, Neuroradiology Section, Duke University Medical Center, Durham, North Carolina

Neurovascular Anatomy

STEVEN C. ROSE, M.D.

Assistant Professor of Radiology, Department of Radiology, University of Utah Medical Center, Salt Lake City, Utah

Arterial Anatomy of the Upper Extremities

MOHSIN SAEED, M.D.

Assistant Clinical Professor of Radiology, UCSD School of Medicine; Staff Physician, Vascular and Interventional Radiology, Scripps Clinic and Research Foundation, La Jolla, California

Celiac, Superior, and Inferior Mesenteric Arteries

ACKNOWLEDGMENTS

We gratefully acknowledge the invaluable help and contributions of our editorial secretary Catherine Manning, the artists Sarah McQueen and Nancy Marshburn, and Drs. William Jones, Marshall Brewer, Nepper Rasmussen, Fred Keller, Carl F. Beckmann, B. K. Janevski, and John Doppman for providing illustrations. The logo was graciously prepared by Ayesha Kadir. We also thank the W. B. Saunders team: Lisette Bralow, senior medical editor, and Lorraine Kilmer, Frank Polizzano, Joan Sinclair, and Edna Dick.

PREFACE

Knowledge of the normal and variant anatomy forms the basis for the interpretation of vascular radiologic studies. The vascular anatomy of the trunk and extremities in anatomic textbooks generally depicts idealized illustrations based on cadaver studies. Consequently, the angiographic appearance frequently differs from that seen in anatomy textbooks and atlases. In addition, variant anatomy is very common.

As the applications of interventional radiologic techniques for the management of disease involving both the large as well as the smaller vessels, microvascular surgical techniques, and the like become more widespread, there is an increasing need for an atlas of angiograms illustrating normal and variant vascular anatomy as seen on in vivo angiographic studies. We hope that the first edition of the "Atlas of Normal and Variant Angiographic Anatomy" will be useful not only for those involved in the management of vascular diseases, i.e., interventional radiologists and surgeons, but also other individuals involved in the study of anatomy, i.e., medical students and radiology and surgery residents.

CONTENTS

Section I

ARTERIAL SYSTEM OF THE TRUNK AND EXTREMITIES

Chapter One

ANGIOGRAPHIC ANATOMY OF THE HEART

STEPHEN W. MILLER, M.D.

Angiographic visualization of the anatomy of the coronary arteries, cardiac chambers, and valves depends on a number of factors, including the proper choice of projection for the particular structure in question, because the resultant image is not tomographic, but a projection silhouette. Factors such as film quality, injection rates, and catheter selection obviously contribute to the quality of the angiographic image. Since the axis of the heart is usually in a leftward, anterior, and inferior direction, compound angulation is necessary to align the x-ray beam with various cardiac structures. Therefore, most cardiac angiography is performed not only in right or left anterior oblique projections but also with the image intensifier in a cranial or caudal position.

THE CORONARY ARTERIES

The right coronary artery originates from the right sinus of Valsalva at an angle varying from roughly 10 to 30 degrees to the right of the sternum. The ostium usually is in the upper third or upper half of the sinus but can be in other parts of the sinus or even above or rarely below the sinus. In bicuspid aortic valve stenosis, in which the heart is horizontal because of left ventricular hypertrophy, the right coronary ostium is directly inferior in the anterior sinus. In most normal hearts, the proximal right coronary artery is horizontal and lies beneath the right atrial appendage in the right atrioventricular groove. In the left anterior oblique view, the right coronary artery has the shape of the letter C and can be subjectively divided into proximal, middle, and distal segments (Figs. 1–1 and 1–2).

The first ventricular branch of the right coronary artery is the conus artery; in many persons this artery has a separate origin from the sinus of Valsalva and therefore is not seen during selective right coronary injection. The conus artery lies on the surface of the right ventricular conus or infundibulum and typically has three distal branches that give it a pitchfork appearance (Fig. 1–3). Right ventricular branches from the middle part of the right coronary artery are called marginal branches and are numbered as they appear distally with the artery—for example, the first, second, etc., right ventricular marginal artery. A common variation is to have a large right ventricular marginal artery near the diaphragm (the acute margin of the heart), and this artery may be called the acute right ventricular marginal artery. This particular branch may continue and give off septal branches as an accessory posterior descending artery.

The sinoatrial nodal artery originates from the proximal part of the right coronary artery in about half of all angiograms. This artery goes posterior to the right atrial wall to end by encircling the superior vena cava at its right atrial junction.

The distal right coronary artery ends by dividing into the posterior descending and posterior left ventricular arteries (Fig. 1–4). The posterior descending artery runs in the inferior interventricular sulcus and is identified by its 1 to 2 cm septal branches, which originate perpendicularly to supply the inferior third of the interventricular septum. The artery that supplies the posterior descending artery is the "dominant" artery. Roughly 80 per cent of subjects have a right dominant coronary artery, and 10 per cent have a left dominant coronary vascular tree, which means that the posterior descending artery comes from the left circumflex artery (Fig. 1–5). The remaining 10 per cent are "codominant," with the posterior descending artery coming from the right coronary artery and the posterior left ventricular artery coming from the left circumflex artery. The posterior left ventricular artery typically consists of a number of branches over the posterolateral left ventricular wall. When this artery is large, the connecting segment between the posterior descending artery and the terminal posterolateral branches is occasionally called the posterolateral left ventricular artery. This segment is frequently marked by a U bend at the crux of the heart. This U bend may be present also when the posterior left ventricular artery comes from the left circumflex artery. The atrioventricular nodal artery originates near this U bend to go superiorly about 1 cm to the atrioventricular node (see Fig. 1–4).

The left main coronary artery originates from the left sinus of Valsalva and ends by bifurcating into the left anterior descending and left circumflex arteries. Occasionally a trifurcation exists in which the middle artery is called an intermediate artery or a ramus medianus. The left main coronary artery is distinctive in that it does not taper; however, its ostium occasionally may have a slight funnel shape. The left main coronary artery lies in a line about 25 degrees posterior to the coronal plane of the aorta. This segment usually is horizontal but may vary from a completely vertical path to a 20-degree inferior path when the heart is vertically oriented.

The left anterior descending artery has epicardial branches over the anterolateral wall of the left ventricle, named diagonal arteries, and septal branches to the interventricular septum (Figs. 1–6 to 1–8). The first septal branch is frequently larger than the others and may itself divide to have multiple tiny branches in the anterior part of the septum. As the left anterior descending artery may occasionally be difficult to identify, the following features are helpful in locating this unique artery: (1) Septal branches originate in a nearly perpendicular direction and are found throughout the length of this artery. Rarely, septal branches can come from a diagonal or circumflex marginal artery near the base of the heart. (2) The anterior descending artery typically terminates in a characteristic inverted Y, with one tiny branch going to the right ventricular side of the septum and the other branch to the left ventricular side. (3) The anterior descending artery usually, but not always, is the longest artery going to the apex. (4) In the right anterior oblique view, the left anterior descending artery is not border-forming except on a near lateral or in a caudal projection.

The left circumflex artery runs in the left atrioventricular groove and typically terminates in a vestigial twig about halfway down this groove. The major branches are called left circumflex marginal arteries and are numbered first, second, etc., depending on the number of branches present. If a major left circumflex marginal artery exists near the diaphragmatic surface, it may be called an obtuse marginal branch. When a left dominant coronary tree is present, the left circumflex artery ends by dividing into a left posterior descending artery and usually several small posterior left ventricular branches (Fig. 1–9).

Atrial branches of the left circumflex artery run posteriorly and are easily identified not only by their direction but also by their motion, which is opposite to the circumflex marginal arteries over the ventricle. About half of coronary angiograms show the sinoatrial nodal artery originating from the left circumflex artery, whereas the other half have this artery coming from the proximal right coronary artery.

Delayed filming is useful to show the coronary sinus (Fig. 1–10), which marks the atrial side of the left atrioventricular groove and is a landmark for the main left circumflex artery position.

Great variability is present in the termination of the right coronary, left anterior descending, and left circumflex arteries. The left anterior descending artery may go around the apex to supply half or all of the inferior septum with additional septal branches. When this occurs, the posterior descending artery from either the right coronary or left circumflex arteries is vestigial. On the other hand, the posterior descending artery may go around the apex to supply part of the anterior interventricular septum with a correspondingly small left anterior descending artery. The posterior left ventricular branches from a dominant right coronary artery may supply a major part of the posterolateral left ventricular wall, with a reciprocal diminution in left circumflex artery size. When the left coronary artery is dominant, the right coronary artery is quite small and may not go to the acute margin of the heart.

THE RIGHT AND LEFT VENTRICLES

Ventricular angiography is performed with biplane right and left anterior oblique projections with cranial angulation in the left anterior oblique view. Atrial angiography is not performed except in the evaluation of congenital heart disease and will not be discussed.

The right ventricle consists of three parts—the inlet segment, the body, and the outlet segment (Fig. 1–11). The inlet or inflow region contains the tricuspid valve, its annulus, and papillary muscles. The anterior, posterior, and septal leaflets of the tricuspid valve are difficult to separate angiographically in the normal heart and are therefore viewed as a unit. The body of the right ventricle has thick, coarse trabeculations. The moderator band is much thicker than most of the trabeculations and runs obliquely leftward and inferior toward the apex. The walls of the right ventricle in the right anterior oblique view include the anteroseptal, apical, and diaphragmatic segments. In the left anterior oblique view, the right ventricular septum and anterior or free wall are profiled. The outflow region of the right ventricle is the conus or infundibulum, which is cylindrical and not trabeculated. The pulmonary valve is considered a part of the pulmonary artery, not the right ventricle. The septal and parietal bands form the lateral and medial walls of the conus on a posteroanterior angiogram. This conal segment is a unique landmark to distinguish the right from left ventricle and is a muscular, contracting segment between the atrioventricular and semilunar valves.

The left ventricle also consists of an inlet segment and body (Fig. 1–12). The naming of the subaortic region as an outlet segment is probably incorrect embryologically but is commonly used in clinical analysis. The walls of the left ventricle in the right anterior oblique view include the apex, anterolateral, and diaphragmatic segments and also the anterior and posterior basal walls near the aortic and mitral valves, respectively. On the left anterior oblique view, the septum occasionally can be separated into a basal and an apical portion. The posterolateral and superior lateral walls comprise the free wall segments on the projection image.

A major feature of the left ventricle is the continuity of the aortic and mitral valves; there is no muscle between the aortic valve and the mitral annulus. In diastole, the left ventricular wall is smooth with minimal trabecu-

TABLE 1–1. Angiographic Characteristics of the Cardiac Chambers*

Right atrium
Connects with the inferior vena cava
Has an appendage with a broad opening
Receives thebesian veins
Has a roughly cylindrical shape except for the inflow region of the tricuspid valve
Crista terminalis and pectinate muscles
Lies on the same side as the trilobed lung and liver and on the opposite side from the stomach
(Connects with the superior vena cava)
(Connects with the coronary sinus)

Left atrium
Has an ellipsoidal shape
Lies in the midline or slightly to the side of the bilobal lung
Has a smooth wall except for the appendage
Has a slender appendage with a narrow opening
(Connects with the pulmonary veins)

Right ventricle
Has a triangular shape on the posteroanterior view and a crescentic shape on the lateral view
Coarse, deep trabeculations, including the septum
Conus (crista supraventricularis) between the tricuspid and pulmonary valves
Tricuspid atrioventricular valve
Occasionally a well-defined septal papillary muscle (moderator band)

Left ventricle
Has an oval shape in diastole (in most projections)
Fine, shallow trabeculations
Mitral-aortic continuity (absence of a subaortic conus)
Bicuspid atrioventricular valve
Absence of septal papillary muscles; smooth septal surface
(Usually two well-defined papillary muscles on the free wall)

*These features are usually found in normal hearts. Those in parentheses may be lacking if congenital anomalies are present. Some characteristics need modification if congenital heart disease is present; e.g., in transposition of the great vessels, there is mitral-pulmonary continuity in the left ventricle.

lations, in contrast to the right ventricle. The anterolateral and posteromedial papillary muscles (Fig. 1–13) are visible in systole and occasionally in diastole. These muscles are easily distinguished from thrombi and tumor because they shorten in length and expand in a radial direction during systole.

The aortic valve is considered part of the aorta (Fig. 1–14). Its three sinuses of Valsalva are named according to the relation of the coronary arteries—the left, right, and noncoronary sinus. The posterior noncoronary sinus is always inferior to the other two sinuses.

The mitral valve (Fig. 1–15) consists of the mitral annulus, leaflets, chordae tendineae, papillary muscles, and adjacent left ventricular wall. The mitral leaflets are easily seen by angiography, but echocardiography remains the preferred imaging modality. The anterior or septal leaflet of the mitral valve is profiled in both right and left anterior oblique projections and is a leaflet that involves about one third of the mitral circumference. This leaflet generally has no scallops and appears as a straight border when seen in systole in the right oblique projection or open in diastole in the left anterior oblique projection. The posterior mitral leaflet typically has a small posterior scallop that is seen angiographically and an anterior scallop that is not. This leaflet, which comprises two thirds of the mitral circumference, is projected through the angiographic contrast material in the right anterior oblique view and is profiled in the left anterior oblique projection. The chordae are poorly seen by angiography.

The angiographic features of the four heart chambers are summarized in Table 1–1.

REFERENCES

1. Baltaxe HA, Amplatz K, Levin DC: Coronary Angiography. Springfield, IL, Charles C Thomas, 1973.
2. Baltaxe HA, Wixson D: The incidence of congenital anomalies of the coronary arteries in the adult population. Radiology 122:47–52, 1977.
3. James TN: Anatomy of the Coronary Arteries. Hagerstown, MD, Harper & Row, 1961.
4. Keith JD: The anomalous origin of the left coronary artery from the pulmonary artery. Br Heart J 21:149–161, 1959.
5. Kimbiris D, Iskandrian AS, Segal BL, et al: Anomalous aortic origin of coronary arteries. Circulation 58:606–615, 1978.
6. Liberthson RR, Dinsmore RE, Fallon JT: Aberrant coronary artery origin from the aorta: Report of 18 patients, review of literature and delineation of natural history and management. Circulation 59:748–754, 1979.
7. Lipton MJ, Barry WA, Obrez I, et al: Isolated single coronary artery: Diagnosis, angiographic classification and clinical significance. Radiology 130:39–47, 1979.
8. Miller SW: Cardiac Angiography. Boston, Little Brown & Company, 1984.
9. Ogden JA: Congenital anomalies of the coronary arteries. Am J Cardiol 25:474–479, 1970.
10. Soto B, Russell RO Jr, Moraski RE: Radiographic Anatomy of the Coronary Arteries: An Atlas. Mount Kisco, NY, Futura Publishing, 1976.
11. Talner NS, Halloran KH, Mahdavy M, et al: Anomalous origin of the left coronary artery from the pulmonary artery. A clinical spectrum. Am J Cardiol 15:689–695, 1965.
12. von Ludinghausen M: Clinical anatomy of cardiac veins: Vv cardiacae. Surg Radiol Anat 9:159–168, 1987.
13. Wesselhoeft H, Fawcett JS, Johnson AL: Anomalous origin of the left coronary artery from the pulmonary trunk. Its clinical spectrum, pathology and pathophysiology based on a review of 140 cases with seven further cases. Circulation 38:403–425, 1968.

Figures 1–1 through 1–15 on following pages.

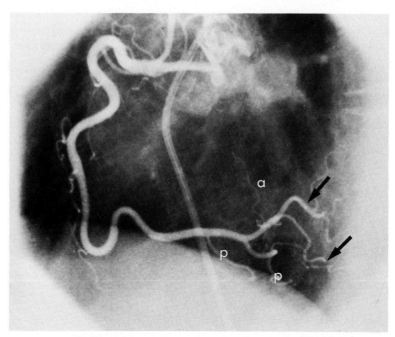

Figure 1–1. Right coronary artery. In the left anterior oblique projection, the right coronary artery projects as a C shape with proximal, middle, and distal segments. This artery has two small posterior descending arteries (p), an atrioventricular nodal artery (a), and two posterior left ventricular arteries *(arrows)*.

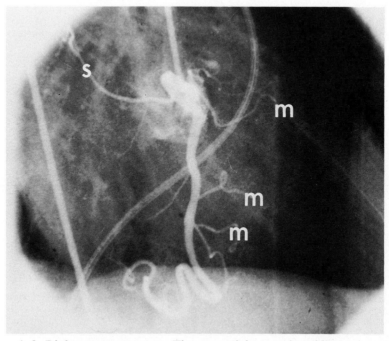

Figure 1–2. Right coronary artery. The steep right anterior oblique view shows mainly the middle segment, as the proximal part is end-on by the tip of the catheter. The distal segment, as seen in Figure 1–1, is tortuous and so hides the posterior descending artery. Right ventricular marginal branches (m) go anterior and the sinoatrial nodal artery (s) goes posterior to the right coronary artery, which is in the right atrioventricular groove.

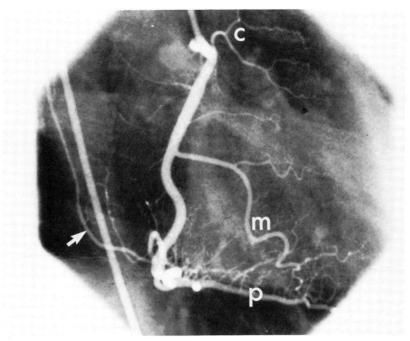

Figure 1–3. Right coronary artery branches. The conus artery (c) in the right anterior oblique view travels above the right coronary ostium and is the epicardial artery over the right ventricular conus. Distal branches are a right ventricular marginal artery (m) and the posterior descending artery (p). The main posterior left ventricular artery *(arrow)* is unusually long in the left atrioventricular groove.

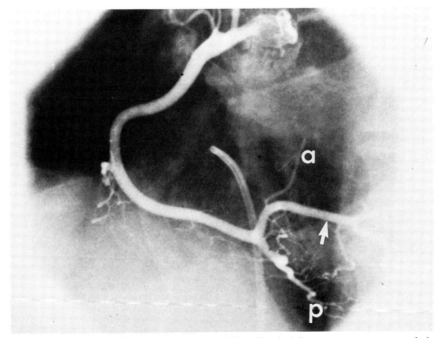

Figure 1–4. Distal right coronary artery. The distal right coronary artery ends by dividing into the posterior descending artery (p) with its tiny septal branches and the posterior left ventricular artery *(arrow)*. The atrioventricular nodal artery (a) originates at the U bend of the posterior left ventricular artery and serves as a marker for that artery.

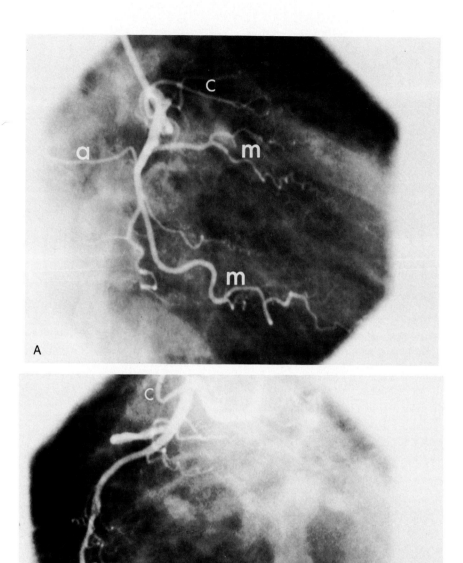

Figure 1–5. Nondominant right coronary artery. *A*, The right and *B*, left anterior oblique angiograms reveal that only the proximal and middle segments of the right coronary artery are present. The posterior descending and posterior left ventricular branches come from the left circumflex artery. The conus artery (c), a right atrial branch (a), and right ventricular marginal branches (m) supply the proximal right atrium and ventricle.

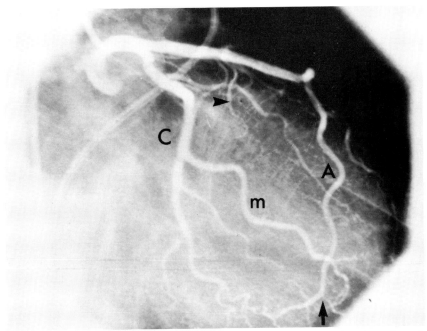

Figure 1–6. Left coronary artery. The left main artery divides after 1 cm into the left anterior descending (A) and left circumflex (C) arteries in this caudal right anterior oblique view. The left anterior descending artery has tiny perpendicular septal branches *(arrowhead)* and terminates in a characteristic inverted Y *(arrow)*. Circumflex marginal arteries (m) supply the lateral left ventricular wall.

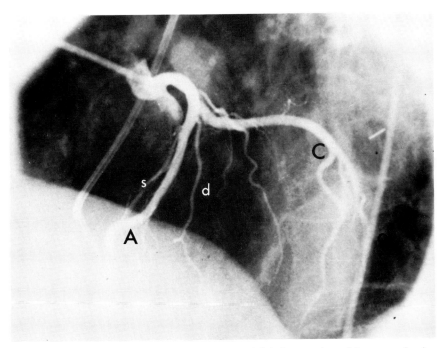

Figure 1–7. Left coronary artery. The cranial left anterior oblique projection separates the bifurcation of the left anterior descending (A) and left circumflex (C) arteries. Septal (s) and diagonal (d) arteries arise from the left anterior descending artery.

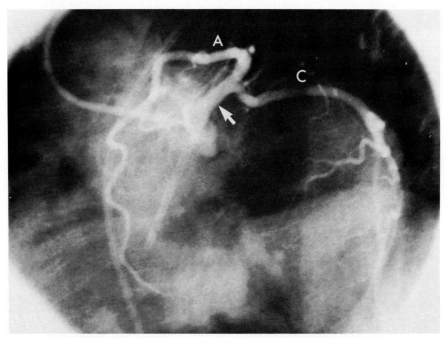

Figure 1–8. Left coronary artery. The caudally angled left anterior oblique projection is designed to show the left main artery *(arrow)* and proximal left circumflex artery (C). Left anterior descending artery (A).

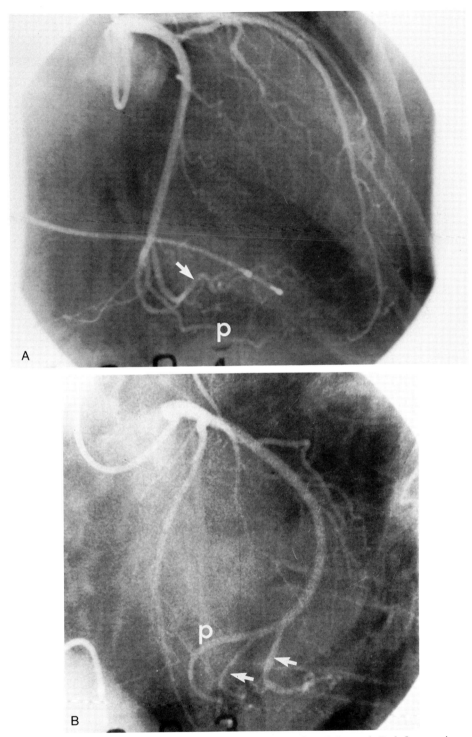

Figure 1–9. Left dominant coronary artery. *A,* The right and *B,* left anterior oblique views illustrate the left circumflex artery terminally dividing into a posterior descending branch (p) and posterior left ventricular branches *(arrows).*

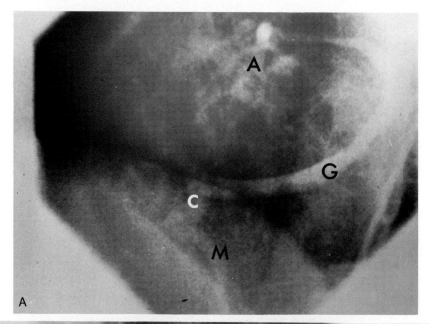

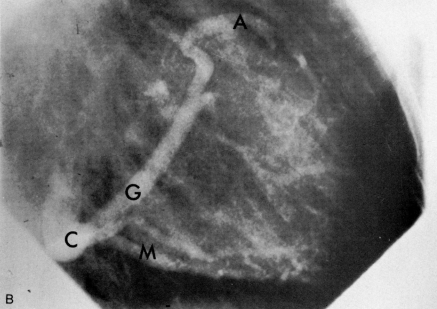

Figure 1–10. Coronary sinus and tributaries. The venous phase of a left coronary angiogram. *A,* Left and *B,* right anterior oblique projections show that the great cardiac vein (G) and the middle cardiac vein (M) join to form the coronary sinus (C). Other marginal veins drain into the great cardiac vein. The anterior interventricular vein (A) runs beside the left anterior descending artery, and the middle cardiac vein lies beside the posterior descending artery.

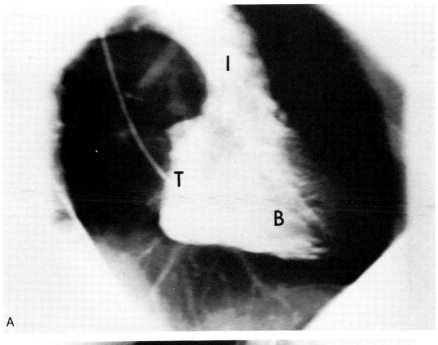

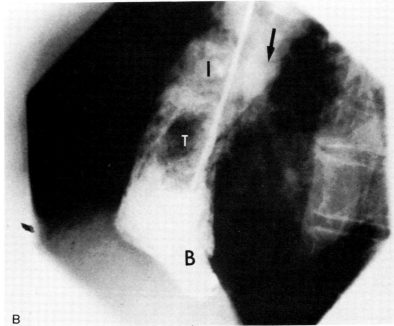

Figure 1–11. Right ventricle. *A,* The right and *B,* left anterior oblique views show the three parts of the right ventricle: the body (B), the tricuspid valve (T), and the cylindrical infundibulum (I). The closed pulmonary valve *(arrow)* is faintly seen in diastole.

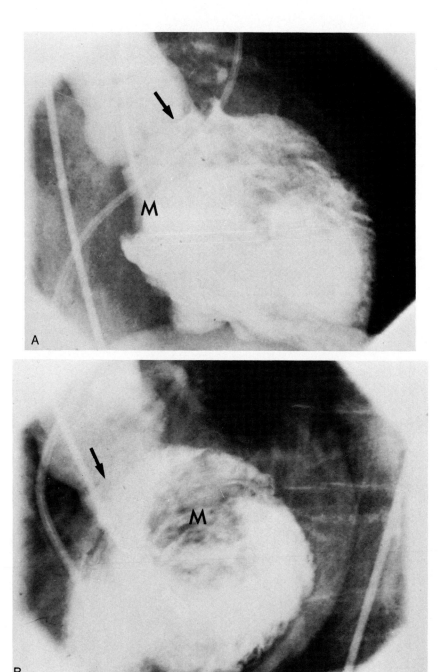

Figure 1–12. Left ventricle. *A,* The right anterior oblique view in diastole shows the aortic valve *(arrow)*, mitral valve (M), and the smooth wall body of the ventricle. *B,* The left anterior oblique view shows the open mitral valve in diastole.

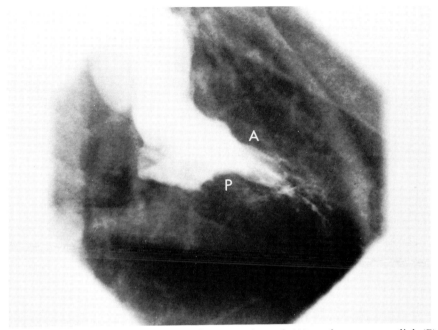

Figure 1–13. Papillary muscles. The anterolateral (A) and posteromedial (P) papillary muscles are usually visible in systole.

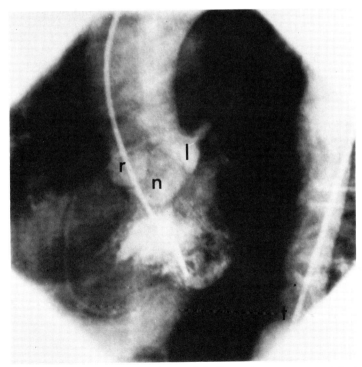

Figure 1–14. Aortic valve. The right (r), left (l), and noncoronary (n) sinuses of Valsalva with the leaflets open in diastole are named by their adjacent coronary arteries.

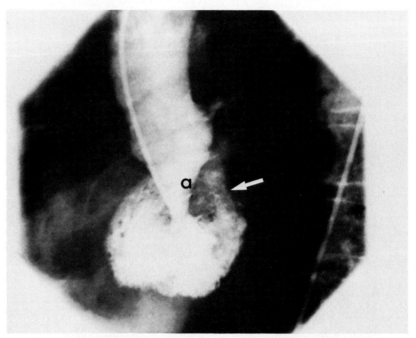

Figure 1–15. Mitral valve. The open mitral valve in diastole shows the anterior (a) leaflet immediately below the aortic valve. The posterior leaflet is not seen, but the posterior part of the mitral annulus *(arrow)* forms the back wall of the ventricle.

Chapter Two

REGIONAL ANATOMY OF THE THORACIC AORTA

SAADOON KADIR, M.D.

EMBRYOLOGY (Fig. 2–1)

The two ventral aortae fuse to form the aortic sac. The dorsal aortae fuse to form the midline descending aorta. Six paired aortic arches develop between the ventral and dorsal aortae. In addition, the dorsal aorta gives off several intersegmental arteries.

The vessels derived from each arch are as follows:

First pair: Contribute to formation of the maxillary and external carotid arteries.

Second pair: Contribute to formation of the stapedial arteries.

Third pair: Proximal segments form the common carotid arteries. Together with segments of the dorsal aortae, the distal portions contribute to formation of the internal carotid arteries.

Fourth pair: The left 4th arch forms the segment of normal left aortic arch between the left common carotid and subclavian arteries.

The right 4th arch forms the proximal right subclavian artery. The distal right subclavian artery is derived from a portion of the right dorsal aorta and the right 7th intersegmental artery.

Fifth pair: Rudimentary vessels that regress early.

Sixth pair: The left 6th arch contributes to the formation of the main and left pulmonary arteries and ductus arteriosus.

The right 6th arch contributes to formation of the right pulmonary artery.

19

With the caudad migration of the heart in the second fetal month, the 7th intersegmental arteries enlarge and migrate cephalad to form the distal subclavian arteries. The left subclavian artery is derived entirely from the left 7th intersegmental artery, while the portions of the right are derived from the right 4th arch and the right dorsal aorta. Malformations of the aortic arch system can be explained by persistence of segments of the aortic arches that normally regress or disappearance of segments that normally remain, or both.

NORMAL ANATOMY (Figs. 2–2 and 2–3)

Regression of the right dorsal aortic root (between the right subclavian artery and the descending aorta) and the right ductus arteriosus leaves the normal left aortic arch. The classic left aortic arch and descending thoracic aorta are seen in approximately 70 per cent of individuals. The three main branches of the aortic arch are (1) the brachiocephalic (innominate) artery; this is usually 3 to 4 cm in length and divides into the right subclavian and common carotid arteries; (2) left common carotid artery; (3) left subclavian artery, the last branch of the aortic arch.

VARIANT ANATOMY OF THE AORTIC ARCH (Figs. 2–4 to 2–6)

The most common variant is a common origin of the brachiocephalic and left common carotid arteries. This occurs in 22 per cent of individuals and accounts for 73 per cent of all arch vessel anomalies. The remaining anomalies of the main branches are shown in Figure 2–4 and account for less than 3 per cent of arch vessel anomalies.

Left Vertebral Artery from the Aortic Arch (Figs. 2–6, 2–7, and 2–10)

This occurs in 6 per cent of individuals and accounts for approximately 14 per cent of arch vessel anomalies. The most frequent location is between the left common carotid and subclavian arteries. Rarely (less than 1 per cent), the proximal left vertebral artery is duplicated or has a bifid origin. In this case, one part arises from the arch and the other from the left subclavian, or both originate from the aortic arch. Occasionally it is the last branch of the aortic arch, after the left subclavian artery (less than 1 per cent of the general population).

Thyroid Ima Artery (Fig. 2–8)

This vessel occurs in 6 per cent of individuals. In approximately 1 per cent it is a branch of the aortic arch between the brachiocephalic and left subclavian arteries. In approximately 3 per cent it is a branch of the brachiocephalic artery, in 1 per cent it is a branch of the right common carotid artery, and in the remainder it may originate from the internal mammary, subclavian, or inferior thyroid arteries.

Aberrant Right Subclavian or Brachiocephalic Artery

(Figs. 2–9 and 2–10)

The right subclavian artery is the last branch of the aortic arch in approximately 1 per cent of individuals. It courses to the right behind the esophagus in 80 per cent of individuals, between the esophagus and trachea in 15 per cent, and anterior to the trachea or mainstem bronchus in 5 per cent of individuals. The aberrant right brachiocephalic artery is rare.

Right Aortic Arch (Fig. 2–9)

This results from the persistence of the right fourth branchial arch. The most common type is the right aortic arch with an aberrant left subclavian artery. The vessels originate in the following order: left common carotid, right common carotid, right subclavian, and left subclavian artery. This type is rarely associated with congenital heart disease. The mirror image type (left brachiocephalic trunk, right common carotid and subclavian arteries) is almost always associated with congenital heart disease, especially the cyanotic type.

Ductus Diverticulum (Figs. 2–5 and 2–11)

This is a fusiform dilatation of the ventromedial portion of the proximal descending thoracic aorta. It represents the most distal segment of the embryonic right arch. The typical and variant angiographic appearances are shown in Figure 2–11.

Miscellaneous Variants and Anomalies (Figs. 2–12 to 2–14)

The double aortic arch is a rare anomaly caused by persistence (to varying degrees) of the fetal double aortic arch system. It is rarely associated with intracardiac defects. The ascending aorta divides into two arches that pass to either side of the esophagus and trachea and reunite to form the descending aorta. The descending aorta is usually on the left side. Most commonly, one arch is dominant, whereas the other may be of small caliber or represented by a fibrous band.

The cervical aortic arch refers to an unusually high location of the aortic arch in the low or mid neck region. There is no association with congenital heart disease, and the anomaly occurs most frequently in association with a right aortic arch. This is also a rare anomaly.

Variations in the sequence of branching of the major arch vessels also occur rarely (less than 0.5 per cent). For example, the left subclavian artery may be the second branch (before the left common carotid), or the internal and external carotid arteries may originate independently from the aortic arch.

DESCENDING THORACIC AORTA

Intercostal and Subcostal Arteries (Figs. 2–15 and 2–16)

The anterior intercostal arteries arise from the internal mammary artery (Fig. 2–15). In 95 per cent of cases, the first, second, and third posterior intercostal arteries originate from the superior intercostal artery, which is a branch of the costocervical trunk. The frequency and variation of the origins of the first through third intercostal arteries are as follows:

1. First posterior intercostal artery from superior intercostal artery: 30 per cent
2. First and second posterior intercostal arteries from the superior intercostal artery: 60 per cent
3. First, second, and third posterior intercostal arteries from the superior intercostal artery: 5 per cent
4. All posterior intercostal arteries from the aorta: approximately 5 per cent.

The remaining intercostal and subcostal spaces are supplied by paired dorsal branches of the thoracic aorta. The origins of the upper intercostal arteries lie closer together and are more commonly involved in the formation of common trunks supplying two or more intercostal spaces. In addition, the upper intercostals show an upward directed course. Figure 2–16 shows the common anatomic variants.

Bronchial Arteries (Figs. 2–17 to 2–19)

The bronchial arteries arise from the third through seventh intercostal spaces. In addition to supplying the major bronchi, the bronchial arteries provide blood supply to the larger bronchopulmonary lymph nodes and have direct anastomoses with the pulmonary and occasionally the coronary arteries.

In approximately 60 per cent of individuals, there is a single right bronchial artery. Overall, a common origin of a right bronchial and intercostal arteries occurs in over 70 per cent of individuals. Multiple bronchial arteries are more common on the left side (approximately 70 per cent). A left intercostal bronchial trunk, usually with a right intercostal artery, occurs infrequently (4 per cent). A common bronchial trunk of left and right bronchial arteries occurs in approximately 45 per cent of individuals.

The most common distribution of the bronchial arteries is as follows:

1. Single bronchial artery bilaterally: approximately 30 per cent of individuals
2. Three bronchial arteries: approximately 45 per cent of individuals
    Two left bronchials and one right bronchial: approximately 40 per cent
    Two right bronchials and one left bronchial: approximately 5 per cent
3. Four bronchial arteries: approximately 24 per cent of individuals
    Two left bronchials and two right bronchials: approximately 20 per cent
    Three left bronchials and one right bronchial: approximately 4 per cent
4. Five or more bronchial arteries: approximately 1 per cent of individuals.

Anomalous origin of the bronchial arteries may be from the internal mammary, superior intercostal, subclavian, brachiocephalic, or inferior thyroid arteries. A left bronchial artery may originate from the concavity of the aortic arch in around 15 per cent of individuals. A left bronchointercostal trunk occurs in only 4 per cent of individuals.

Spinal Arteries (Figs. 2–20 to 2–23)

The anterior 70 to 80 per cent of the spinal cord is supplied by the anterior spinal artery (ASA). The posterior 20 to 30 per cent is supplied by the paired posterior spinal arteries (PSA).

The ASA is formed near the vertebrobasilar junction from branches of the vertebral arteries. The posterior spinal arteries are formed by posterior branches of the vertebral or posterior inferior cerebellar arteries. Both the PSAs and ASA receive branches from extraspinal arteries (e.g., intercostal, bronchial, lumbar, internal iliac, vertebral, subclavian). Those branches that supply the spinal cord are termed radioculomedullary arteries. On arteriography these are recognized by their characteristic hairpin loop.

Tributaries contributing to the formation of the anterior spinal artery are the following (Fig. 2–21):

1. Anterior spinal branches of the vertebral arteries
2. C_2–C_3: Radiculomedullary branches from the vertebral artery
3. C_5–C_6: Radiculomedullary branches from the costal, cervical, or thyrocervical trunk. Also called the artery of cervical enlargement (see Fig. 2–22)
4. C_8: Radiculomedullary branch from the first intercostal or the costocervical trunk
5. T_4–T_5: Radiculomedullary branch from a posterior intercostal artery
6. T_9–T_{12}: Arteria radicularis magna
7. Lumbar or lateral sacral branches

In 75 per cent of individuals the arteria radicularis magna (artery of Adamkiewicz) arises between T_9 and T_{12} from the left side. Its origin can vary from between T_5 and L_2.

Esophageal Arteries (Figs. 2–24 and 2–25)

These are approximately four to five in number and form a longitudinal vascular chain along the esophagus. The esophageal vascular supply can be divided into three segments:

Cervical: From the inferior thyroid artery, mostly from the right, or from the subclavian and common carotid arteries

Thoracic: From bronchial and intercostal arteries or directly from the thoracic aorta

Abdominal: From two to three branches of the left gastric artery or accessory left hepatic artery or left inferior phrenic arteries

REFERENCES

1. Blake HA, Manion WC: Thoracic arterial arch anomalies. Circulation 26:251–265, 1962.
2. Boechat MI, Gilsanz V, Fellows KE: Subclavian artery as the first branch of the aortic arch: A normal variant in two patients. Am J Roentgenol 131:721–722, 1978.
3. Caix M, Descottes B, Rousseau DG, Rousseau D: The arterial vascularization of the middle thoracic and lower esophagus. Anat Clin 3:95–106, 1981.
4. Chiras J, Morvan G, Merland JJ, Bories J: Blood supply to the thoracic (dorsal) and lumbar

spine. Normal angiographic appearances with comparative anatomy. Anat Clin 4:23–31, 1982.

5. Grollman JH Jr, Harris CH, Hamilton LC: Congenital diverticula of the aortic arch. N Engl J Med 276:1178–1182, 1969.
6. Klinkhamer AC: Aberrant right subclavian artery: Clinical and roentgenologic aspects. AJR 97–438–446, 1966.
7. McDowell DE, Grant MA, Gustafson RA: Single arterial trunk arising from the aortic arch. Circulation 62:181–182, 1980.
8. Moncada R, Shannon M, Miller R, White H, Friedman J, Shuford WH: The cervical aortic arch. AJR 125:591–601, 1975.
9. Shuford WH, Sybers RG, Milledge RD, Brinsfield D: The cervical aortic arch. AJR 116:519–527, 1972.
10. van der Horst RL, Fisher EA, DuBrow IW, Hastreiter AR: Right aortic arch, right patent ductus arteriosus, and mirror-image branching of the brachiocephalic vessels. Cardiovasc Radiol 1:147–149, 1978.

Figures 2–1 through 2–25 on following pages.

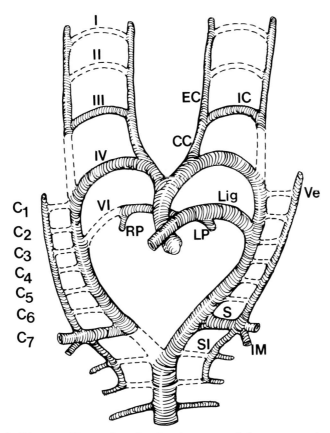

Figure 2–1. Diagram illustrating the development of the aorta and pulmonary, brachial, and cerebral arteries. Unshaded areas represent segments that normally regress.

I, II, III, IV, VI	Paired branchial arches between the ventral and dorsal aortae
C_1–C_7	Cervical intersegmental arteries
CC	Common carotid artery
EC	External carotid artery
IC	Internal carotid artery
IM	Internal mammary artery
Lig	Ligamentum arteriosum
LP	Left pulmonary artery
RP	Right pulmonary artery
S	Subclavian artery
SI	Superior intercostal artery
Ve	Vertebral artery

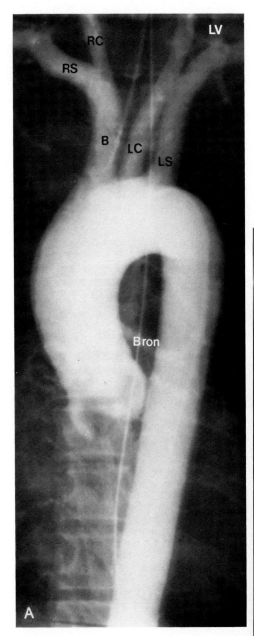

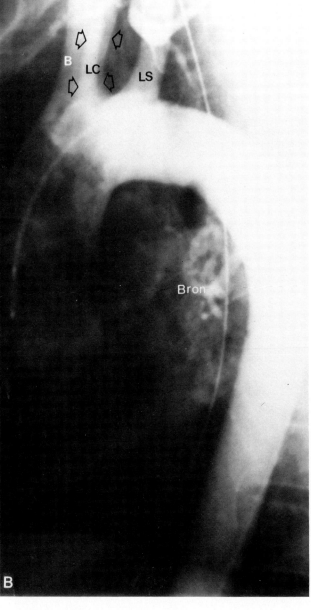

Figure 2–2. *A,* Anteroposterior and *B,* lateral arch aortogram. In *B,* the left common carotid artery is outlined by the open arrows.

B	Brachiocephalic artery
Bron	Bronchial artery
LC	Left common carotid artery
LS	Left subclavian artery
LV	Left vertebral artery
RC	Right common carotid artery
RS	Right subclavian artery

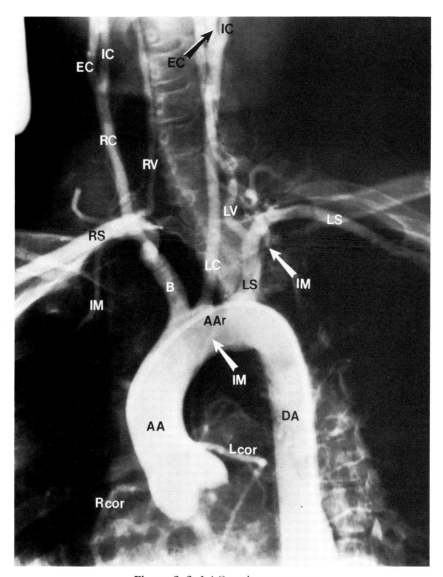

Figure 2–3. LAO arch aortogram.

AA	Ascending aorta
AAr	Aortic arch
B	Brachiocephalic artery
DA	Descending aorta
EC	External carotid artery
IC	Internal carotid artery
IM	Internal mammary artery
LC	Left common carotid artery
Lcor	Left coronary artery
LS	Left subclavian artery
LV	Left vertebral artery
RC	Right common carotid artery
Rcor	Right coronary artery
RS	Right subclavian artery
RV	Right vertebral artery

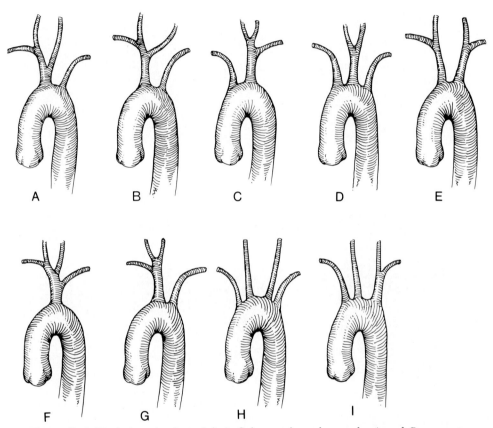

Figure 2–4. Variations in the origins of the aortic arch vessels. *A* and *B* account for 73 per cent of all arch vessel anomalies.

A   Common origin of left common carotid and brachiocephalic arteries (approximately 15 per cent of individuals)

B   Left common carotid originating from mid to upper brachiocephalic artery (approximately 7 per cent of individuals)

C   Common carotid trunk giving off the left subclavian artery

D   Common carotid trunk

E   Left and right brachiocephalic arteries

F   Single arch vessel (the brachiocephalic artery) gives off the left common carotid and left subclavian arteries

G   Common carotid trunk gives off the right subclavian artery, or origin of left common carotid artery from the right common carotid artery

H   Independent origin of all vessels; i.e., no brachiocephalic artery is present

I   Left brachiocephalic artery

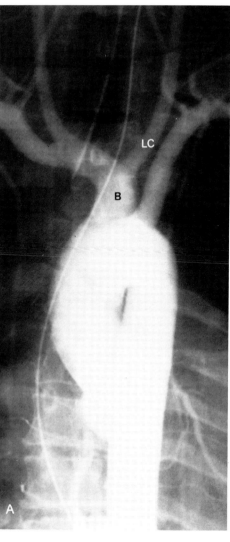

Figure 2–5. *A,* AP arch aortogram shows left common carotid artery originating from the brachiocephalic artery. *B,* LAO arch aortogram showing a common origin of the left common carotid and brachiocephalic arteries. NOTE: There is a fusiform widening of the proximal descending aorta *(arrows).* This is a normal variant caused by the presence of a ductus diverticulum (also see Fig. 2–11*B*).

B	Brachiocephalic artery
LC	Left common carotid artery
LS	Left subclavian artery
RC	Right common carotid artery
RS	Right subclavian artery

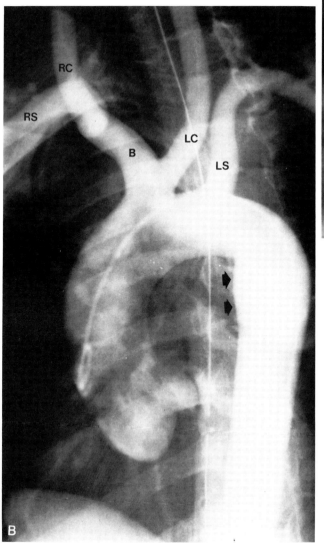

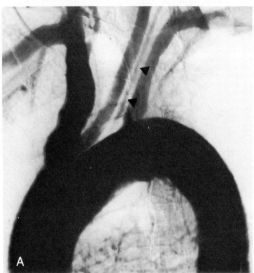

Figure 2–6. *A,* Left anterior oblique arch aortogram shows the left vertebral artery *(arrowheads)* originating from the aortic arch between the common trunk of the brachiocephalic and left common carotid arteries and the left subclavian artery. *B,* Lateral arch aortogram showing the left vertebral artery as the fourth branch of the aortic arch. (*A* from Kadir S: Diagnostic Angiography. Philadelphia, WB Saunders Company, 1986.)

B   Brachiocephalic artery
LC   Left common carotid artery
LS   Left subclavian artery
LV   Left vertebral artery

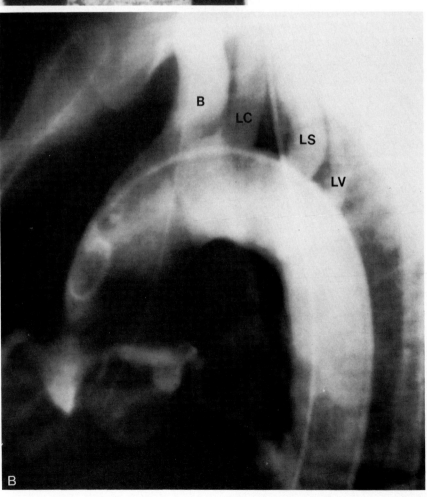

Figure 2–7. Intravenous DSA of the neck vessels shows a bifid proximal left vertebral artery *(open arrows)*.

LC   Left common carotid artery
LV   Left vertebral artery
RC   Right common carotid artery
RC   Right vertebral artery

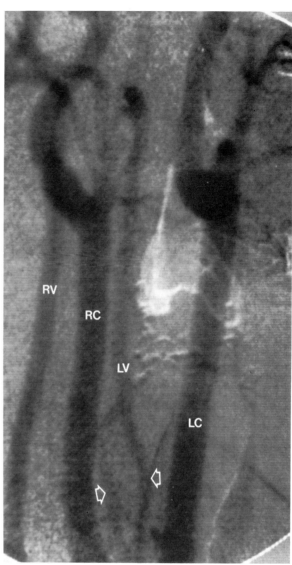

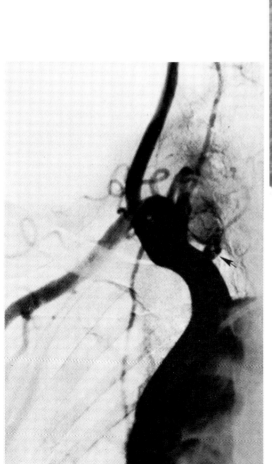

Figure 2–8. RPO arch aortogram shows the thyroid ima artery arising from the brachiocephalic artery *(arrow)*. (From Janevski BK: Angiography of the Upper Extremity. The Hague, Martinus Nijhoff Publishers, 1982; used with permission.)

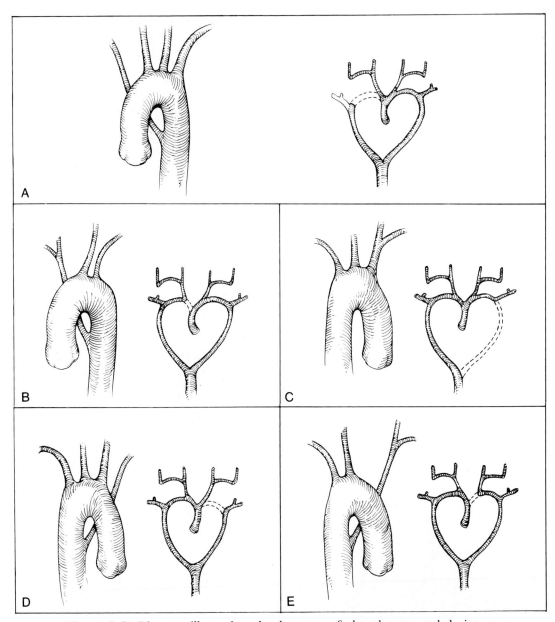

Figure 2–9. Diagram illustrating development of the aberrant subclavian or brachiocephalic artery and the right aortic arch.

- *A* Interruption of the embryonic right arch proximal to the seventh cervical intersegmental artery gives rise to the aberrant right subclavian artery. This can also be associated with other anomalies of the arch vessels.
- *B* Interruption at a more central level gives rise to the aberrant right brachiocephalic artery.
- *C* Persistence of the right fourth arch and regression of the left aorta give rise to the right aortic arch.
- *D* Interruption of the left fourth arch proximal to the seventh cervical intersegmental artery gives rise to the aberrant left subclavian artery seen with a right aortic arch.
- *E* Interruption of the left fourth arch at a more central location results in the formation of aberrant left brachiocephalic artery.

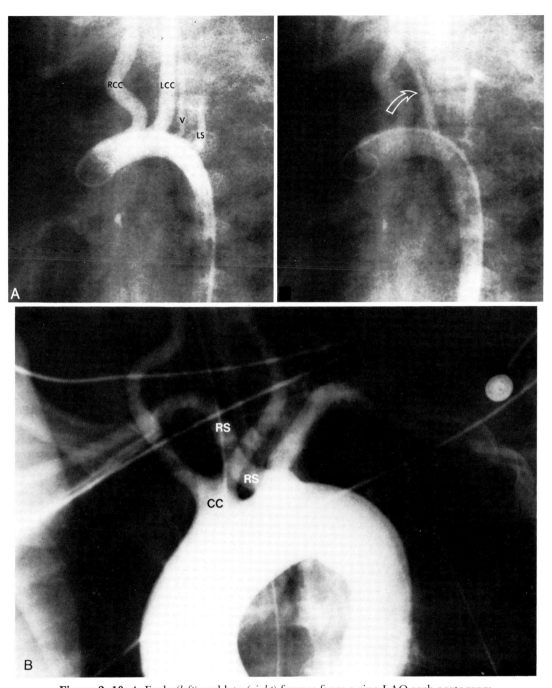

Figure 2–10. *A,* Early *(left)* and late *(right)* frames from a cine LAO arch aortogram show a left arch and aberrant right subclavian artery *(arrow).* The left vertebral arises directly from the aortic arch. (From Kadir S: Diagnostic Angiography. Philadelphia, WB Saunders Company, 1986.) *B,* LAO arch aortogram from another patient shows an aberrant right subclavian artery and a common carotid trunk.

CC	Common carotid trunk
LCC	Left common carotid artery
LS	Left subclavian artery
RCC	Right common carotid artery
RS	Right subclavian artery
V	Vertebral artery

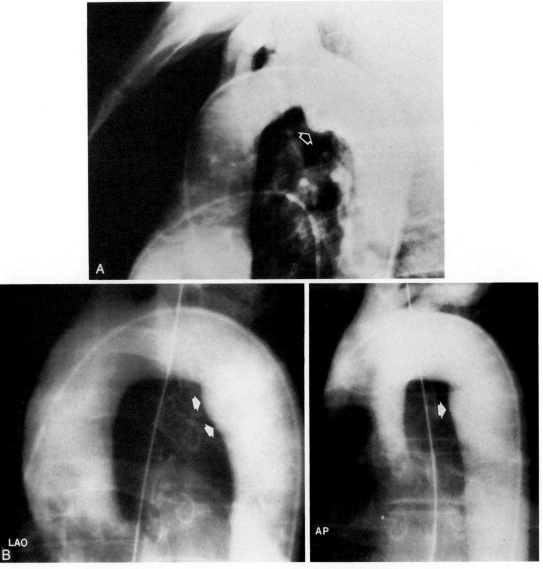

Figure 2–11. *A–E,* The normal ductus (aortic) diverticulum *(arrows).*

Illustration continued on opposite page.

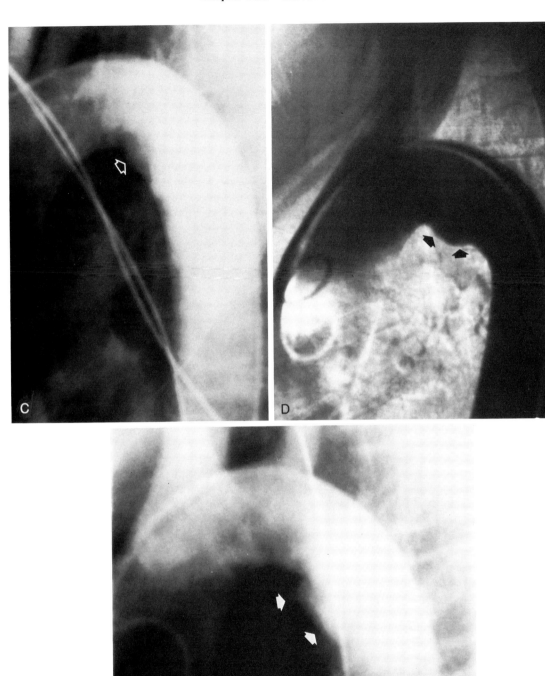

Figure 2–11. *Continued.*

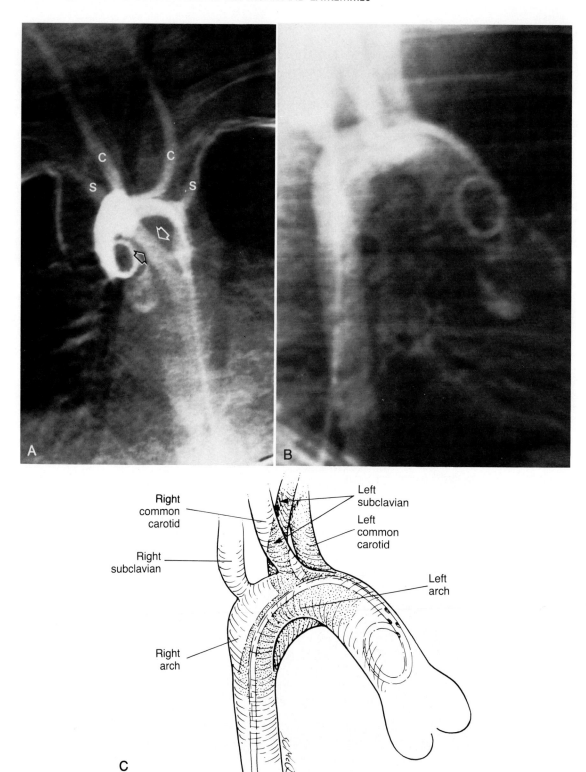

Figure 2–12. Double aortic arch. *A*, AP intra-arterial DSA. C = common carotid; S = subclavian. Open arrows point to the right aorta. *B*, Lateral intra-arterial DSA. *C*, Drawing of *B* illustrating the vascular anatomy. NOTE: The right arch is higher than the left.

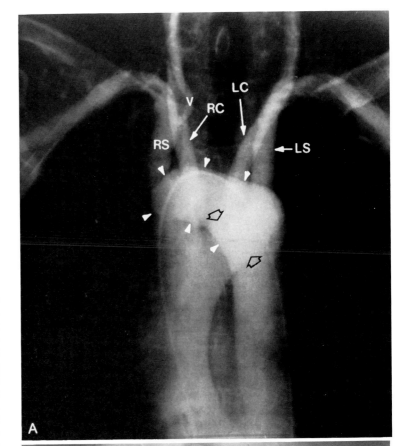

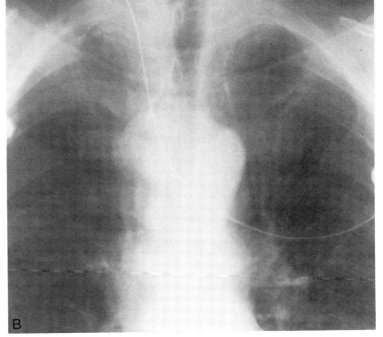

Figure 2–13. Double aortic arch with a large ductus diverticulum arising off the left arch.

A Anteroposterior aortogram. The right subclavian and right common carotid arteries arise independently off the right arch. The left common carotid and left subclavian arteries arise from the left arch. In addition, there is a large ductus diverticulum *(arrowheads)*. Open arrows outline the left ascending aorta. The catheter lies in the right arch.

B Corresponding posteroanterior chest radiograph. The ductus diverticulum forms the right arch contour.

Illustration continued on following page.

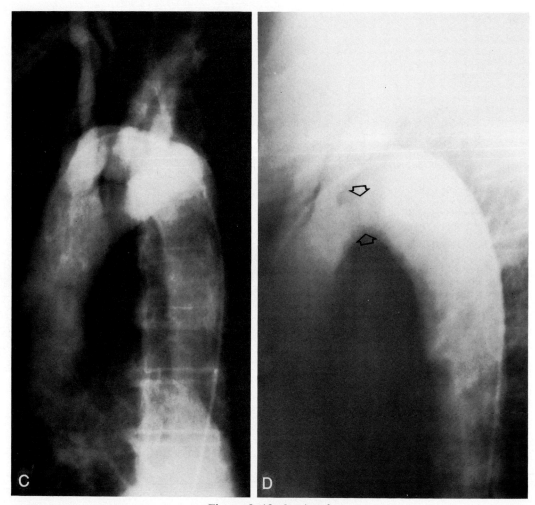

Figure 2–13. *Continued.*

C   Slight left anterior oblique aortogram shows both arches.
D   Lateral arch aortogram. The left arch is outlined by open arrows.
E–J Ten-millimeter coronal magnetic resonance scans show the
       ascending aorta divide into the left and right arches and
       continue as a left descending aorta.

Illustration continued on opposite page.

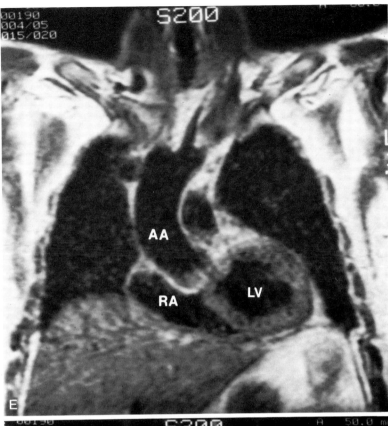

Figure 2–13. *Continued.*

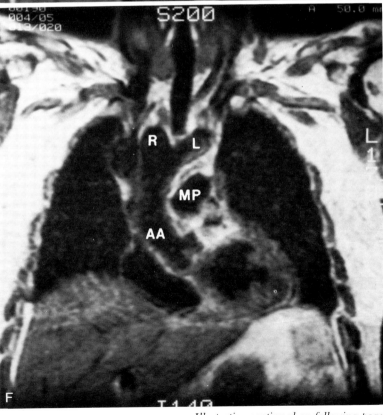

Illustration continued on following page.

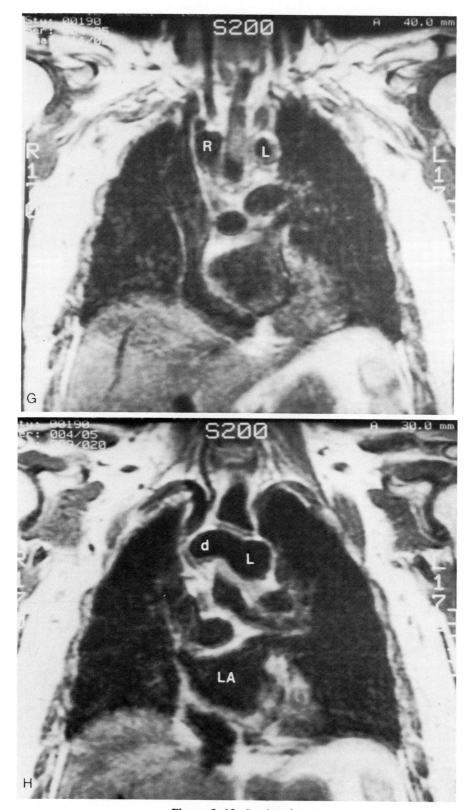

Figure 2–13. *Continued.*

Illustration continued on opposite page.

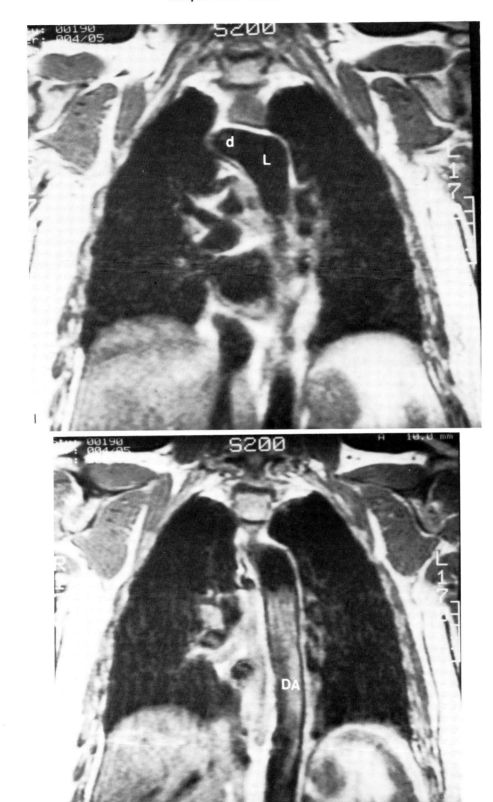

Figure 2–13. *Continued.*

Illustration continued on following page.

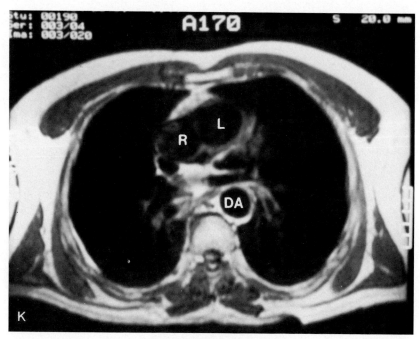

Figure 2–13. *Continued.*

K   Sagittal magnetic resonance scan shows the two aortic arches.

AA	Ascending aorta
d	Aortic diverticulum
DA	Descending aorta
L	Left arch
LA	Left atrium
LC	Left common carotid artery
LS	Left subclavian artery
LV	Left ventricle
MP	Main pulmonary artery
R	Right arch
RA	Right atrium
RC	Right common carotid artery
RS	Right subclavian artery
V	Vertebral artery

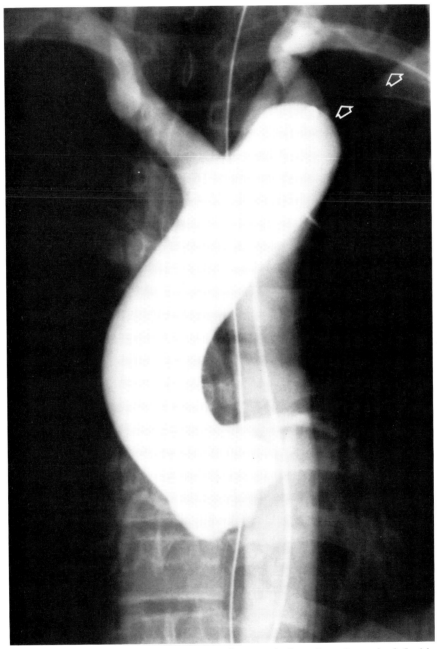

Figure 2–14. AP arch aortogram shows a low cervical aortic arch on the left side. Note the position of the arch convexity above the left clavicle *(open arrows)*.

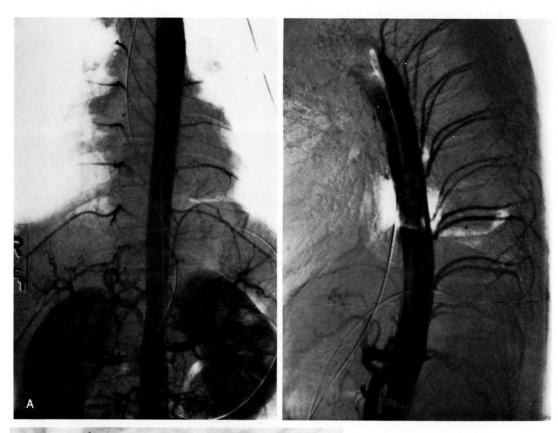

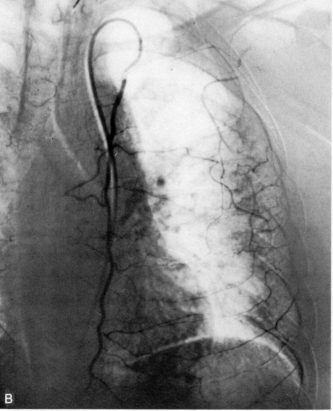

Figure 2–15. *A*, AP and lateral descending thoracic aortogram showing the intercostal arteries. *B*, Left internal mammary arteriogram showing the anterior intercostal arteries. (From Kadir S: Diagnostic Angiography. Philadelphia, WB Saunders Company, 1986.)

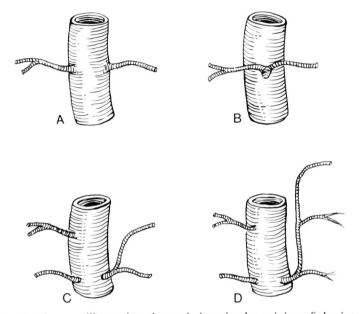

Figure 2–16. Diagram illustrating the variations in the origins of the intercostal arteries. Numbers listed below apply to each segment.

A	Separate origins of left and right intercostal arteries occur in over 80 per cent.
B	Common origin of left and right intercostal arteries.
C and *D*	Unilateral trunk formation. This occurs in 10 to 15 per cent.

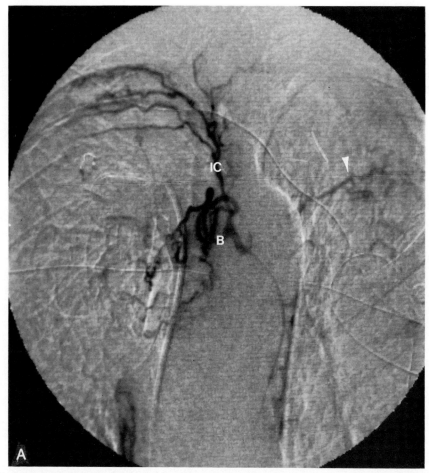

Figure 2–17. Bronchial arteries. *A*, Bronchial arteriogram shows a right intercostal–bronchial trunk. This occurs in more than 70 per cent of individuals. There is flash filling of the left bronchial artery (arrowhead). *B*, Right intercostal–bronchial trunk in another individual. *C*, Left bronchial artery.

    B   Bronchial artery
    IB   Intercostobronchial trunk
    IC   Intercostal artery

Illustration continued on opposite page.

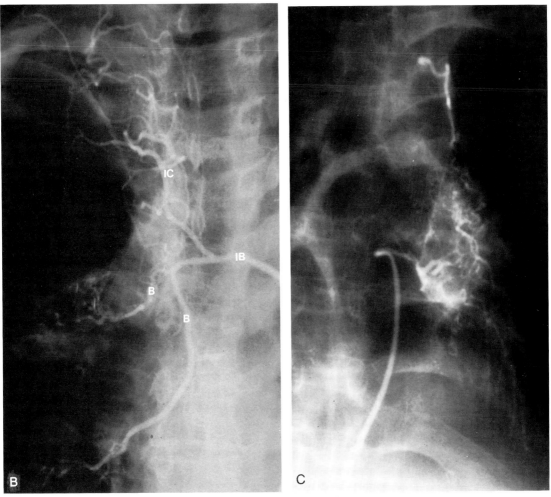

Figure 2–17. *Continued.*

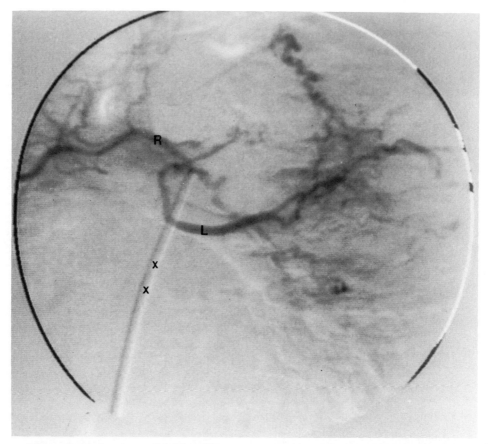

Figure 2–18. Intra-arterial DSA shows a common bronchial trunk. This occurs in approximately 45 per cent of individuals.

L   Left bronchial artery
R   Right bronchial artery
xx   Catheter

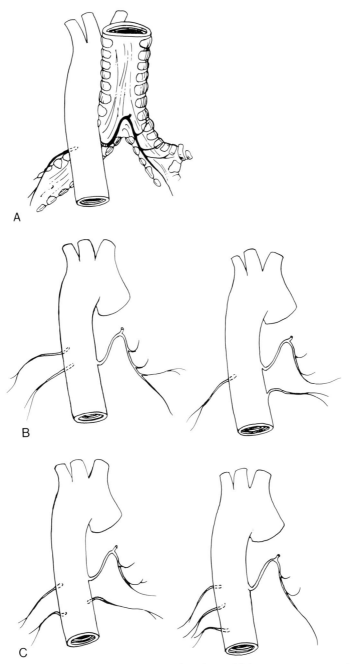

Figure 2–19. Drawing illustrating the variant bronchial artery anatomy visualized from behind. A single bronchial artery occurs most frequently on the right side.

A Single bronchial arteries bilaterally (approximately 30 per cent).

B Two bronchial arteries on one side and a single bronchial artery on the contralateral side (approximately 45 per cent).

C Four bronchial arteries (approximately 24 per cent): two on each side (approximately 20 per cent); three left and one right (approximately 4 per cent).

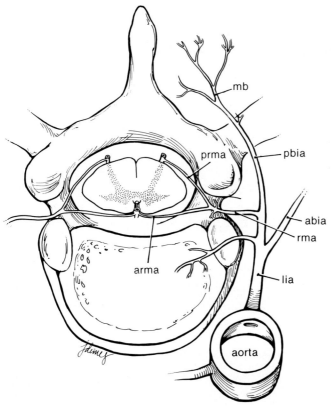

Figure 2–20. Diagram illustrating segmental (intercostal or lumbar) artery branching. The posterior branch supplies the spinal cord and paravertebral muscles. (From Kadir S: Diagnostic Angiography. Philadelphia, WB Saunders Company, 1986.)

abia	Anterior branch of intercostal/lumbar artery
arma	Anterior radiculomedullary artery
lia	Left intercostal/lumbar artery
mb	Muscular branches
pbia	Posterior branch of intercostal/lumbar artery
prma	Posterior radiculomedullary artery
rma	Radiculomedullary artery

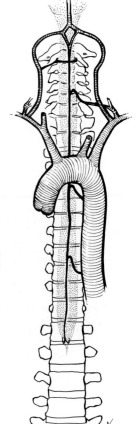

Figure 2–21. Diagram illustrating anatomy of the anterior spinal arteries. (From Kadir S: Diagnostic Angiography. Philadelphia, WB Saunders Company, 1986.)

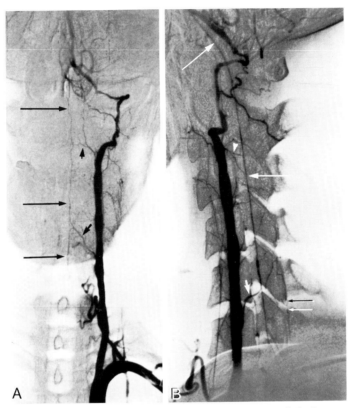

Figure 2–22. *A,* Anteroposterior and *B,* lateral views from a subclavian arteriogram show the anterior spinal artery *(long arrows).* Lower short arrows point to the artery of cervical enlargement, which is seen arising from the ascending cervical artery. Arrowheads point to another small radiculomedullary artery at C_2–C_3. Double arrows *(B)* point to the posterior spinal artery. (From Kadir S: Diagnostic Angiography. Philadelphia, WB Saunders Company, 1986.)

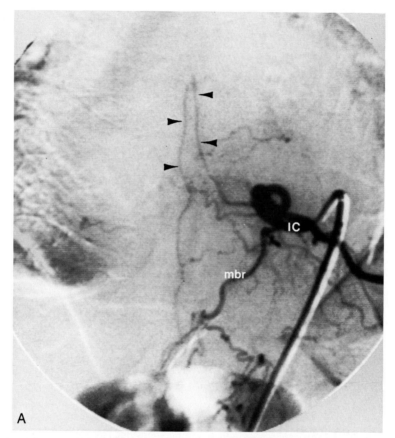

Figure 2–23. Arteria radicularis magna. Intercostal arteriograms in different individuals *(A–C)* show the arteria radicularis magna *(arrowheads)* with a typical hairpin loop.

IC   Posterior intercostal artery
mbr   Muscular branch

Illustration continued on opposite page.

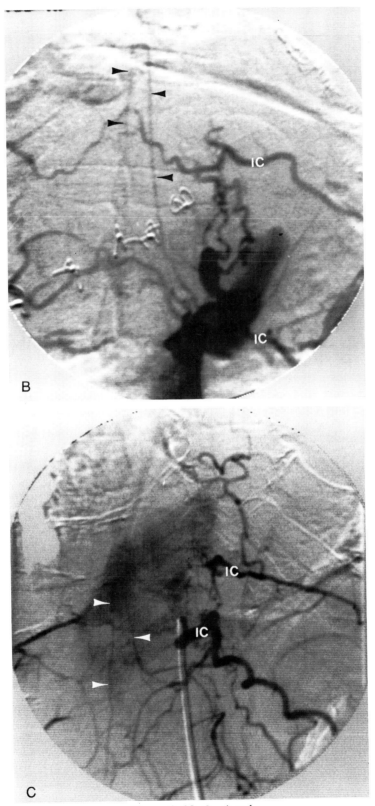

Figure 2–23. *Continued.*

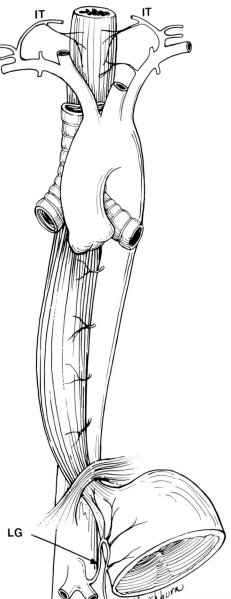

Figure 2–24. Diagram illustrating arterial blood supply to the esophagus. The cervical esophagus is supplied by branches of the inferior thyroid artery (IT), the midportion by esophageal branches from the aorta and bronchial arteries, and the lower portion by esophageal branches of the left gastric artery (LG).

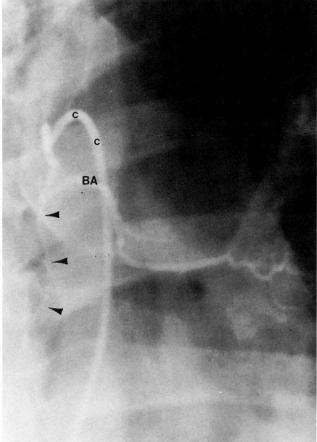

Figure 2–25. Esophageal branch *(arrowheads)* arising from the left bronchial artery.

BA   Left bronchial artery
c   Catheter

Chapter Three

ARTERIAL ANATOMY OF THE UPPER EXTREMITIES

STEVEN C. ROSE, M.D.
SAADOON KADIR, M.D.

SUBCLAVIAN AND AXILLARY ARTERIES

Embryology (see Fig. 2–1)

The proximal right subclavian artery is derived from the distal right fourth branchial arch and a portion of the dorsal aorta. The right seventh intersegmental artery forms the distal right subclavian and axillary arteries. The left subclavian and axillary arteries are derived from the left seventh intersegmental artery. Longitudinal anastomoses between various intersegmental arteries contribute to the formation of axially oriented arteries (e.g., internal mammary) and arterial trunks (e.g., thyrocervical and costocervical).

Subclavian Artery (Figs. 3–1 to 3–7)

The right subclavian artery originates from the brachiocephalic artery. The left subclavian artery arises from the aortic arch as the last major branch. The subclavian artery continues as the axillary artery after crossing the lateral margin of the first rib. The axillary artery becomes the brachial artery after coursing beyond the inferior lateral margin of the teres major muscle.

The first, i.e., intrathoracic, segment of each subclavian artery (proximal to the anterior scalene muscle) sequentially gives rise to the following vessels:

Vertebral Artery: See Chapter 2

Thyrocervical Trunk: This divides into the inferior thyroid artery (supplies inferior portion of the thyroid and lower parathyroid glands), the superficial cervical artery (to anterior and lateral neck musculature), and the suprascapular (transverse scapular) artery to the superior shoulder musculature. In approximately one third of individuals the superficial cervical and dorsal scapular (descending scapular) arteries have a common origin from the thyrocervical trunk, which is called the transverse cervical artery.

Internal Mammary Artery: This vessel courses caudally adjacent to the sternum and dorsal to the anterior ribs and continues as the superior epigastric artery in the abdomen.

The second segment of the subclavian artery lies posterior to the anterior scalene muscle and gives rise to the

Costocervical Trunk (Figs. 3–2, 3–4, and 3–6):   On the left side, the costocervical trunk may arise from the first portion of the subclavian artery. The costocervical trunk branches include the superior (highest) intercostal artery (supplies the upper two or three posterior intercostal spaces), the deep cervical artery (supplies the posterior neck musculature), and frequently a small radiculomedullary branch to the spinal cord.

The third segment of the subclavian artery distal to the anterior scalene muscle does not have any named branches. Table 3–1 lists the variant anatomy of the subclavian artery branches and the frequency of such variations. Variant anatomy of the brachiocephalic, subclavian, and vertebral arteries is discussed in Chapter 2. Anatomy of the intracranial vertebral artery is discussed in Chapter 17.

TABLE 3–1. Variant Anatomy of the Subclavian Artery Branches and their Frequency

Artery	Frequency (%)	Illustrations
Vertebral	See Chapter 2	
Thyrocervical trunk		
Single trunk (inferior thyroid, superficial cervical, and suprascapular arteries)	52%	Fig. 3–2
Independent origin of all branches	31%	
Main trunk with one independent branch	16%	Fig. 3–3
Independent transverse cervical artery	8%	
Independent inferior thyroid artery	2%	Fig. 3–6
Independent suprascapular artery	4%	
Miscellaneous	2%	
Internal mammary		
Lateral costal branch	10%	Fig. 3–7
Costocervical trunk		
Single trunk	88%	Fig. 3–2
Independent origin of superior intercostal and deep cervical arteries	12%	

Axillary Artery (Figs. 3–1 to 3–3 and 3–8 to 3–12)

The first portion of the axillary artery lies proximal to the pectoralis minor muscle and gives rise to the superior thoracic artery, which supplies the three upper intercostal spaces anteriorly (Fig. 3–8). The second portion of the axillary artery lies posterior to the pectoralis minor muscle and gives rise to the thoracoacromial and lateral thoracic arteries (supplies lateral chest wall). The former bifurcates into a descending branch to the clavicle and anterior chest wall and an ascending branch to the acromion and deltoid muscles.

The third portion of the axillary artery (lateral to the pectoralis minor muscle) gives rise to the large subscapular and the humeral circumflex arteries. The former branches into the scapular circumflex artery, which courses around the lateral margin of the scapula to supply the posterior shoulder musculature, and the thoracodorsal artery, which continues to the tip of the scapula. The humeral circumflex artery bifurcates into anterior and posterior humeral circumflex arteries, which supply the shoulder joint and lateral shoulder

TABLE 3–2. Variant Anatomy of the Axillary Artery Branches and their Frequency

Artery	Frequency (%)	Illustrations
Superior (highest) thoracic		
Absent	~16%	
Single trunk, from axillary artery	76%	
Single trunk, from thoracoacromial artery	4%	Fig. 3–6
Two vessels	4%	
Three vessels	1%	
Thoracoacromial		
Separate origin	72%	
Common origin with lateral thoracic artery	28%	
Lateral thoracic		
Separate origin from the axillary artery	64%	
Single trunk	38%	Fig. 3–9
Two vessels	22%	Fig. 3–8
Three vessels	3%	
More than 3 vessels	1%	
Common origin with thoracoacromial artery	28%	
Common origin with subscapular artery	7%	
Subscapular		
Absent (independent origin of the scapular circumflex and thoracodorsal arteries)	2%	
Independent origin	80%	Fig. 3–8
Gives off lateral thoracic artery	7%	
Common origin with humeral circumflex artery	10%	Fig. 3–9
Common trunk: subscapular, humeral circumflex, and profunda brachial arteries	1%	
Circumflex humeral		
Common trunk branching into anterior and posterior humeral circumflex arteries	70%	Fig. 3–10
Separate origins of anterior and posterior humeral circumflex arteries	2%	
Common origin with profunda brachial artery	12%	Fig. 3–10
Common origin with subscapular artery	10%	Fig. 3–9
Common origin with subscapular, thoracoacromial, and profunda brachial arteries	4%	
Multiple small branches	2%	
Large trunk branching into thoracoacromial, thoracodorsal, or subscapular, anterior, and posterior humeral circumflex arteries	4%	
Radial artery originates from distal axillary artery	2–5%	Fig. 3–11
Ulnar artery originates from distal axillary artery	1%	Fig. 3–12

musculature. Table 3–2 lists the variant anatomy of the axillary artery branches and the frequency with which these variants are observed.

THE UPPER ARM

Embryology (Fig. 3–13)

The seventh intersegmental artery hypertrophies to form the axial artery, which courses down the arm as the brachial artery proximally and the interosseous artery distal to the elbow. Later a superficial brachial artery arises from the axillary region and extends peripherally to the palmar arch in the hand; the segment distal to the elbow remains as the radial artery, whereas the proximal segment usually involutes.

Brachial Artery (Figs. 3–14 to 3–17)

The axillary becomes the brachial artery at the lateral margin of the teres major muscle. The brachial artery courses along the medial aspect of the arm, and anteriorly in the antecubital fossa it divides into radial and ulnar arteries. Major branches of the brachial artery include the deep brachial (A. profunda brachii), superior, and inferior ulnar collateral arteries. The larger deep brachial artery arises in the proximal upper arm and passes posterolaterally to supply the deep and posterior musculature of the upper arm. It bifurcates distally into the laterally located radial collateral artery (anastomoses with the radial recurrent artery) and the middle collateral branch posteromedially (anastomoses with the interosseous recurrent artery and the posterior ulnar recurrent artery [Fig. 3–15]). The superior ulnar collateral artery is usually small and arises at the midhumerus level. It anastomoses with the posterior ulnar recurrent artery. The inferior ulnar collateral artery (supratrochlear artery) arises in the distal upper arm and courses medially to bifurcate into one branch that anastomoses with both the superior ulnar collateral artery and the middle collateral artery and another branch that anastomoses distally with the anterior ulnar recurrent artery. Variant anatomy of the brachial artery is listed in Table 3–3.

TABLE 3–3. Variant Anatomy of the Brachial Artery and its Branches and their Frequency

Arterial Variants	Frequency (%)	Illustrations
Persistent superficial brachial artery	1–2%	Fig. 3–16A
Radial artery origin from proximal brachial artery (above the humeral intercondylar line)	12%	Fig. 3–17
Ulnar artery origin from proximal brachial artery	1–2%	
Common interosseous artery origin from proximal brachial artery	Rare	
Accessory brachial artery (duplication of the brachial artery; rejoins the distal brachial artery in the antecubital fossa)	0.1%	Fig. 3–16B

TABLE 3–4. Variant Anatomy of the Forearm Arteries and their Frequency

Artery	Frequency (%)	Illustrations
Radial		
High origin (brachial or axillary)	14–17%	Figs. 3–11, 3–17
Aplasia or hypoplasia	0.1%	Fig. 3–19
Partial duplication	0.8%	Fig. 3–20
Complete duplication	0.1%	
Dorsal continuation (a large branch, arising in the distal forearm, courses to the dorsum of the hand)	1%	Fig. 3–20
Ulnar		
High origin (brachial or axillary)	2–3%	Fig. 3–12
Low origin (5–7 cm below elbow)	1%	
Aplasia	0.1%	
Persistent median artery (from common or anterior interosseous artery; may contribute to superficial palmar arch)	2–4%	Fig. 3–21*A*
Persistent interosseous artery	<0.1%	Fig. 3–21*B*

THE FOREARM

Embryology (Fig. 3–13)

Distal to the elbow, the axial artery remains as the interosseous artery. A median artery arises from the proximal segment of the interosseous artery and fuses with the distal interosseous artery and also supplies the digits. The ulnar artery arises from the distal brachial artery, courses along the ulna to join the distal median artery in the hand, and forms the superficial palmar arch.

The superficial brachial artery arises from the proximal brachial artery, courses along the radial aspect, and terminates in a deep palmar arch. The proximal segment atrophies, whereas the segment distal to the elbow fuses with the distal brachial artery and forms the radial artery. Simultaneously, the median artery atrophies.

Normal Anatomy (Figs. 3–18 to 3–21)

The brachial artery bifurcates a few centimeters below the elbow joint into the radial and ulnar arteries. Table 3–4 lists the variant anatomy of the forearm arteries and their frequency.

THE HAND

Embryology (Fig. 3–13)

During early development the axial artery terminates in the hand as a capillary network. This network later develops into the various digital arteries to the fingers. The ulnar artery anastomoses with the median artery to form the superficial palmar arch. The superficial brachial artery, which persists as the radial artery, provides a deep branch that forms the deep palmar arch and a more distal superficial branch that anastomoses with the superficial palmar arch. As the median artery involutes, it leaves the ulnar artery as the dominant arterial supply to the superficial palmar arch.

TABLE 3–5. Variant Anatomy of the Hand: Deep Palmar Arch

Artery	Frequency (%)	Illustrations
Complete arch	95–97%	Fig. 3–23
A. Formed by deep palmar branch of radial artery and superior deep palmar branch of ulnar artery	35%	Fig. 3–24*A*
B. Deep palmar branch of radial artery and inferior deep palmar branch of ulnar artery	49%	Fig. 3–24*B*
C. Deep palmar branch of radial artery communicates with both superior and inferior deep palmar branches of ulnar artery	13%	Fig. 3–24*C*
D. Formed by superior deep branch of ulnar artery, communicates with radial artery via enlarged perforating artery of the second digital interspace	0.5%	
Incomplete arch	3–5%	
A. Deep palmar branch of radial artery supplies thumb and radial aspect of index fingers while inferior deep branch of ulnar artery communicates with a perforating artery of the second interspace	1.5%	Fig. 3–25*A* Fig. 3–28
B. Deep palmar branch of radial artery supplies thumb and radial aspect of index fingers, then terminates as perforating artery of the second interspace; deep branch of ulnar artery terminates as perforating artery of the third interspace	1.5%	Fig. 3–25*B*

Normal Anatomy (Figs. 3–22 and 3–24)

At the radial styloid process, the radial artery divides into a smaller superficial palmar branch that anastomoses with the superficial palmar arch and a larger deep palmar branch that continues along the base of the first metacarpals to form the deep palmar (volar) arch (Table 3–5). The deep palmar arch gives off four palmar (volar) metacarpal arteries, which lie in the corresponding interosseous spaces. At the interdigital webspace, each palmar metacarpal artery anastomoses with a common palmar digital artery from the superficial arch (Table 3–6), then promptly bifurcates into proper digital arteries that supply appositional surfaces of adjacent digits (e.g., ulnar aspect of the index finger and radial aspect of the middle finger).

The deep branch of the radial artery gives off small branches that unite with branches of the distal ulnar artery to form the dorsal carpal rete. The small dorsal metacarpal arteries that supply the dorsum of the hand and proximal fingers may arise either from the dorsal carpal rete or as small superficial perforating arteries from the deep palmar arch.

At the pisiform bone, the ulnar artery gives off a small deep palmar branch that anastomoses with the deep palmar arch and a larger superficial palmar branch that forms the superficial palmar arch. The latter lies distal to the deep palmar arch and gives rise to four common palmar (volar) digital arteries (Table 3–7) that travel in the interosseous space to join the palmar metacarpal arteries (Table 3–8) from the deep palmar arch. Additionally, the superficial arch provides the proper digital artery to the ulnar aspect of the fifth finger. In general, an inverse relationship exists between the caliber of the common palmar digital arteries and the corresponding palmar metacarpal arteries.

TABLE 3–6. Variant Anatomy of the Hand: Superficial Palmar Arch

Artery	Frequency (%)	Illustrations
Complete arch	78% (anatomic) 42% (angiographic)	
A. Classic radioulnar arch	35%	Fig. 3–26*A*
B. Ulnar artery is the main contributor to the superficial arch, giving rise to all four common palmar digital arteries. It anastomoses with small branches of the deep arch in the first digital interspace	37%	Fig. 3–29*B*
C. Mediano-ulnar arch formed from the ulnar and median arteries	4%	Fig. 3–26*C*
D. Radio-mediano-ulnar arch formed from the radial, median, and ulnar arteries	1%	Fig. 3–26*D*
E. Superficial arch formed from ulnar artery and an anastomosis with a large unnamed artery from the deep arch.	2%	Fig. 3–26*E*
Incomplete arch	22% (anatomic) 58% (angiographic)	
A. The superficial palmar branch of the radial artery and the ulnar branch fail to anastomose, yet each supplies common palmar digital arteries	3%	Fig. 3–27 Fig. 3–28
B. Ulnar artery is the sole contributor to the superficial arch. The thumb is supplied by the radial artery	13%	Fig. 3–29*A*
C. The median and ulnar arteries fail to anastomose; each supplies common palmar digital arteries	4%	Fig. 3–29*B*
D. The radial, median, and ulnar arteries fail to anastomose; each gives rise to common palmar digital arteries	1%	

*Frequency as seen in anatomical or angiographic studies. Percentages listed are from angiographic studies.

TABLE 3–7. Common Palmar (Volar) Digital Arteries (CPDA's)

Artery	Frequency (%)	Illustrations
A. Four CPDA's; one to each digital interosseous space	77%	Fig. 3–22,
B. Three CPDA's; supply the second, third, fourth interosseous spaces	9%	Fig. 3–23 and 3–30
C. Three CPDA's as in B, with an additional artery to the thumb	3%	
D. Three CPDA's as in B, with an additional artery to the radial aspect of the index finger	3%	
E. Three CPDA's; supply the first, second, and fourth interosseous spaces	2%	
F. Two CPDA's; supply the second and third interosseous spaces	2%	
G. Two CPDA's; supply the third and fourth interosseous spaces	1%	

TABLE 3–8. Palmar (Volar) Metacarpal Arteries

Artery	Frequency (%)	Illustrations
A. Palmar metacarpal artery to the first interosseous space	98%	Fig. 3–22
1. Principal artery of the thumb and radial artery to the index finger arise from a common trunk	48–52%	and 3–30
2. Each arises independently from the deep palmar arch	48–52%	
B. Palmar metacarpal artery to the second interosseous space	97%	
C. Palmar metacarpal arteries to other interosseous spaces highly variable with regard to sites of origin and number		

REFERENCES

1. Coleman SS, Anson BJ: Arterial patterns in the hand based on a study of 650 specimens. Surg Gynecol Obstet 119:409–424, 1961.
2. Daseler EH, Anson BJ: Surgical Anatomy of the Subclavian Artery and Its Branches. Surg Gynecol Obstet 108:149–174, 1959.
3. Gainor BJ, Jeffries JT: Pronator syndrome associated with a persistent median artery. J Bone Joint Surg 69-A:303–304, 1987.
4. Ikeda A, Ugawa A, Kazihara Y, Hamada N: Arterial patterns in the hand based on a three-dimensional analysis of 220 cadaver hands. J Hand Surg 13A:501–509, 1988.
5. Janevski BK: Angiography of the Upper Extremity. The Hague, Martinus Nijhoff Publishers, 1982, pp 37–122.
6. Jonsson K, Karlsson S: Angiography of the internal mammary artery. Acta Radiol 26:113–120, 1985.
7. Lippert H, Pabst R: Arterial Variations in Man. Classification and Frequency. Munich, JF Bergman Verlag, 1985.
8. McCormack LJ, Cauldwell EW, Anson BJ: Brachial and antebrachial arterial patterns: A study of 750 extremities. Surg Gynecol Obstet 96:43–54, 1953.
9. Simmons JT, Doppman JL, Norton J: Inferior thyroid artery from common carotid artery with abberant right subclavian artery. Cardiovasc Intervent Radiol 10:150–152, 1987.
10. Uglietta JP, Kadir S: Arteriographic study of variant arterial anatomy of the upper extremities. J Cardiovasc Intervent Radiol 12:145–148, 1989.

Figures 3–1 through 3–30 on following pages.

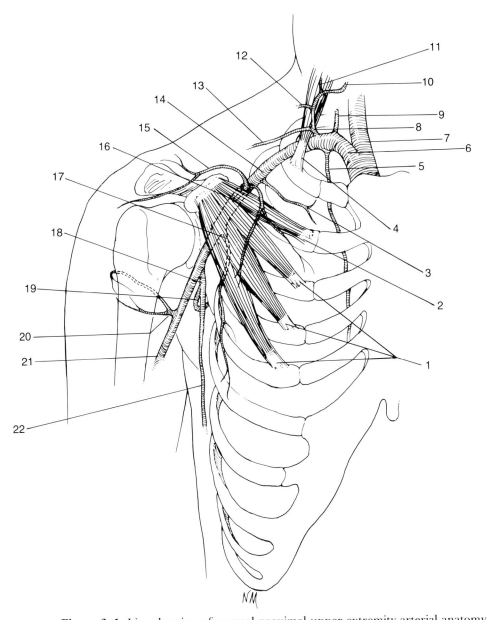

Figure 3–1. Line drawing of normal proximal upper extremity arterial anatomy.

1	Pectoralis minor muscle	12	Superficial cervical
2	Pectoral branch of thoracoacro- mial	13	Suprascapular
		14	Axillary
3	Superior (highest) thoracic	15	Acromial branch of thoracoacro- mial
4	Anterior scalene muscle		
5	Internal mammary	16	Thoracoacromial
6	Right subclavian	17	Lateral thoracic
7	Right common carotid	18	Subscapular
8	Thyrocervical trunk	19	Circumflex scapular
9	Vertebral	20	Circumflex humeral
10	Inferior thyroid	21	Brachial
11	Ascending cervical	22	Thoracodorsal

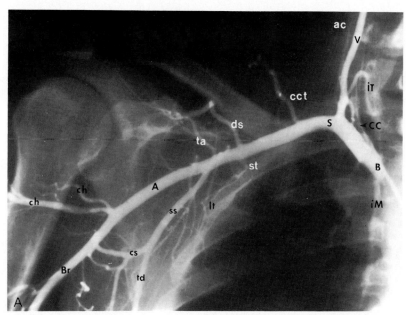

Figure 3–2. Normal right *(A)* and left *(B)* subclavian arteriograms. *(A* reproduced from Kadir S: Diagnostic Angiography. Philadelphia, WB Saunders Company, 1986.)

A	Axillary	mbr	Mammary branch of lateral
Abr	Acromial branch		thoracic
Ac	Ascending cervical	S	Subclavian
B	Brachiocephalic	sc	Superficial cervical
Br	Brachial	ss	Subscapular
CC	Common carotid	st/si	Superior (highest) thoracic
cct	Costocervical trunk	ta	Thoracoacromial
ch	Circumflex humeral	td	Thoracodorsal
cs	Circumflex scapular	ts	Transverse scapular (suprascapular)
ds	Dorsal (descending) scapular		
iM	Internal mammary	V	Vertebral
IT	Inferior thyroid		
lt	thoracic		

Illustration continued on opposite page.

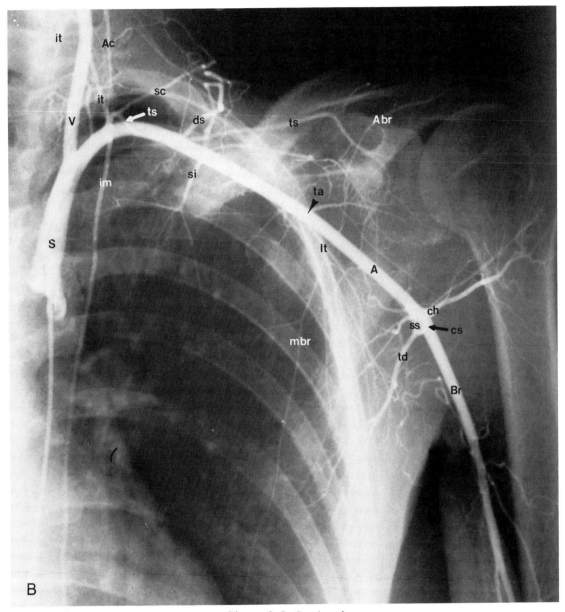

Figure 3–2. *Continued.*

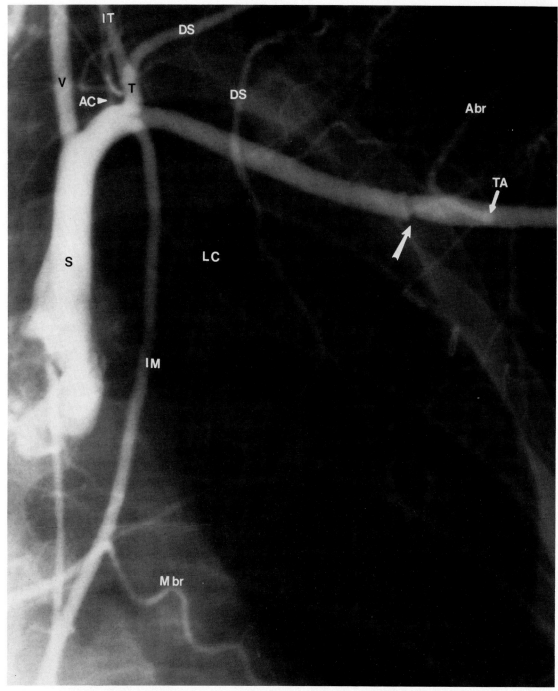

Figure 3–3. Left subclavian arteriogram in a patient with prior injury to the axillary artery *(arrow)*.

Abr	Acromial branch of thoraco-acromial		Mbr	Mammary branch of internal mammary
AC	Ascending cervical		S	Subclavian
DS	Dorsal (descending) scapular		T	Thyrocervical trunk
IM	Internal mammary		TA	Thoracoacromial
IT	Inferior thyroid		V	Vertebral
LC	Lateral costal branch of internal mammary			

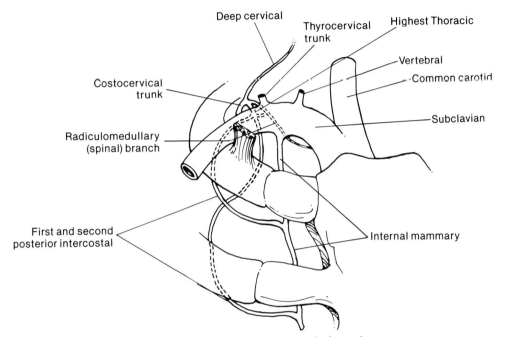

Figure 3–4. Line drawing of the costocervical trunk anatomy.

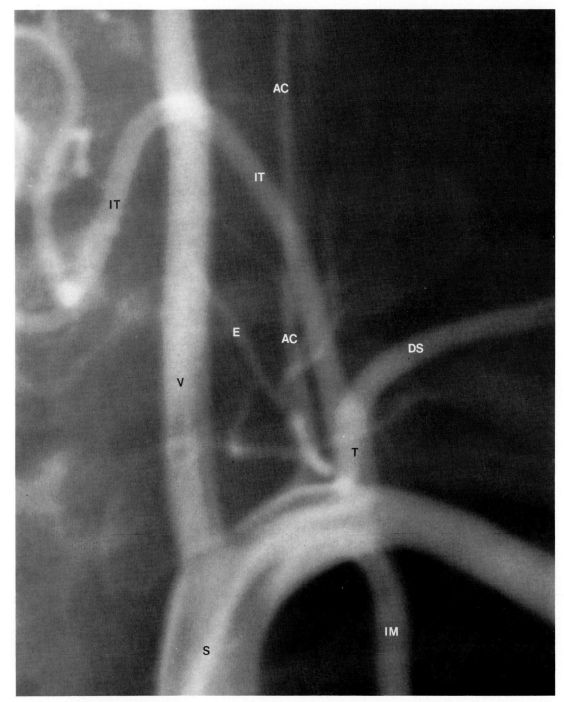

Figure 3–5. Left subclavian arteriogram showing the proximal branches (same patient as in Figure 3–3).

AC   Ascending cervical (arising independently from subclavian artery)
DS   Dorsal scapular
E   Esophageal
IM   Internal mammary
IT   Inferior thyroid
S   Subclavian
T   Thyrocervical trunk
V   Vertebral

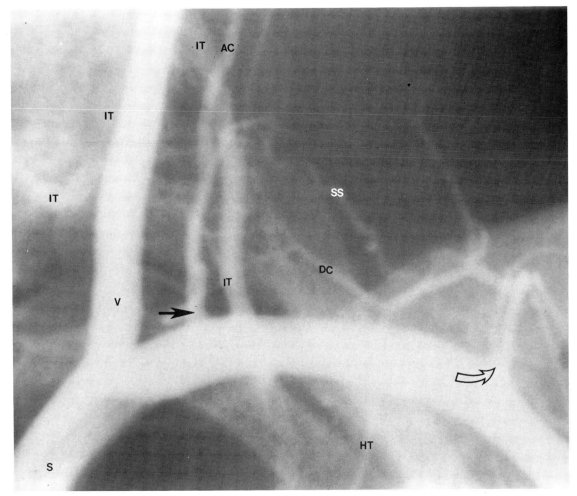

Figure 3–6. Left subclavian arteriogram showing independent origin of thyrocervical branches. The ascending cervical and transverse cervical arteries *(straight arrow)* and the costocervical and thoracoacromial and highest thoracic arteries *(open arrow)* form a common trunk.

AC	Ascending cervical
DC	Deep cervical
HT	Highest thoracic
IT	Inferior thyroid
S	Subclavian
SS	Suprascapular
V	Vertebral

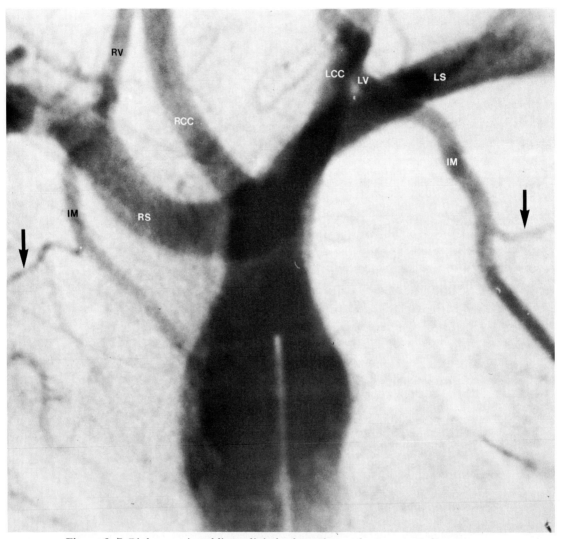

Figure 3–7. Right anterior oblique digital subtraction arch aortogram demonstrates the lateral costal branches of the internal mammary arteries *(arrows)*.

IM	Internal mammary
LCC	Left common carotid
LS	Left subclavian
LV	Left vertebral
RCC	Right common carotid
RS	Right subclavian
RV	Right vertebral

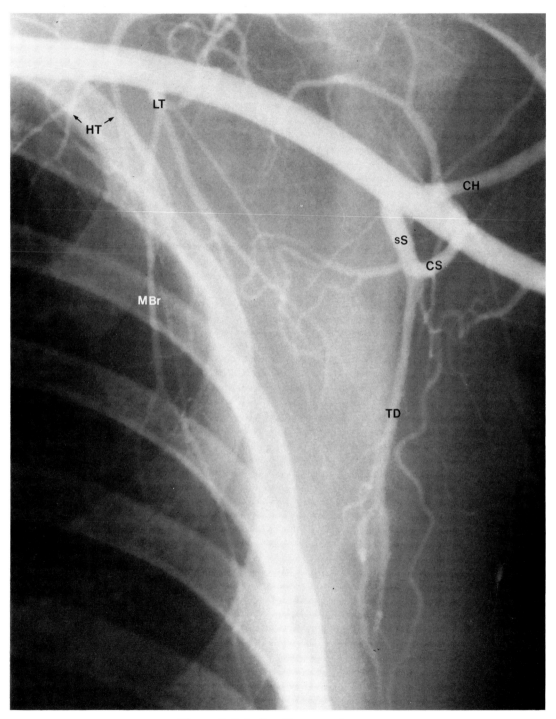

Figure 3–8. Left axillary arteriogram.

CH   Circumflex humeral
CS   Circumflex scapular
HT   Superior (highest) thoracic
LT   Lateral thoracic
MBr Lateral mammary branch of lateral thoracic
sS   Subscapular
TD   Thoracodorsal

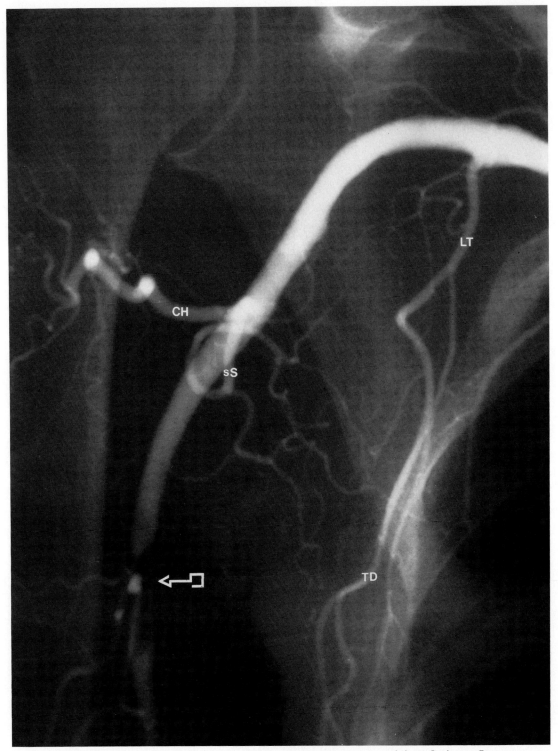

Figure 3–9. Right axillary arteriogram shows common origin of circumflex humeral and subscapular arteries. Incidental thrombus in brachial artery *(arrow)*.

CH   Circumflex humeral
LT   Lateral thoracic
sS   Subscapular
TD   Thoracodorsal

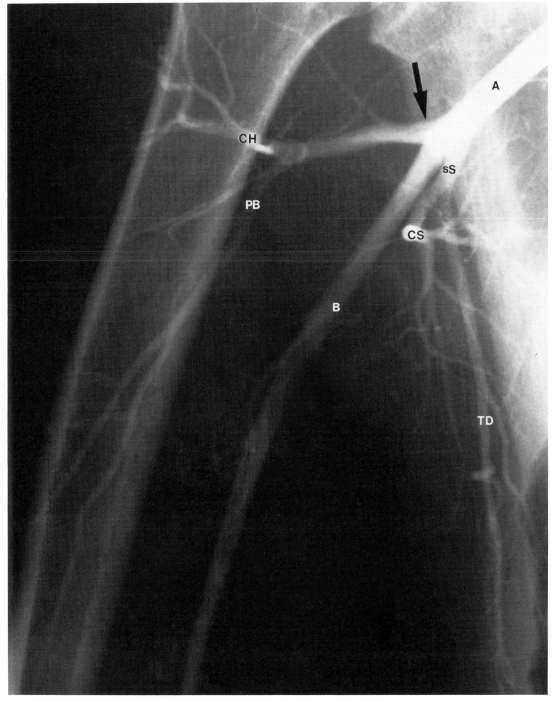

Figure 3–10. Axillary arteriogram shows a high origin of the profunda brachial artery together with the circumflex humeral *(arrow)*.

A	Axillary
B	Brachial
CH	Circumflex humeral
CS	Circumflex scapular
PB	Profunda (deep) brachial
sS	Subscapular
TD	Thoracodorsal

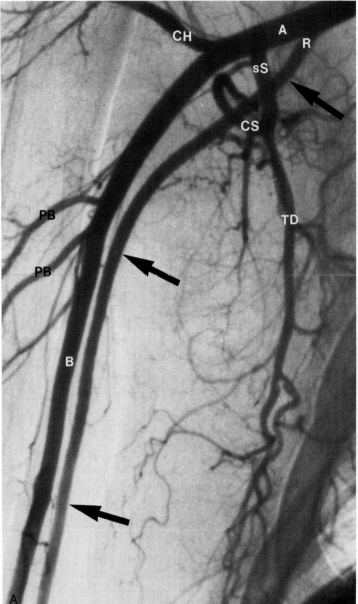

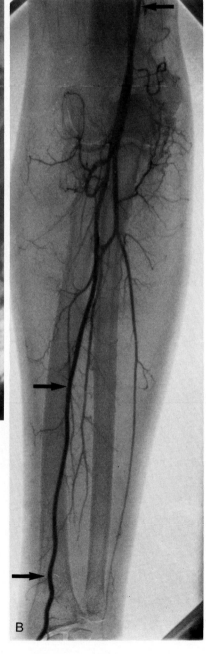

Figure 3–11. Axillary artery origin of the right radial artery (*arrows*).

A   Axillary
B   Brachial
CH   Circumflex humeral
CS   Circumflex scapular
PB   Profunda brachial
R   Radial
sS   Subscapular
TD Thoracodorsal

Figure 3–12. Axillary artery origin of the left ulnar artery *(arrows)*.

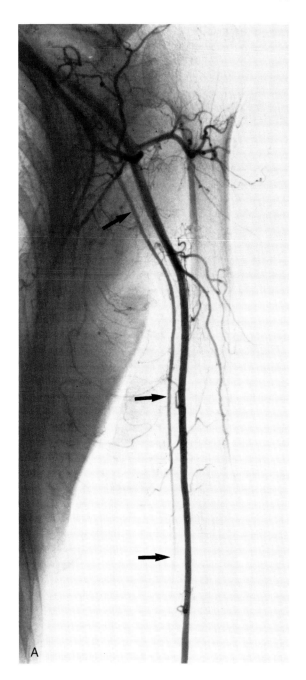

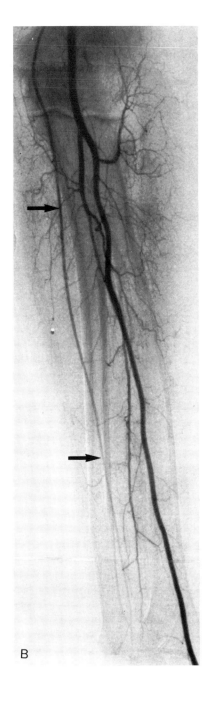

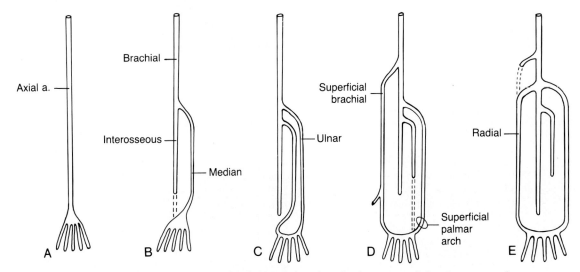

Figure 3–13. Line drawing depicting the embryologic stages of development of the upper extremity arteries. (After Piersol, from Singer E: Embryological pattern persisting in the arteries of the arm. Anat Rec 55:403–409, 1933.)

A   The axial artery extends to the wrist. Digital arteries develop from the capillary network of the wrist.

B   Development of the median artery, which takes over the blood supply to the digits.

C   Development of the ulnar artery. Together with the median artery, this forms the superficial palmar arch.

D   Development of the superficial brachial artery and regression of the distal median artery.

E   The proximal superficial brachial artery regresses and the distal segment becomes the radial artery.

Figure 3–14. Line drawing of the classic upper arm arterial anatomy.

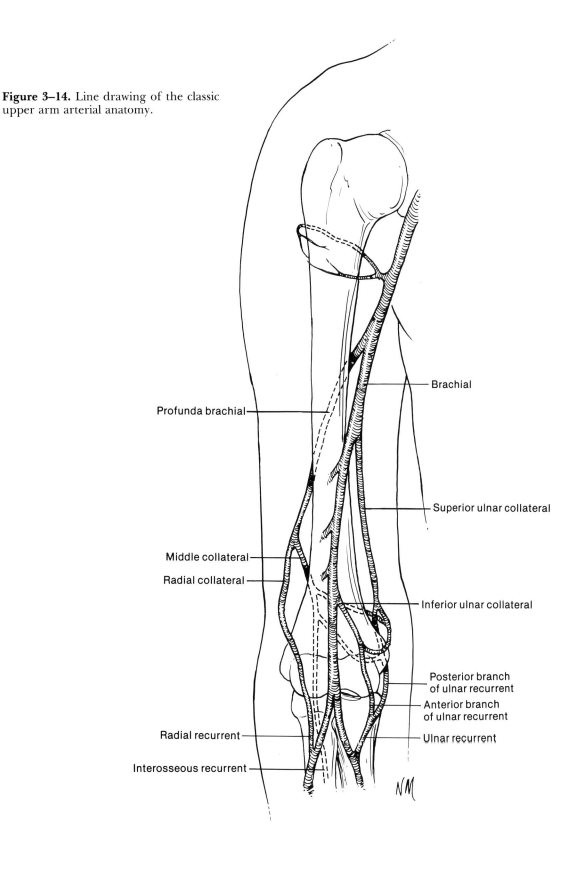

Brachial

Profunda brachial

Superior ulnar collateral

Middle collateral

Radial collateral

Inferior ulnar collateral

Posterior branch of ulnar recurrent

Anterior branch of ulnar recurrent

Radial recurrent

Ulnar recurrent

Interosseous recurrent

NM

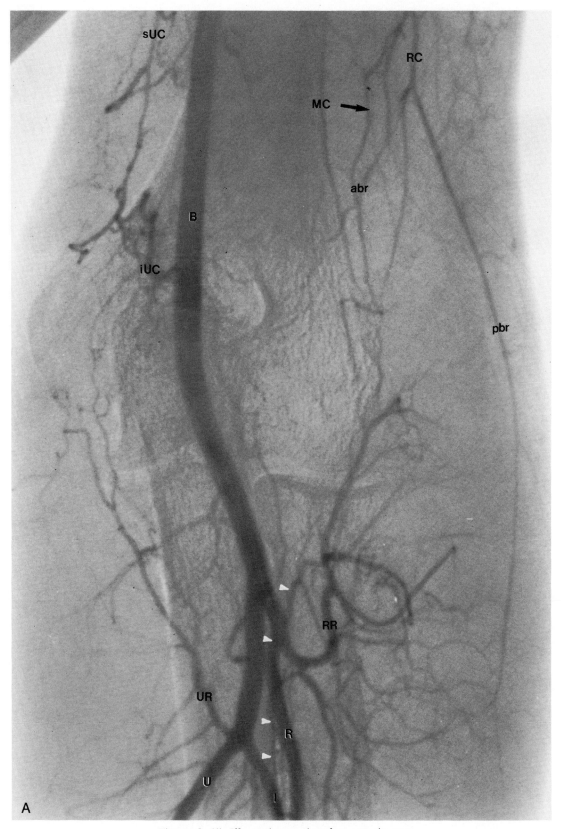

Figure 3–15. *Illustration continued on opposite page.*

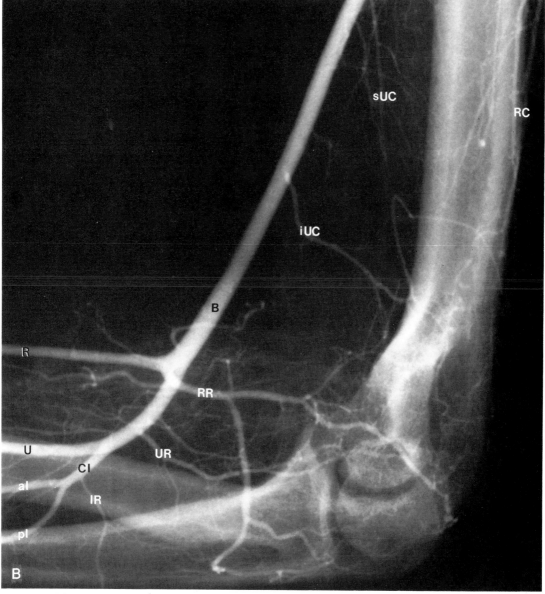

Figure 3–15. *A*, AP and *B*, lateral brachial arteriograms showing the normal anatomy around the elbow.

abr	Anterior (deep) branch of radial collateral
aI	Anterior interosseous
B	Brachial
CI	Common interosseous
I	Interosseous
IR	(and *arrowheads*) Interosseous recurrent
iUC	Inferior ulnar collateral
MC	Middle collateral
pbr	Posterior (superficial) branch of radial collateral
pI	Posterior interosseous
R	Radial
RC	Radial collateral
RR	Radial recurrent
sUC	Superior ulnar collateral
U	Ulnar
UR	Ulnar recurrent

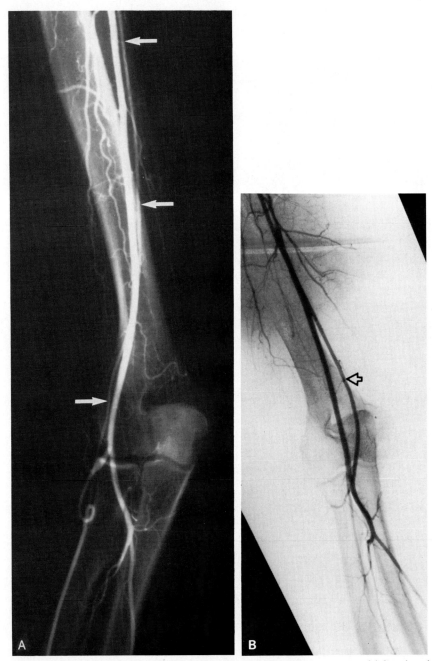

Figure 3–16. *A*, Persistent superficial brachial artery *(white arrows)*, which arises in the proximal portion of the brachial artery, continues as the radial artery. *B*, Accessory brachial artery *(arrow)*.

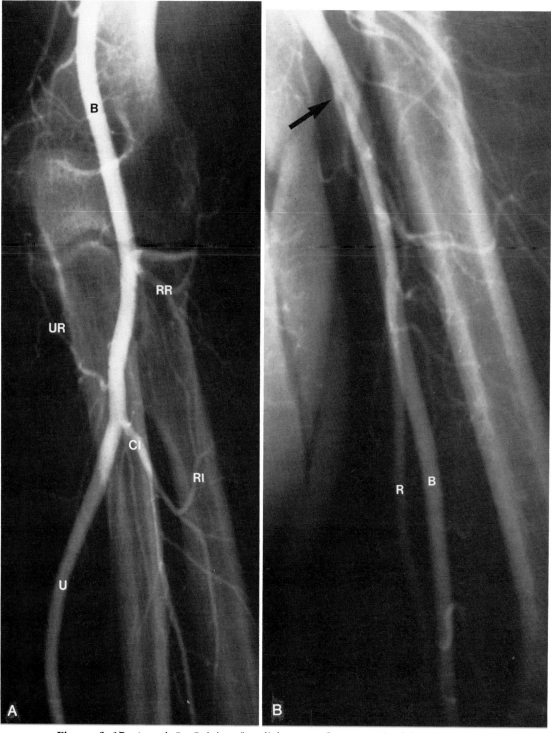

Figure 3–17. *A* and *B*, Origin of radial artery from proximal brachial artery *(arrow)*. NOTE: The recurrent radial artery arises from the brachial artery.

B	Brachial	RR	Radial recurrent
CI	Common interosseous	UR	Ulnar recurrent
R	Radial	U	Ulnar
RI	Recurrent interosseous		

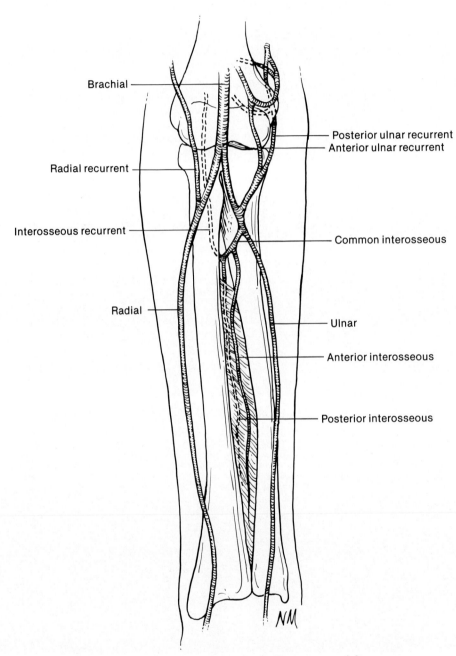

Figure 3–18. Line drawing of the classic forearm arterial anatomy.

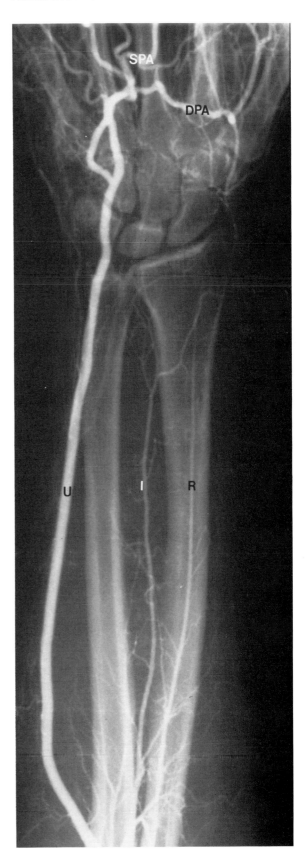

Figure 3–19. Hypoplastic radial artery. Radial artery is diminutive and terminates proximal to the wrist. There is compensatory enlargement of the ulnar artery which supplies both the deep and superficial palmar arches. NOTE: Hypoplasia or aplasia of the radial artery is seen in association with Down's syndrome.

DPA	Deep palmar arch
I	Interosseous
R	Radial
SPA	Superficial palmar arch
U	Ulnar

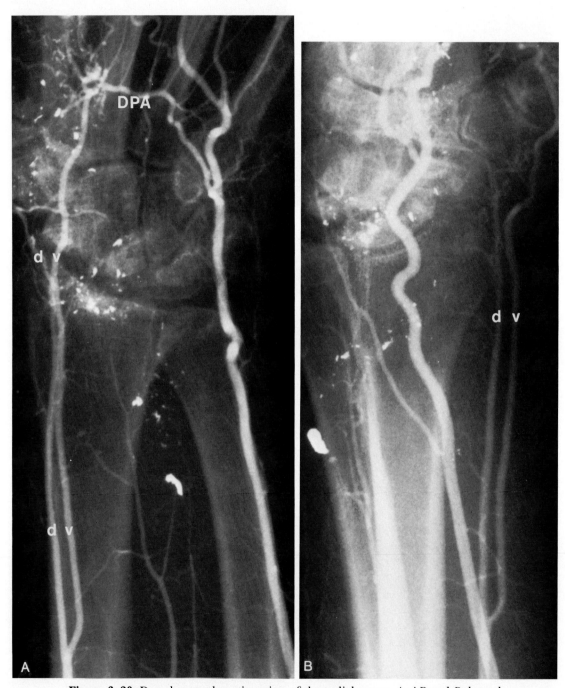

Figure 3–20. Dorsal manual continuation of the radial artery. *A,* AP and *B,* lateral wrist arteriogram in a patient with a bullet injury. The distal radial artery bifurcates. The ventral branch (v) forms the deep palmar arch (DPA), and the dorsal branch (d) is occluded in the dorsum of the hand.

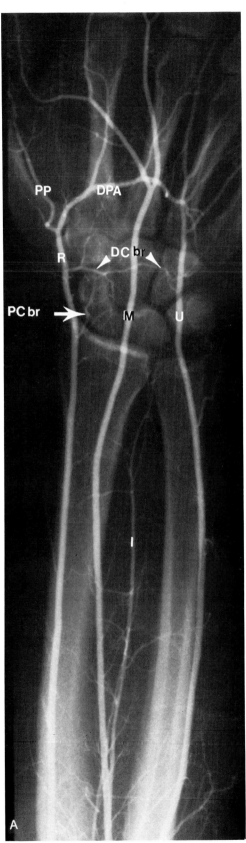

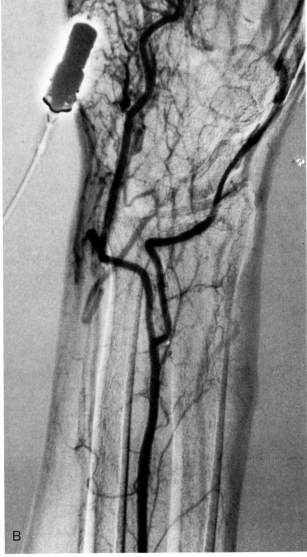

Figure 3–21. Persistent median and interosseus arteries. *A,* Persistent median artery. This vessel arises from the common interosseous artery and supplies some common palmar digital arteries normally supplied by the superficial palmar arch. Occasionally, the persistent median artery may arise from the anterior interosseous artery. *B,* Persistent interosseous artery and absent radial and ulnar arteries.

DCbr	Dorsal carpal branch
DPA	Deep palmar arch
I	Interosseous
M	Median
PCbr	Palmar carpal branch of radial artery
PP	Princeps pollicis artery (main artery to thumb)
R	Radial
U	Ulnar

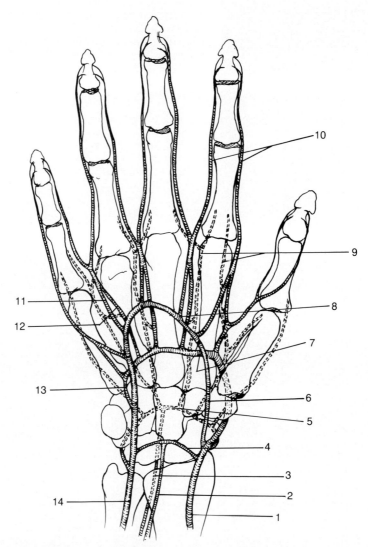

Figure 3–22. Line drawing of the classic arterial anatomy of the hand.

    1 Radial
    2 Anterior interosseous
    3 Posterior interosseous
    4 Palmar carpal branch
    5 Dorsal carpal branch forming the dorsal carpal rete
    6 Superficial palmar branch of radial artery
    7 Deep palmar arch
    8 Superficial palmar arch
    9 Dorsal metacarpal arteries
  10 Proper palmar digital arteries
  11 Common palmar digital arteries
  12 Palmar metacarpal
  13 Deep palmar branch of ulnar artery
  14 Ulnar artery

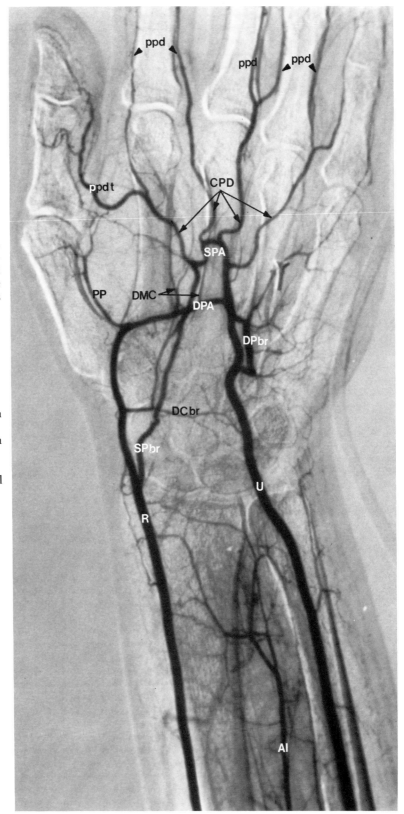

Figure 3–23. Normal hand arteriogram showing complete deep and superficial palmar arches. NOTE: The superficial palmar arch is dominant in this individual.

AI   Anterior interosseous
CPD Common palmar digital
DCbr Dorsal carpal branch
DMC Dorsal metacarpal
DPA Deep palmar arch
DPbr Deep palmar branch of ulnar
PP   Princeps pollicis (main artery to thumb)
ppd Palmar proper digital
ppdt Palmar proper digital to thumb
R   Radial
SPA Superficial palmar arch
SPbr Superficial palmar branch of radial
U   Ulnar

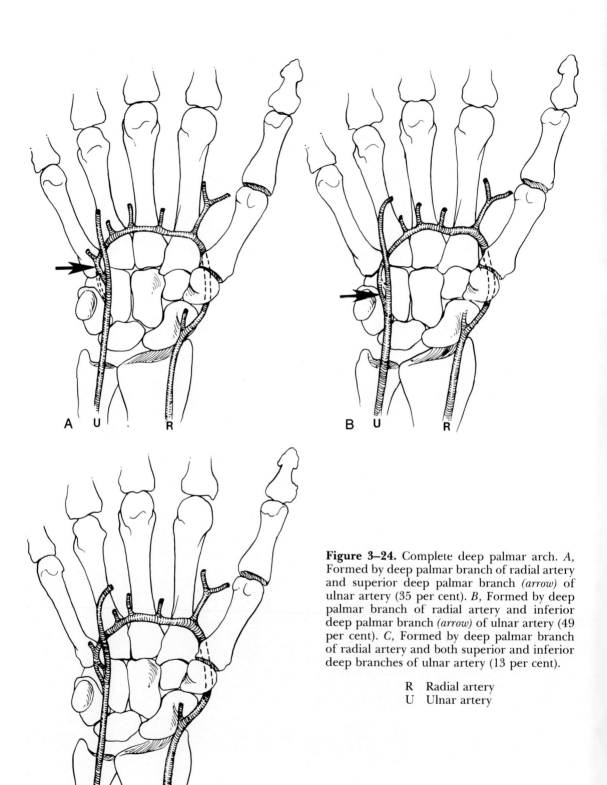

Figure 3–24. Complete deep palmar arch. *A,* Formed by deep palmar branch of radial artery and superior deep palmar branch *(arrow)* of ulnar artery (35 per cent). *B,* Formed by deep palmar branch of radial artery and inferior deep palmar branch *(arrow)* of ulnar artery (49 per cent). *C,* Formed by deep palmar branch of radial artery and both superior and inferior deep branches of ulnar artery (13 per cent).

R Radial artery
U Ulnar artery

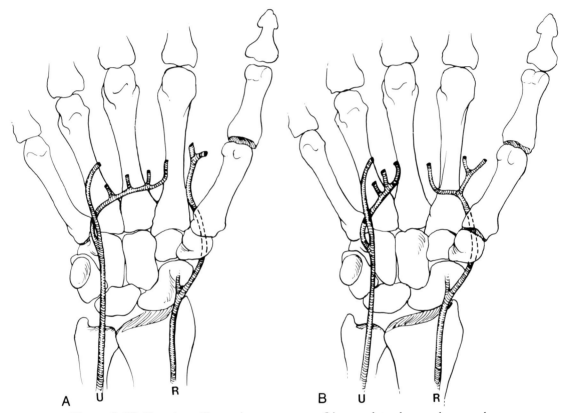

Figure 3–25. Drawings illustrating two types of incomplete deep palmar arches. Each occurs in 1.5 per cent of individuals.

R   Radial artery
U   Ulnar artery

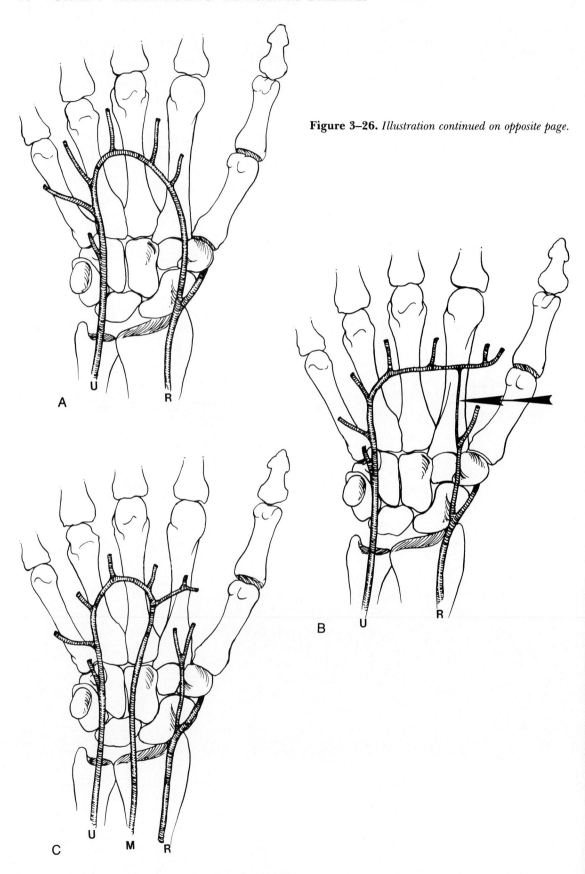

Figure 3–26. *Illustration continued on opposite page.*

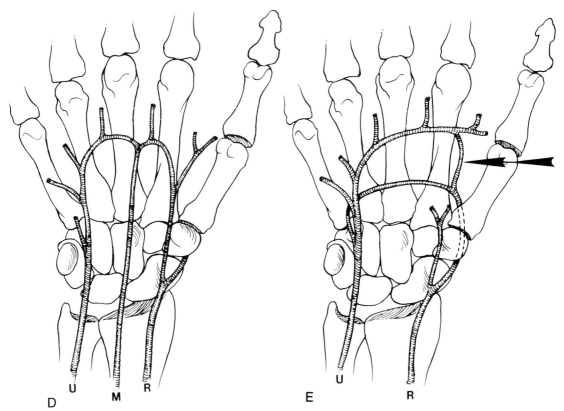

Figure 3–26. Complete superficial palmar arch. *A*, Classic radioulnar arch (35 per cent). *B*, Ulnar artery is the main contributor that anastomoses with small branch(es) *(arrow)* of the deep arch in the first digital interspace (37 per cent). *C*, Mediano-ulnar arch (4 per cent). *D*, Radio-mediano-ulnar arch (1 per cent). *E*, Formed by ulnar artery and a large unnamed branch *(arrow)* from the deep arch (2 per cent).

M   Median artery
R   Radial artery
U   Ulnar artery

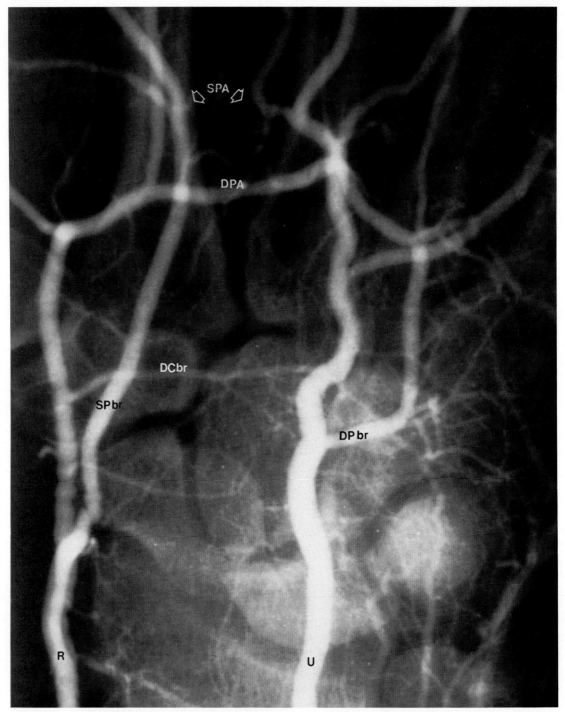

Figure 3–27. Arteriogram showing an incomplete superficial palmar arch.

DCbr	Dorsal carpal branch
DPA	Deep palmar arch
DPbr	Deep palmar branch of ulnar artery
R	Radial
SPA	Superficial palmar arch
SPbr	Superficial palmar branch of radial artery
U	Ulnar

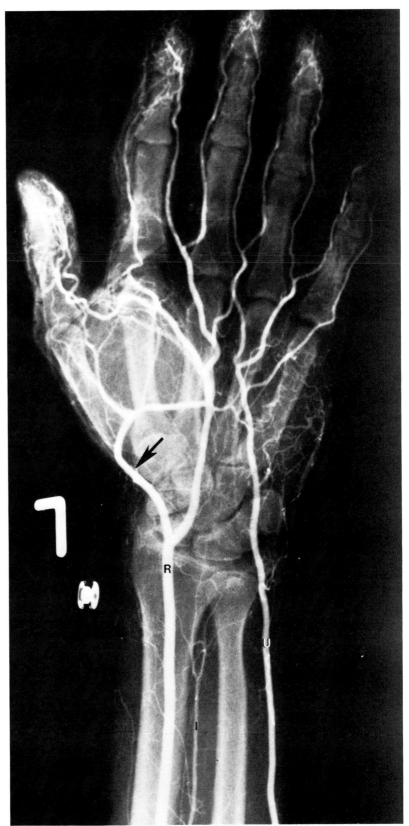

Figure 3–28. Incomplete deep and superficial palmar arches. Arrow points to deep palmar branch at radial artery.

CPD   Common palmar
         digital
DPbr Deep palmar branch
         of ulnar artery
I   Interosseous
R   Radial
U   Ulnar

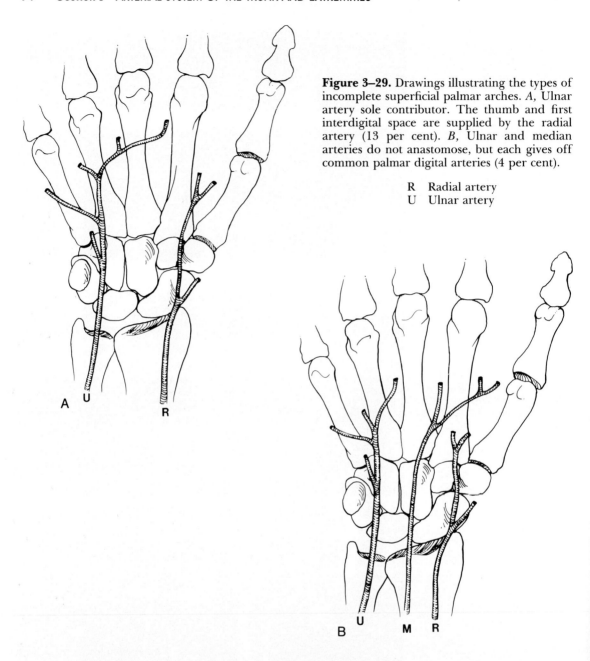

Figure 3–29. Drawings illustrating the types of incomplete superficial palmar arches. *A,* Ulnar artery sole contributor. The thumb and first interdigital space are supplied by the radial artery (13 per cent). *B,* Ulnar and median arteries do not anastomose, but each gives off common palmar digital arteries (4 per cent).

R   Radial artery
U   Ulnar artery

Figure 3–30. Subtraction film showing the hand arteries. The deep palmar arch is absent. The deep palmar branch of the radial artery terminates in a palmar metacarpal artery.

CPD	Common palmar digital arteries
DPbr	Deep palmar branch of ulnar artery
DR	Deep palmar branch of radial artery
PM	Palmar metacarpal artery
PP	Princeps pollicis artery
ppd	Proper palmar digital arteries
R	Radial
SPA	Superficial palmar arch
SPbr	Superficial palmar branch of radial artery
U	Ulnar

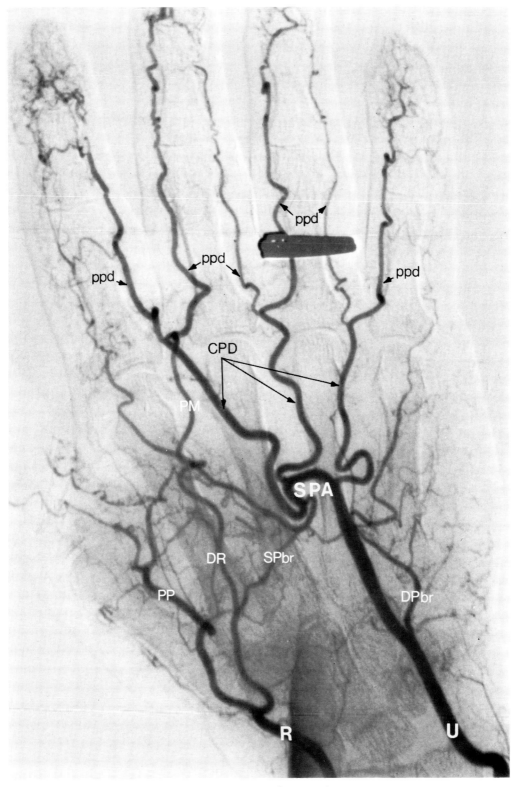

Figure 3–30. *See legend on opposite page.*

Chapter Four

ABDOMINAL AORTA AND PELVIS

SAADOON KADIR, M.D.

ABDOMINAL AORTA (Figs. 4–1 to 4–4)

The abdominal aorta bifurcates at L_4 or L_5. Occasionally, the aortic bifurcation is higher or lower. It is frequently lower in older individuals and those with tortuous and ectatic vessels.

PHRENIC ARTERIES (Figs. 4–5 and 4–6)

The superior phrenic arteries are small branches of the descending thoracic aorta.

The inferior phrenic arteries supply the abdominal side of the diaphragm. The origin of the inferior phrenic arteries is from one of the following:

1. Celiac artery or one of its branches, i.e., left hepatic or left gastric arteries
2. Abdominal aorta
3. Renal arteries, mostly the right.

Both left and right inferior phrenic arteries arise separately in 67 per cent of individuals and form a common trunk in 33 per cent. Rarely the origin of the inferior phrenic artery may be from the common hepatic, superior mesenteric, or gonadal vessels. A detailed description follows in Chapter 16.

97

COMMON AND EXTERNAL ILIAC ARTERIES
(Figs. 4–7 to 4–11)

Absent or very short common iliac arteries are rare. In such situations, the internal iliac arteries arise at or close to the aortic bifurcation. Branches off the common iliac arteries occur in one third of cadaver dissections. These consist mainly of lumbar and/or aberrant renal arteries. The latter is usually associated with a horseshoe or ectopic kidney. Important branches of the external iliac artery are the deep iliac circumflex and inferior epigastric arteries. These arise behind the inguinal ligament. Distal to this ligament, it continues as the common femoral artery.

INTERNAL ILIAC ARTERY (Figs. 4–12 to 4–21)

The internal iliac artery branching pattern can be quite variable. There are four larger branches: superior and inferior gluteal, obturator, and internal pudendal arteries. In 60 per cent of individuals, the internal iliac arteries divide into two main trunks—the anterior and posterior divisions. In approximately 10 per cent of individuals, there is only one trunk. Figure 4–14 illustrates the main branching patterns.

The superior gluteal artery forms the terminal branch of the posterior division, and the internal pudendal artery is the terminal branch of the anterior division.

Anterior Division of the Internal Iliac Artery

There are three main parietal branches—obturator, inferior gluteal, and internal pudendal arteries—and several visceral arteries. Each of these branches may show considerable variation in origin.

Obturator Artery (Figs. 4–7, 4–12, and 4–14 to 4–18)

In 75 per cent of individuals, the obturator artery is a branch of the internal iliac artery. It arises from one of the following:

1. Anterior division in approximately 25 per cent of individuals (Fig. 4–12)

2. From the superior gluteal artery or rarely from another branch of the posterior division in approximately 20 per cent of individuals (Fig. 4–7)

3. From the main trunk of the internal iliac artery in 15 per cent of individuals

4. From the inferior gluteal artery in approximately 10 per cent of individuals (Fig. 4–18)

5. From the internal pudendal artery in approximately 5 per cent of individuals (Fig. 4–16).

In 25 per cent of individuals, it is a branch of the common femoral or external iliac artery (approximately 2 per cent) (Fig. 4–17). Frequently, it arises together with or from the inferior epigastric artery (approximately 22 per cent). The obturator artery terminates in an anterior and posterior branch. The former courses along the medial margin and the latter along the lateral margin of the obturator foramen.

Inferior Gluteal Artery (Figs. 4–10 to 4–12 and 4–14 to 4–19)

This vessel is a branch of the anterior division in 75 per cent of individuals, and in 25 per cent it arises from the superior gluteal artery (Fig. 4–19). In the embryo, this vessel forms a segment of the primitive axial artery which supplies the lower extremity. Persistence of the embryonic vessel (called the sciatic artery) is observed in fewer than 0.1 per cent of individuals.

The inferior gluteal artery provides one or more branches to the sciatic nerve in its extrapelvic course. Rarely it is duplicated.

Internal Pudendal Artery (Figs. 4–7 and 4–11 to 4–16)

This is usually a branch of the anterior division and frequently arises together with the inferior gluteal artery. In 6 to 10 per cent of individuals, there is an accessory pudendal artery from the main internal iliac artery or one of its other branches. The main branches of the internal pudendal artery are the inferior hemorrhoidal and penile arteries (to the corpus cavernosum and the dorsal artery of the penis) (see Chapter 12).

Visceral Branches

1. Superior vesical arteries (Figs. 4–12 and 4–14 to 4–16): These are two or three arteries that provide the major amount of blood supply to the urinary bladder. These are best identified when the bladder is distended (Fig. 4–15).
2. Inferior vesical arteries (Fig. 4–12).
3. Internal genital arteries (Figs. 4–12 and 4–15): In the male, these are the arteries to the prostate, seminal vesicles, and vas deferens; in the female, they are the uterine arteries (see Chapter 12).
4. Middle hemorrhoidal artery (Fig. 4–12): This is usually a branch of the anterior division (from the obturator or internal pudendal arteries) and is occasionally duplicated (see Chapter 13).

Posterior Division of the Internal Iliac Artery

There are three consistent branches of the posterior division of the internal iliac artery:

Superior Gluteal Artery (Figs. 4–7, 4–12, and 4–14 to 4–19)

In 25 per cent of individuals, this gives off the inferior gluteal artery and in 20 per cent, the obturator artery (Figs. 4–7 and 4–19).

Iliolumbar Artery (Figs. 4–13, 4–14, 4–16, and 4–18 to 4–20)

This artery is most frequently a branch of the posterior division, but occasionally it is a branch of the main internal iliac or the common iliac artery. Rarely, it is absent. The iliac and lumbar branches can have independent origins from the internal iliac artery. In addition, the lumbar branch may originate from the common iliac or a lumbar artery (see Fig. 4–20).

Lateral Sacral Arteries (Figs. 4–7, 4–12 to 4–14, 4–16, 4–18, and 4–21)

These are usually two in number, the superior and inferior lateral sacral arteries, but may be as many as four. Their origins can be variable, but most commonly they arise from the posterior division of the internal iliac artery.

REFERENCES

1. Braithwaite JL: Variations in origin of the parietal branches of the internal iliac artery. J Anat 86:423–430, 1952.
2. El Mamoun BA, Demmel U: The lateral branches of the common iliac artery. Surg Radiol Anat 10:161–164, 1988.
3. Hassen-Khodja R, Batt M, Michetti C, et al: Radiologic anatomy of the anastomotic systems of the internal iliac artery. Surg Radiol Anat 9:135–140, 1987.
4. Lippert H, Pabst R: Arterial Variations in Man. Classification and Frequency. Munich, JF Bergman Verlag, 1985.
5. Merland J-J, Chiras J: Arteriography of the Pelvis. Diagnostic and Therapeutic Procedures. New York, Springer Verlag, 1981.
6. Páč L, Hamplová M, Pelcova O: An atypical case of arising of some parietal branches of the arteria iliaca interna in man. Anat Anz 141:450–454, 1977.

Figures 4–1 through 4–21 on following pages.

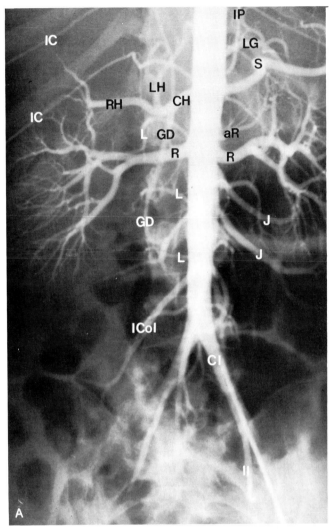

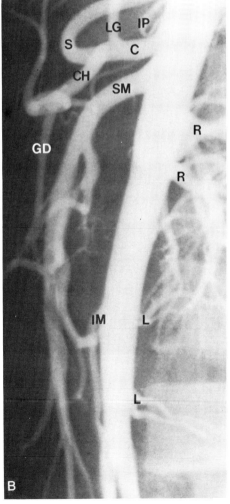

Figure 4–1. *A,* AP and *B,* lateral abdominal aortogram.

aR	Accessory renal artery to upper pole
C	Celiac
CH	Common hepatic
CI	Common iliac
GD	Gastroduodenal
IC	Intercostal
ICol	Ileocolic
II	Internal iliac
IM	Inferior mesenteric
IP	Inferior phrenic
J	Jejunal
L	Lumbar
LG	Left gastric
LH	Left hepatic
R	Renal
RH	Right hepatic
S	Splenic
SM	Superior mesenteric

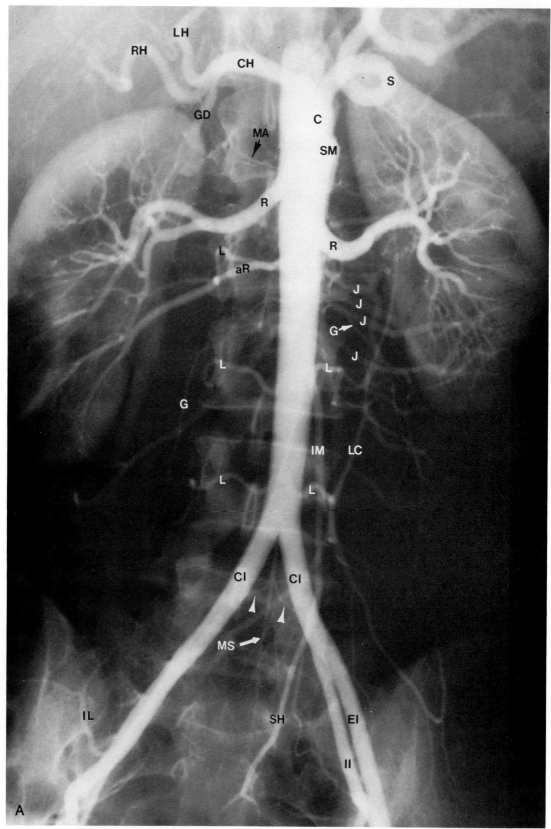

Figure 4–2. *A*, AP and *B*, lateral abdominal aortograms from different individuals. Arrowheads in *A* point to small lumbar branches originating from the middle sacral artery.

Illustration continued on opposite page.

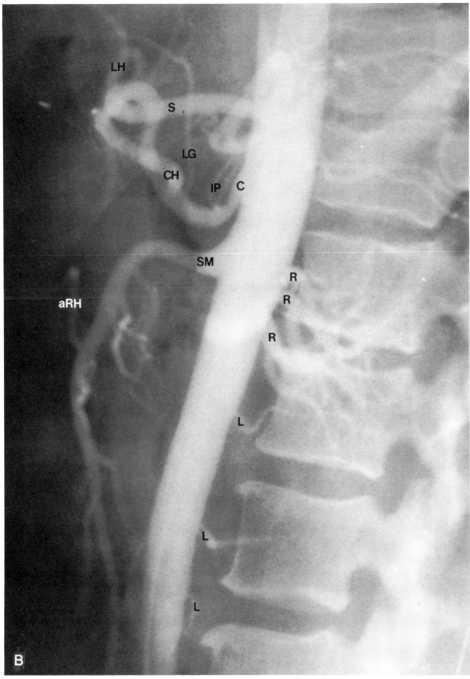

Figure 4–2. *Continued.*

aR	Accessory lower pole renal artery	J	Jejunal
aRH	Accessory right hepatic	L	Lumbar
C	Celiac	LC	Left colic
CH	Common hepatic	LH	Left hepatic
CI	Common iliac	MA	Middle adrenal
EI	External iliac	MS	Middle sacral
G	Gonadal	R	Renal
GD	Gastroduodenal	RH	Right hepatic
II	Internal iliac	S	Splenic
IL	Ileolumbar	SH	Superior hemorrhoidal
IM	Inferior mesenteric	SM	Superior mesenteric

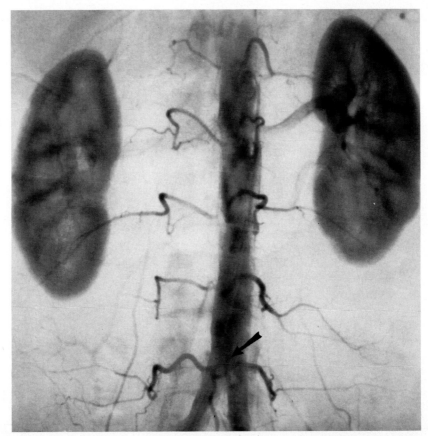

Figure 4–3. Subtraction of a late film from an abdominal aortogram shows five pairs of lumbar arteries. The lowest pair forms a common trunk and gives off the middle sacral artery *(arrow)*.

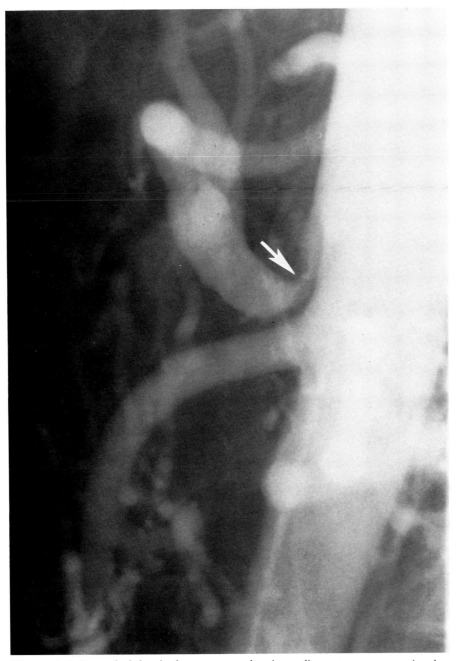

Figure 4–4. Lateral abdominal aortogram showing celiac artery compression by diaphragmatic crux (*arrow*).

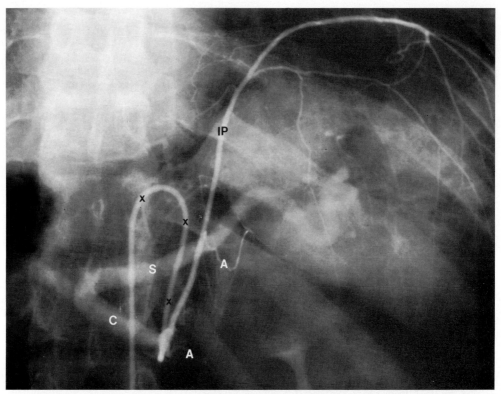

Figure 4–5. Left inferior phrenic artery arises from the proximal celiac artery.

A	Superior adrenal arteries
C	Celiac
IP	Inferior phrenic
S	Splenic
× × ×	Catheter

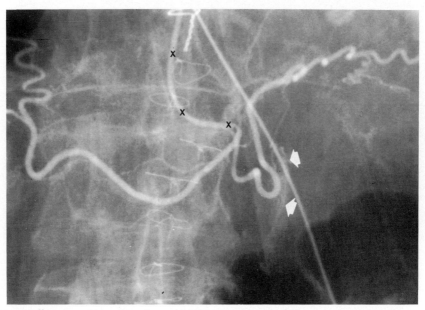

Figure 4–6. Common phrenic trunk. Arrows point to left adrenal gland. × × × = Catheter.

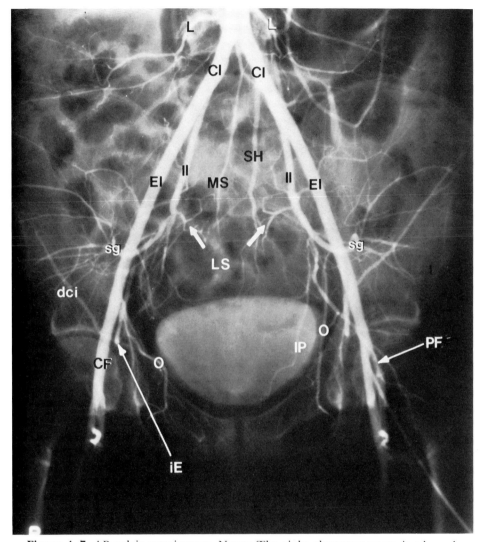

Figure 4–7. AP pelvic arteriogram. NOTE: The right obturator artery is a branch of the inferior epigastric artery, and the left obturator is a branch of the left superior gluteal artery. The left common femoral artery bifurcates early.

CF	Common femoral
CI	Common iliac
dci	Deep circumflex iliac
EI	External iliac
iE	Inferior epigastric
II	Internal iliac
IP	Internal pudendal
L	Lumbar
LS	Lateral sacral
MS	Middle sacral
O	Obturator
PF	Profunda femoris
sg	Superior gluteal
SH	Superior hemorrhoidal

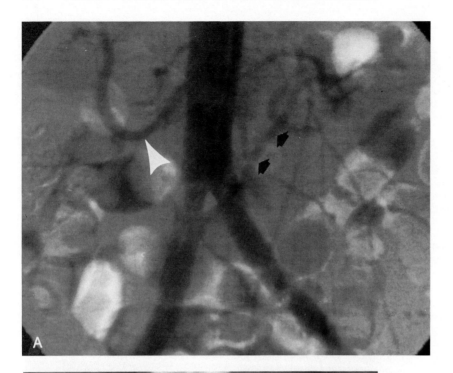

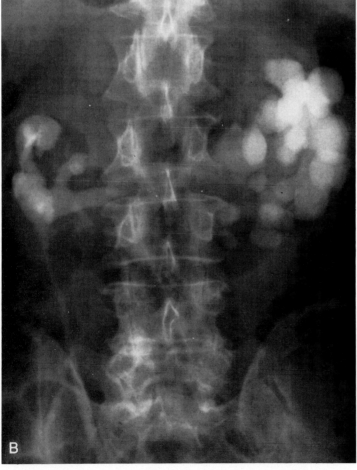

Figure 4–8. Aberrant origin of renal artery from common iliac artery in a patient with a horseshoe kidney. *A*, AP abdominal aortogram (DSA) shows a lower pole artery to the left kidney arising from the right common iliac artery *(black arrows)*. The white arrowhead points to the right lower renal artery. *B*, Intravenous urogram from the same patient as in *A* showing the horseshoe kidney and obstruction of the left collecting system.

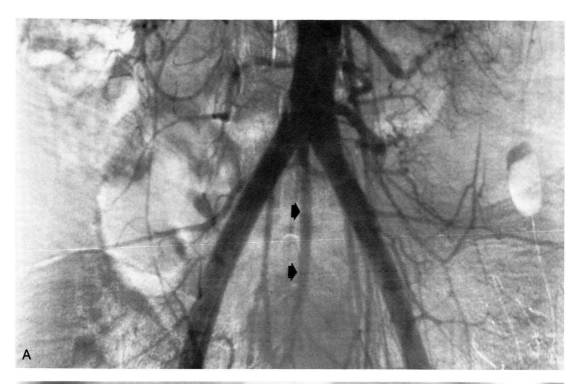

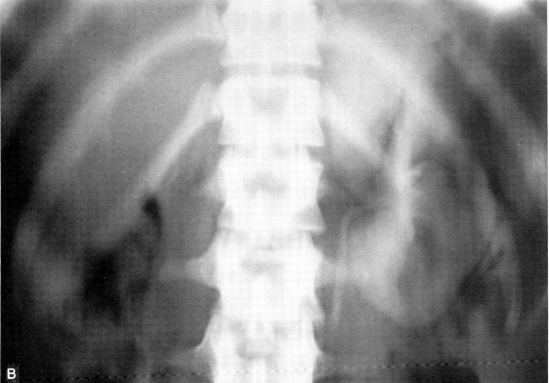

Figure 4–9. Aberrant origin of renal artery from lower aorta in an individual with a pelvic kidney. *A,* AP aortogram shows a large midline vessel (renal artery to pelvic kidney) descending into the pelvis *(arrows)* from the aortic bifurcation. *B,* Nephrotomogram shows absence of the right kidney in its normal location.

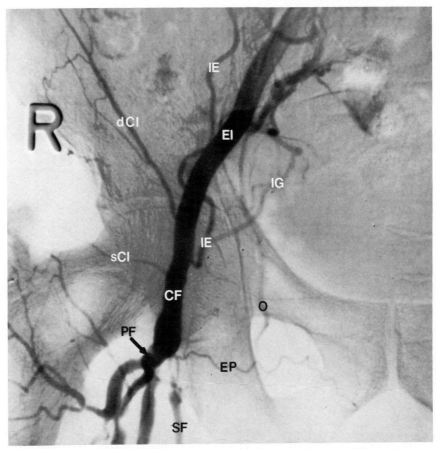

Figure 4–10. Right external iliac–common femoral arteriogram. There is severe stenosis of the proximal superficial femoral artery.

CF	Common femoral
dCI	Deep circumflex iliac
EP	External pudendal
EI	External iliac
IE	Inferior epigastric
IG	Inferior gluteal
O	Obturator
PF	Profunda femoris
sCI	Superficial circumflex iliac
SF	Superficial femoral

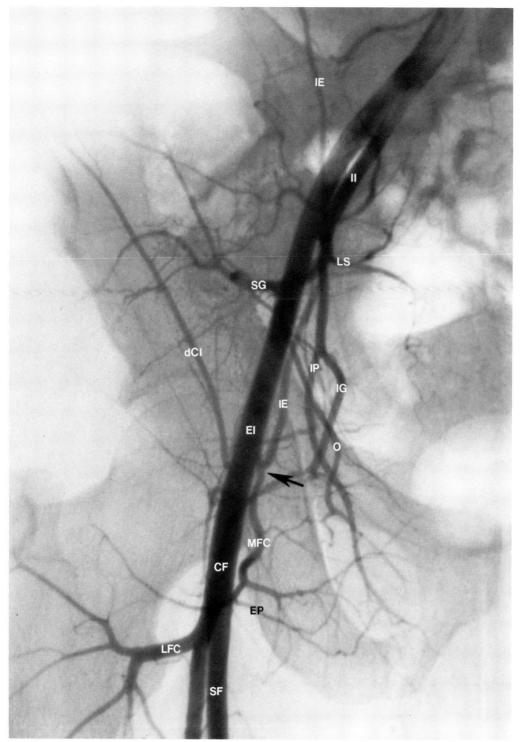

Figure 4–11. Right common iliac arteriogram. The medial femoral circumflex artery arises together with the inferior epigastric artery *(arrow)*.

CF	Common femoral	IP	Internal pudendal
dCI	Deep circumflex iliac	LFC	Lateral femoral circumflex
EI	External iliac	LS	Lateral sacral
EP	External pudendal	MFC	Medial femoral circumflex
IE	Inferior epigastric	O	Obturator
II	Internal iliac	SF	Superficial femoral
IG	Inferior gluteal	SG	Superior gluteal

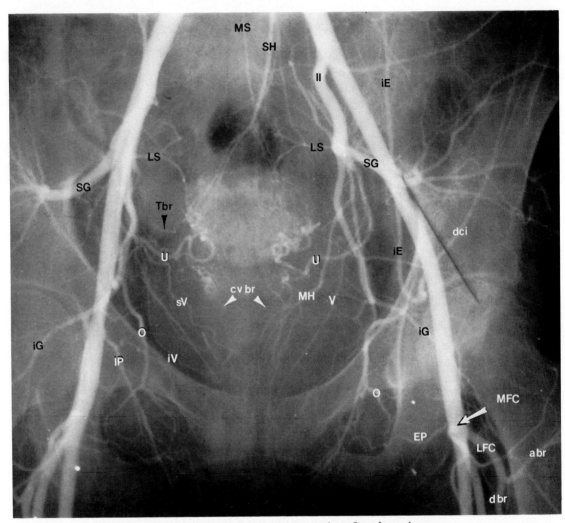

Figure 4–12. AP pelvic arteriogram in a female patient.

abr	Ascending branch of LFC	LFC	Lateral femoral circumflex
dbr	Descending branch of LFC	LS	Lateral sacral
cvbr	Cervicovaginal branches of uterine artery	MFC	Medial femoral circumflex
		MH	Middle hemorrhoidal
dci	Deep circumflex iliac	MS	Middle sacral
EP	External pudendal	SG	Superior gluteal
iE	Inferior epigastric	SH	Superior hemorrhoidal
iG	Inferior gluteal	sV	Superior vesical
II	Internal iliac	Tbr	Tubal branch of uterine artery
IP	Internal pudendal	U	Uterine
iV	Inferior vesical	V	Vaginal
LFC	Lateral femoral circumflex		

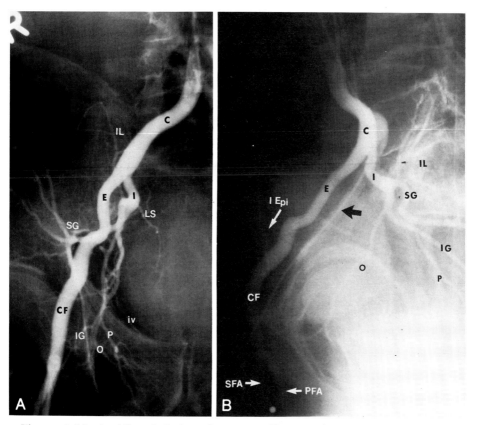

Figure 4–13. *A,* AP and *B,* lateral common iliac arteriogram. (From Kadir S: Diagnostic Angiography. Philadelphia, WB Saunders Company, 1986.)

C	Common iliac
CF	Common femoral
E	External iliac
I	Internal iliac
IEpi	Inferior epigastric
IG	Inferior gluteal
IL	Iliolumbar
iv	Inferior vesical
LS	Lateral sacral
O	Obturator
P	Internal pudendal
PFA	Profunda femoris
SFA	Superficial femoral
SG	Superior gluteal

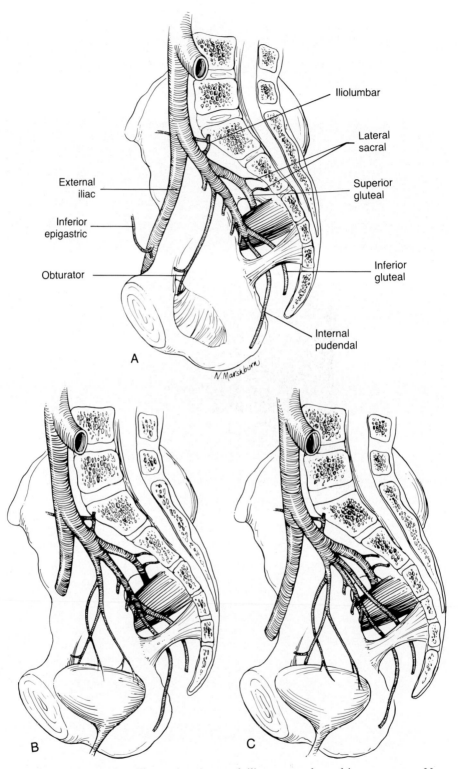

Figure 4–14. Drawing illustrating internal iliac artery branching patterns. Not shown on these illustrations, 10 per cent of individuals have one trunk. *A*, Divides into two trunks: anterior and posterior divisions (60 per cent of individuals). *B*, Divides into three trunks (20 per cent of individuals). *C*, Divides into four or more trunks (10 per cent of individuals).

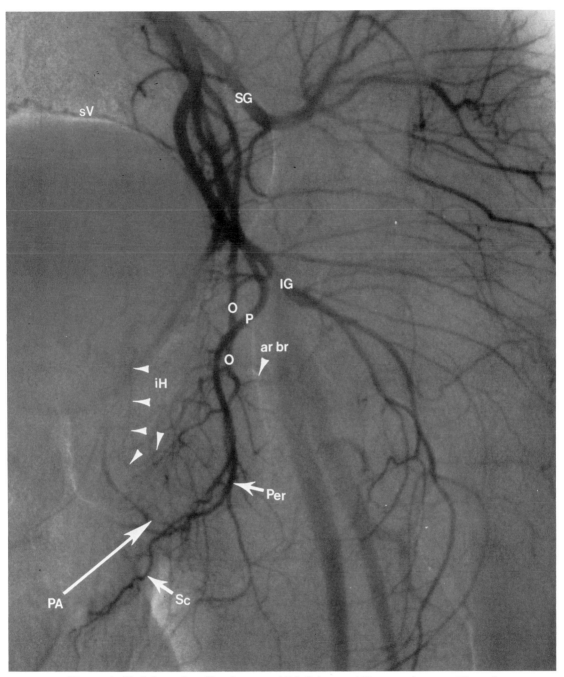

Figure 4–15. Subtraction film from an AP left internal iliac arteriogram. There is flash filling of the superficial femoral and profunda femoris arteries.

arbr	Articular branch of obturator artery	P	Internal pudendal
IG	Inferior gluteal	PA	Penile artery
iH	Inferior hemorrhoidal (course of distal rectum outlined by arrowheads)	Per	Perineal artery
		Sc	Posterior scrotal branches
		SG	Superior gluteal
O	Obturator	sV	Superior vesical

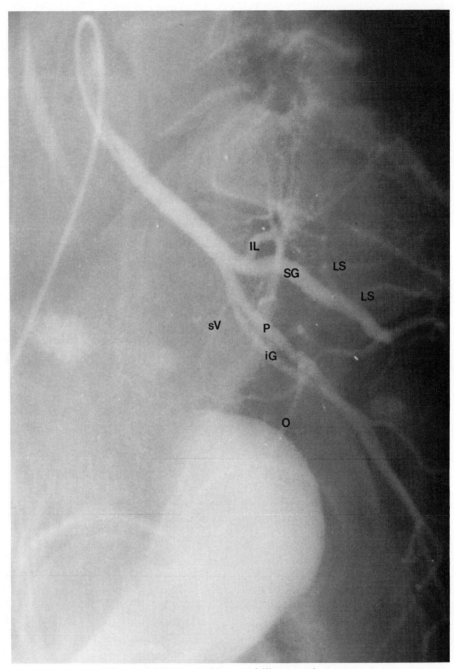

Figure 4–16. Lateral internal iliac arteriogram.

iG	Inferior gluteal
IL	Iliolumbar
LS	Lateral sacral
O	Obturator
P	Internal pudendal
SG	Superior gluteal
sV	Superior vesical

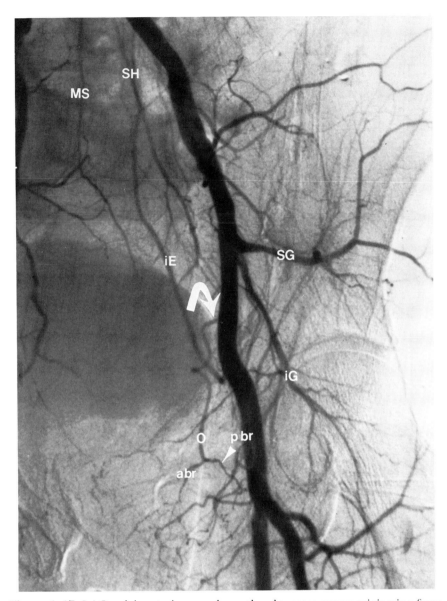

Figure 4–17. LAO pelvic arteriogram shows the obturator artery originating from the external iliac artery *(curved arrow).*

abr	Anterior branch of obturator
iE	Inferior epigastric
iG	Inferior gluteal
MS	Middle sacral
O	Obturator
pbr	Posterior branch of obturator
SG	Superior gluteal
SH	Superior hemorrhoidal

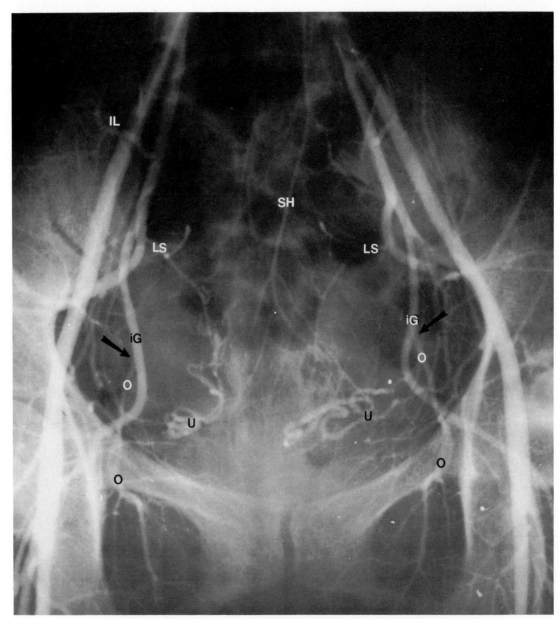

Figure 4–18. Pelvic arteriogram showing bilateral obturator arteries orginating from the inferior gluteal arteries *(arrows).*

iG	Inferior gluteal
IL	Iliolumbar
LS	Lateral sacral
O	Obturator
SH	Superior hemorrhoidal
U	Uterine

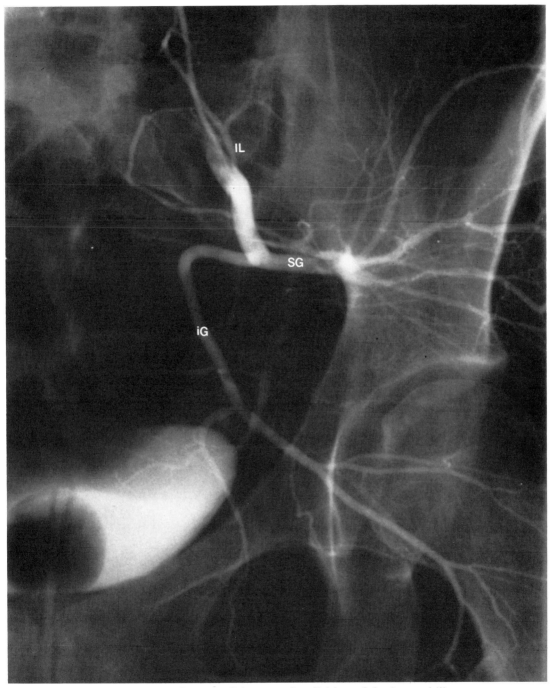

Figure 4–19. AP arteriogram of the posterior division of the internal iliac artery, showing the inferior gluteal artery arising from the superior gluteal artery.

iG   Inferior gluteal
IL   Iliolumbar
SG   Superior gluteal

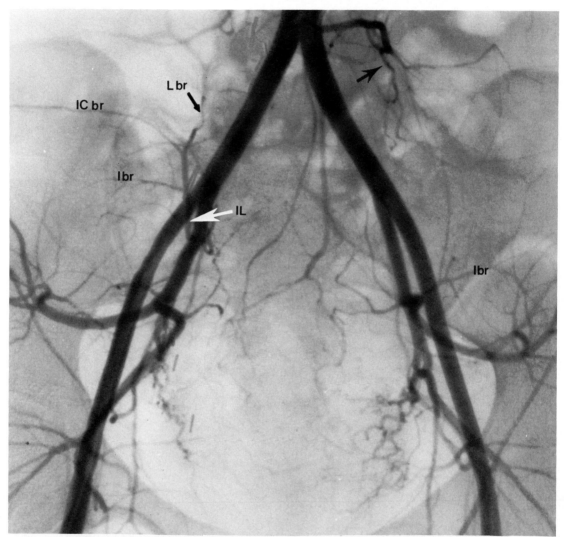

Figure 4–20. Subtraction from AP pelvic arteriogram shows the right iliolumbar artery. On the left, the iliac branch originates from the internal iliac artery, and the other branches originate from the 4th lumbar artery *(arrow)*.

Ibr	Iliac branch
ICbr	Iliac crest branch
IL	Iliolumbar artery
Lbr	Lumbar branch

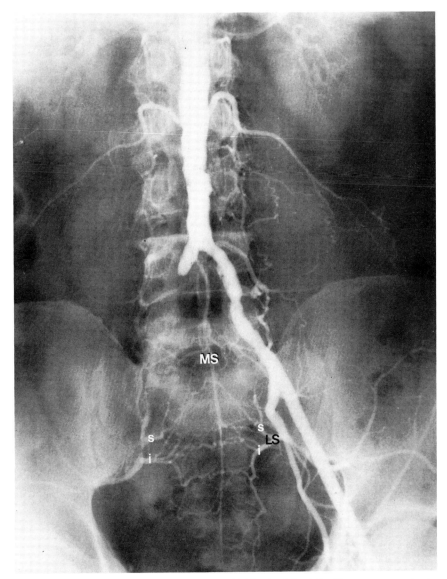

Figure 4–21. Pelvic arteriogram in an individual with right iliac artery occlusion showing the sacral arteries.

MS	Middle sacral
i	Inferior lateral sacral
LS	Lateral sacral
s	Superior lateral sacral

Chapter Five

ARTERIAL ANATOMY OF THE LOWER EXTREMITIES

SAADOON KADIR, M.D.

EMBRYOLOGY

In the embryo, the axial artery supplying the lower limb arises as a dorsal branch of the umbilical artery and courses dorsally into the thigh, lying between the tibia and the popliteus muscle at the knee. The primitive posterior tibial and peroneal arteries branch off above the popliteus muscle and continue dorsally into the lower leg. The anterior tibial artery originates at the inferior margin of the popliteus muscle. The femoral artery, arising from the external iliac artery, lies ventrally in the thigh and communicates distally with the embryonic axial artery of the leg.

As the embryo develops, the femoral artery increases in size and the axial artery regresses. The most proximal segments of the latter persist as the inferior gluteal artery and also as arterial branches to the sciatic nerve. Fusion of the primitive posterior tibial and peroneal arteries gives rise to the popliteal artery, located posterior to the popliteus muscle. Further distally, segments of the primitive axial artery regress while others are incorporated into the peroneal artery. Aberrations in the pattern of regression and fusion of the primitive axial artery and its branches account for the variant arterial anatomy of the lower extremity.

FEMORAL ARTERIES (Figs. 5–1 to 5–8)

Below the inguinal ligament, the external iliac artery continues as the common femoral artery (CFA). The CFA varies in length between 2 and 6 cm and bifurcates into the superficial femoral (SFA) and profunda femoris arteries (PFA). Infrequently, the common femoral artery is absent, and both SFA and

123

PFA originate from the external iliac artery. More commonly, the common femoral artery is very short, giving rise to the "high bifurcation" (Fig. 5–2; also see Fig. 4–4). Rarely, the PFA is absent and its branches originate independently from the SFA (Fig. 5–7).

The variations in the location of the PFA relative to the SFA are shown in Figure 5–3. In about 40 per cent of individuals, the PFA lies immediately behind the SFA. This location is of particular significance when antegrade femoral artery puncture is attempted using the double wall technique. The PFA exists as a single trunk in approximately 60 per cent of individuals. Figure 5–4 illustrates the frequent branching patterns of this vessel. Figure 5–8 shows the normal arterial supply to the hip.

POPLITEAL AND LOWER LEG ARTERIES (Figs. 5–9 to 5–20)

Major variations in the popliteal artery branching pattern are observed in up to 12 per cent of individuals. The popliteal artery divides at the lower margin of the popliteus muscle in 95 per cent of individuals. In the remainder, one or more branches originate above the upper margin of this muscle, i.e., at or above the level of the knee joint space (Figs. 5–13 to 5–15). Very rarely, there is a very low origin of one of the branches (Fig. 5–16).

In 7 per cent of individuals, the peroneal artery is a major source of blood supply to the foot (Fig. 5–18). It is congenitally absent in less than 0.1 per cent of individuals. The anterior tibial artery is absent or terminates early in 2 per cent of individuals (Figs. 5–19 and 5–28). The perforating branch of the peroneal artery may continue as the dorsalis pedis artery. In up to 5 per cent of individuals, the posterior tibial artery is either absent or terminates early (Fig. 5–20). In this situation, the communicating branch of the peroneal artery gives origin to the plantar arteries. Variant arterial anatomy of the lower leg is bilateral in approximately 28 per cent of such cases.

NUTRIENT ARTERY OF THE FIBULA (Fig. 5–21)

The nutrient artery enters the fibula via the nutrient foramen, which is located in the middle third of this bone. In most individuals, this vessel is demonstrated on nonselective lower extremity arteriograms. It is around 1 mm in diameter and originates from the proximal peroneal artery within the first 10 cm of the peroneal artery origin and occasionally from the tibioperoneal trunk. In addition, there are several periosteal branches, arising from muscular branches of the peroneal artery, which are considered essential for viability of the bone in patients undergoing vascularized fibular grafts.

ARTERIES OF THE FOOT (Figs. 5–22 to 5–28)

The anterior tibial artery continues as the dorsalis pedis artery, gives rise to the lateral and medial tarsal arteries, and forms the arcuate artery of the foot. The latter gives off four dorsal metatarsal arteries. In 20 per cent of individuals, all dorsal metatarsal arteries originate from the arcuate artery. In the remainder, one or more have a plantar origin. The major arterial variants are illustrated in Figure 5–25.

The plantar arch is analogous to the deep palmar arch and is formed by the lateral plantar artery (from the posterior tibial artery) and the deep plantar branch from the dorsalis pedis artery. The predominant blood supply to the plantar arch is from the dorsalis pedis artery. The area supplied by each artery can usually be distinguished anatomically but may be difficult to determine on nonselective lower extremity arteriography. The major arterial variants are illustrated in Figure 5–26.

SCIATIC AND SAPHENOUS ARTERIES (Figs. 5–7 and 5–29 to 5–31)

The sciatic artery is a rare anomaly observed in less than 0.1 per cent of individuals. It originates from the anterior division of the internal iliac artery and exits the pelvis together with the sciatic nerve and continues as the popliteal artery. In such individuals, the femoral artery is small and supplies the upper thigh but may continue distally and anastomose with the sciatic artery to form the popliteal artery. The saphenous artery is observed much less frequently. This vessel is usually small and runs along the saphenous vein.

REFERENCES

1. Bonnel F, Lesire M, Gomis R, et al: Arterial vascularization of the fibula. Micro-surgical transplant techniques. Diaphysis-superior epiphysis. Anat Clin 3:13–22, 1981.
2. Golan JF, Garrett WV, Smith BL, et al: Persistent sciatic artery and vein: An unusual case. J Vasc Surg 3:162–165, 1986.
3. Lippert H, Pabst R: Arterial Variations in Man. Classification and Frequency. Munich, JF Bergmann Verlag, 1985.
4. Müssbichler H: Arteriographic investigations of the normal hip in adults. Evaluation of methods and vascular findings. Acta Radiol 11:195–215, 1971.
5. Nabatoff RA: Anomalies encountered during varicose vein surgery. Arch Surg 113:586–588, 1978.
6. Nepper-Rasmusen J, Henneberg EW: Persisterende arteria ischiadica. Ugeskr Laeger 149:710—712, 1987.
7. Theron J: Superselective angiography of the hip. Radiology 124:649–657, 1977.

Figures 5–1 through 5–31 on following pages.

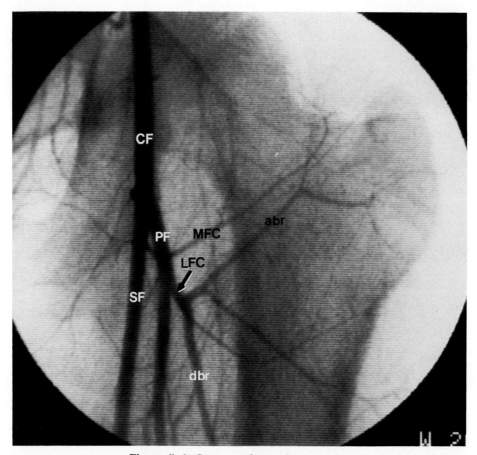

Figure 5–1. Common femoral arteriogram.

abr	Ascending branch of lateral femoral circumflex
CF	Common femoral
dbr	Descending branch of lateral femoral circumflex
LFC	Lateral femoral circumflex
MFC	Medial femoral circumflex
PF	Profunda femoris
SF	Superficial femoral

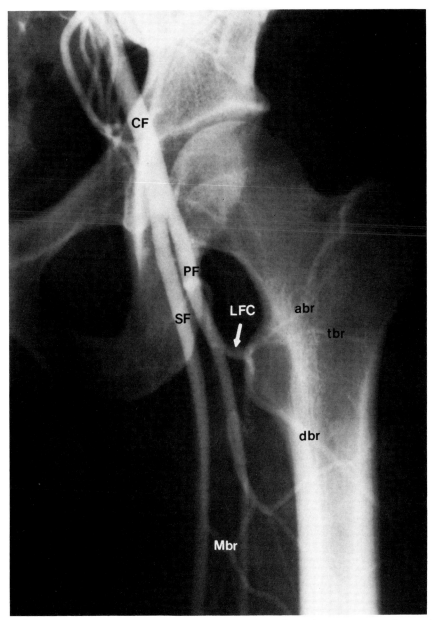

Figure 5–2. Common femoral arteriogram. There is a short common femoral artery (or the so-called high bifurcation). *Note:* The common femoral artery is located medially to the femoral head.

abr	Ascending branch of lateral femoral circumflex
CF	Common femoral
dbr	Descending branch of lateral femoral circumflex
LFC	Lateral femoral circumflex
Mbr	Muscular branch of superficial femoral
PF	Profunda femoris
SF	Superficial femoral
tbr	Transverse branch of lateral femoral circumflex

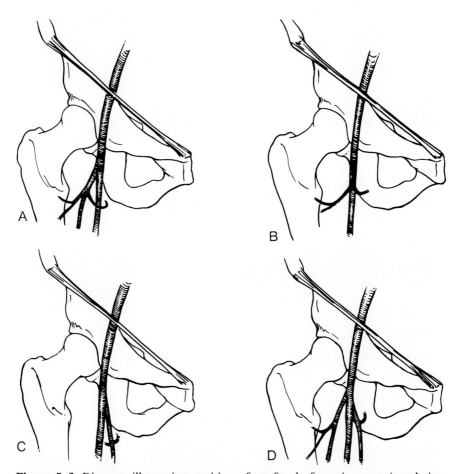

Figure 5–3. Diagram illustrating position of profunda femoris artery in relationship to the superficial artery.

A   The profunda femoris artery lies posterior lateral to the superficial femoral artery (45 per cent of individuals).

B   The profunda femoris is located directly posterior to the superficial femoral artery (40 per cent of individuals).

C   The main trunk of the profunda femoris artery lies posterior medial to the superficial femoral artery (approximately 10 per cent of individuals).

D   Larger trunks constituting the main branches of the profunda femoris artery lie posterior medial and posterior lateral to the superficial femoral artery (approximately 5 per cent of individuals).

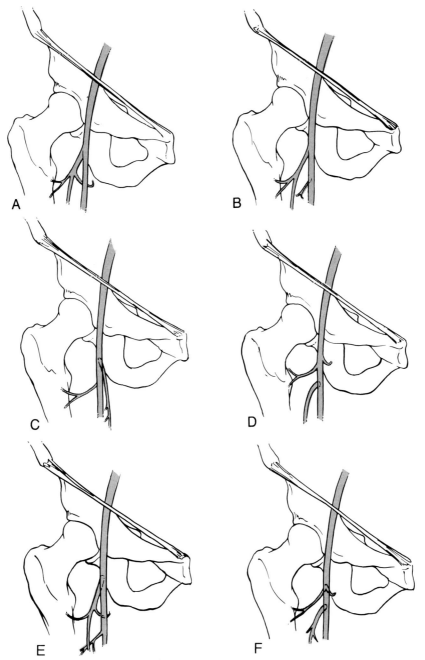

Figure 5–4. Diagram illustrating branching patterns of the profunda femoris artery. (Redrawn after Lippert H and Pabst R: Arterial Variations in Man. Classification and Frequency. Munich, JF Bergmann Verlag, 1985.)

A   A single trunk that gives rise to both femoral circumflex arteries (60 per cent of individuals).

B   The medial femoral circumflex artery arises as an independent branch from the superficial femoral artery (20 per cent of individuals).

C   The lateral femoral circumflex arises independently from the superficial femoral artery (approximately 15 per cent of individuals).

D   Both medial and lateral femoral circumflex arteries arise independently from the common femoral artery (approximately 3 per cent of individuals).

E   A large branch of the lateral femoral circumflex arises directly from the superficial femoral artery (approximately 1 per cent of individuals).

F   Both femoral circumflex arteries arise from a common trunk from the common femoral artery (approximately 1 per cent of individuals).

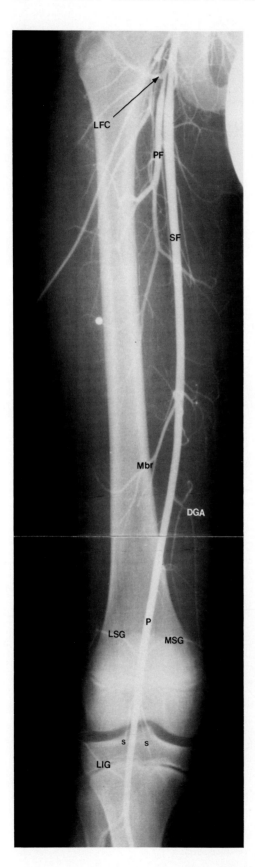

Figure 5–5. The superficial femoral and popliteal arteries.

DGA	Descending genicular
LFC	Lateral femoral circumflex
LIG	Lateral inferior genicular
LSG	Lateral superior genicular
Mbr	Muscular branch of superficial femoral
MSG	Medial superior genicular
P	Popliteal
PF	Profunda femoris
s	Sural
SF	Superficial femoral

Figure 5–6. Superficial femoral and popliteal arteries.

DGA   Descending genicular
LIG   Lateral inferior genicular
Mbr   Muscular branch of super-
          ficial femoral
MIG   Medial inferior genicular
P   Popliteal
s   Sural
SF   Superficial femoral

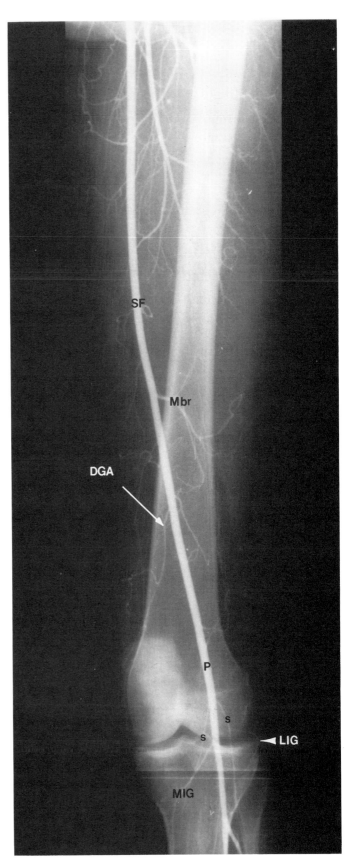

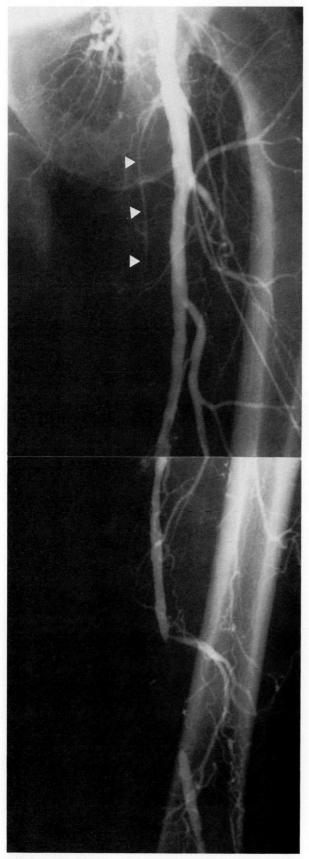

Figure 5–7. Absent profunda femoris artery. There is a single artery originating from the common femoral and extending to the distal lower extremity and giving off the profunda femoris branches. There is a segmental occlusion at the adductor canal. Arrowheads point to a saphenous artery. (Courtesy of Dr. Marshall Brewer.)

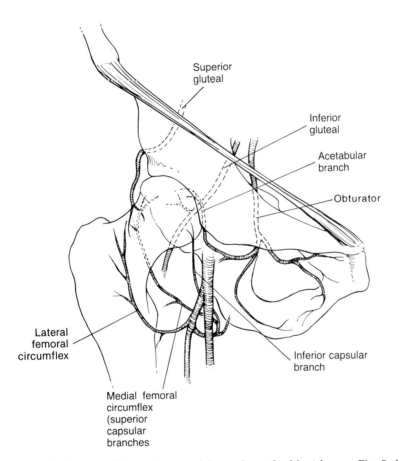

Figure 5–8. Drawing illustrating arterial supply to the hip (also see Fig. 5–1).

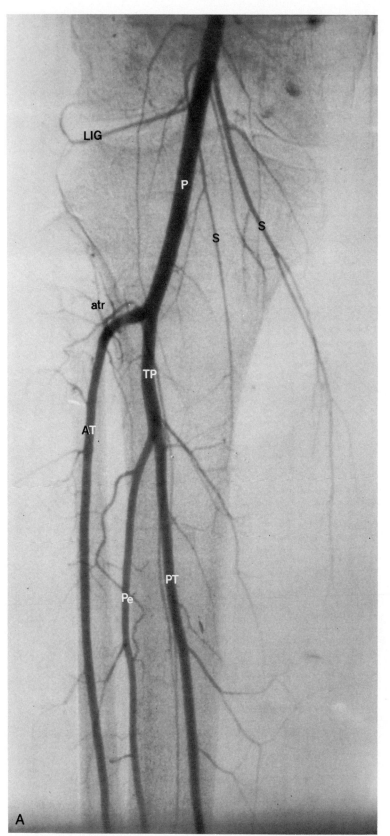

Figure 5–9. *Illustration continued on opposite page.*

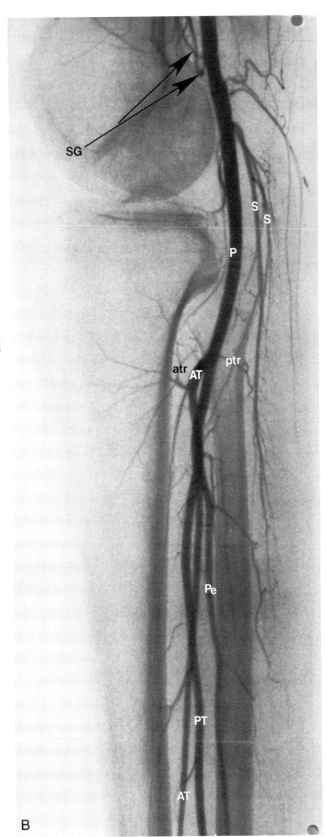

Figure 5–9. *A*, AP and *B*, lateral popliteal and proximal tibioperoneal arteriogram.

AT	Anterior tibial
atr	Anterior tibial recurrent
LIG	Lateral inferior genicular
P	Popliteal
Pe	Peroneal
PT	Posterior tibial
ptr	Posterior tibial recurrent
S	Sural
SG	Superior genicular
TP	Tibioperoneal trunk

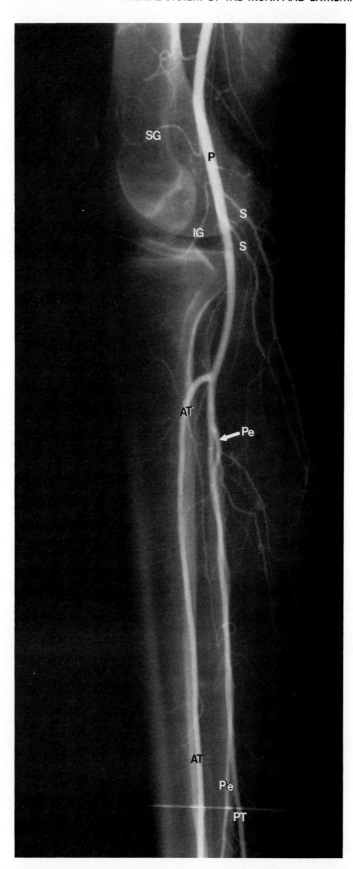

Figure 5–10. Lateral popliteal and tibioperoneal arteriogram.

AT   Anterior tibial
IG   Inferior genicular
P   Popliteal
Pe   Peroneal
PT   Posterior tibial
S   Sural
SG   Superior genicular

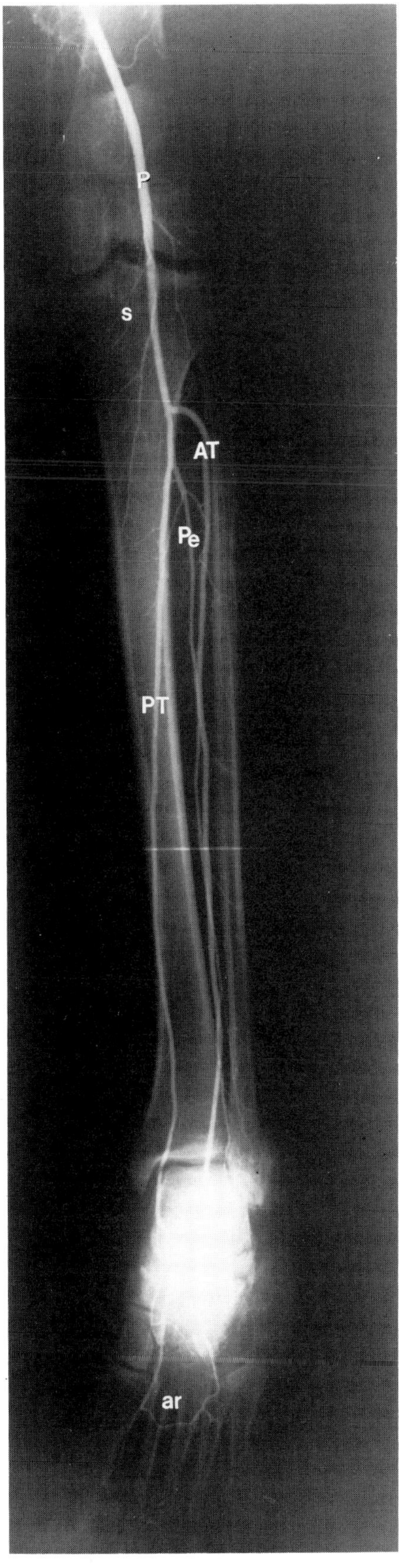

Figure 5–11. Normal AP distal lower extremity arteriogram.

ar	Arcuate
AT	Anterior tibial
P	Popliteal
Pe	Peroneal
PT	Posterior tibial
s	Sural

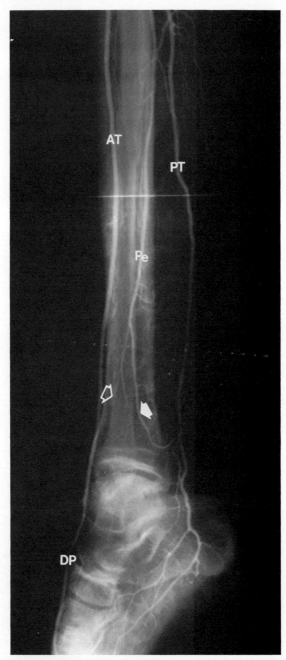

Figure 5–12. Lateral distal leg arteriogram shows the communicating branch *(closed arrow)* and the perforating branch *(open arrow)* of the peroneal artery.

AT	Anterior tibial
DP	Dorsalis pedis
Pe	Peroneal
PT	Posterior tibial

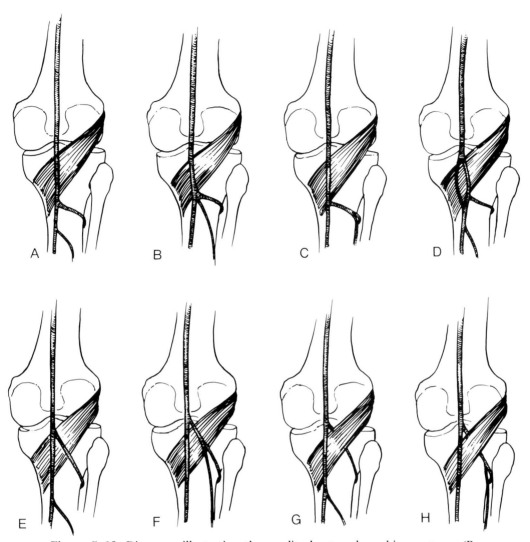

Figure 5–13. Diagrams illustrating the popliteal artery branching pattern. (Redrawn after Lippert H and Pabst R: Arterial Variations in Man. Classification and Frequency. Munich, JF Bergmann Verlag, 1985.)

A–D Major branches occur at or below the lower margin of the popliteus muscle.

A Classic textbook description (93 per cent).

B True trifurcation (less than 1 per cent).

C Bifurcation into anterior tibial-peroneal trunk and posterior tibial arteries (approximately 1 per cent).

D Duplication of lower half of the popliteal artery (less than 0.1 per cent).

E–H Popliteal artery branches originate above the upper margin of the popliteus muscle.

E High origin of anterior tibial artery (3 per cent).

F High origin of anterior tibial-peroneal artery trunk (approximately 1 per cent).

G Ventral course (to popliteus muscle) of anterior tibial artery (approximately 1 per cent).

H Ventral location (to popliteus muscle) of anterior tibial-peroneal trunk. This occurs in less than 0.1 per cent of individuals.

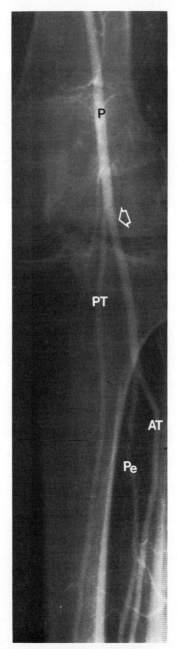

Figure 5–14. AP popliteal arteriogram shows high origin of the anterior tibioperoneal trunk *(open arrow)*.

AT	Anterior tibial
P	Popliteal
Pe	Peroneal
PT	Posterior tibial

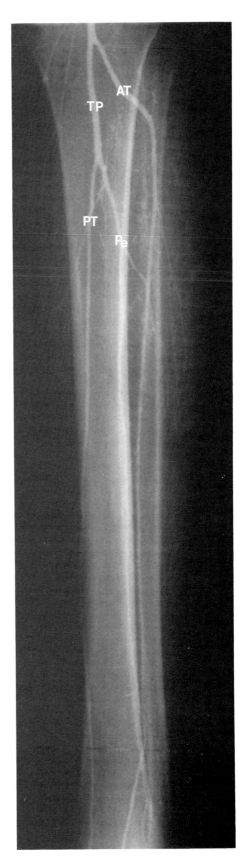

Figure 5–15. High origin of the anterior tibial artery (compare with Fig. 5–11).

    AT   Anterior tibial
    Pe   Peroneal
    PT   Posterior tibial
    TP   Posterior tibial peroneal trunk

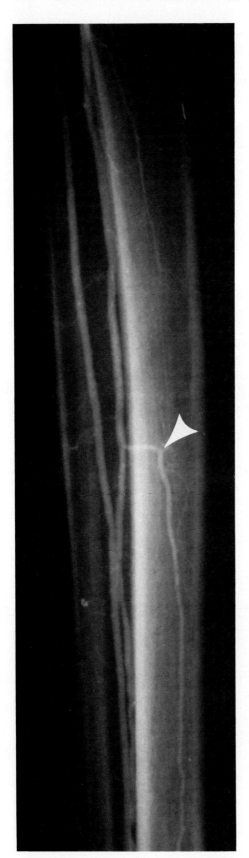

Figure 5–16. Very low origin of the posterior tibial artery at the mid-calf level *(arrowhead)*.

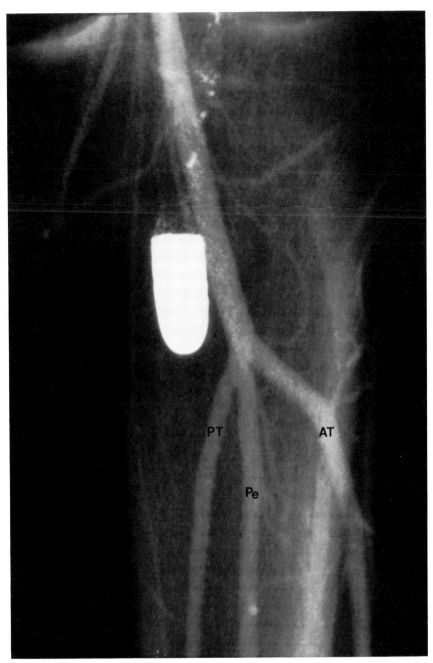

Figure 5–17. Popliteal artery trifurcation. This is seen in less than 1 per cent of individuals.

AT   Anterior tibial
Pe   Peroneal
PT   Posterior tibial

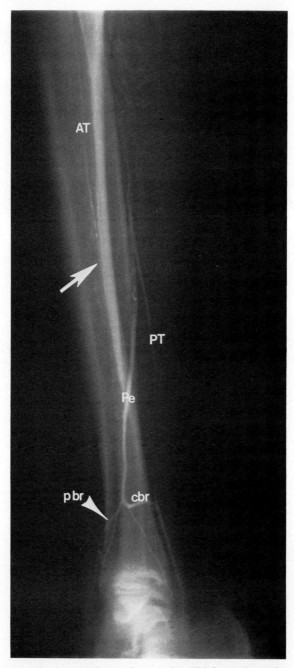

Figure 5–18. Hypoplastic anterior and posterior tibial arteries. The anterior tibial artery terminates early *(arrow)*. The peroneal artery is the dominant source of supply to the foot via the communicating and the perforating branches.

AT	Anterior tibial
cbr	Communicating branch
pbr	Perforating branch
Pe	Peroneal
PT	Posterior tibial

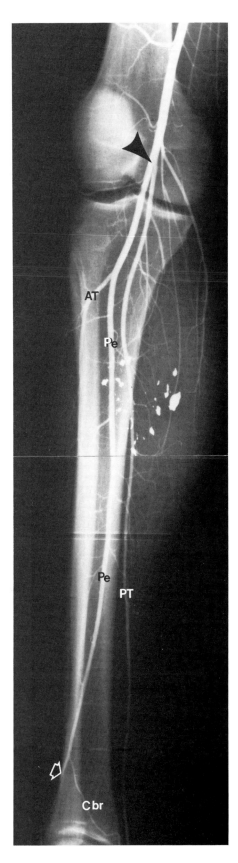

Figure 5–19. High origin of the posterior tibial artery *(black arrowhead)* with hypoplasia of the distal anterior tibial artery. The peroneal artery perforating branch *(open arrow)* continues as the dorsalis pedis artery.

AT Anterior tibial
Cbr Communicating branch of peroneal
Pe Peroneal
PT Posterior tibial

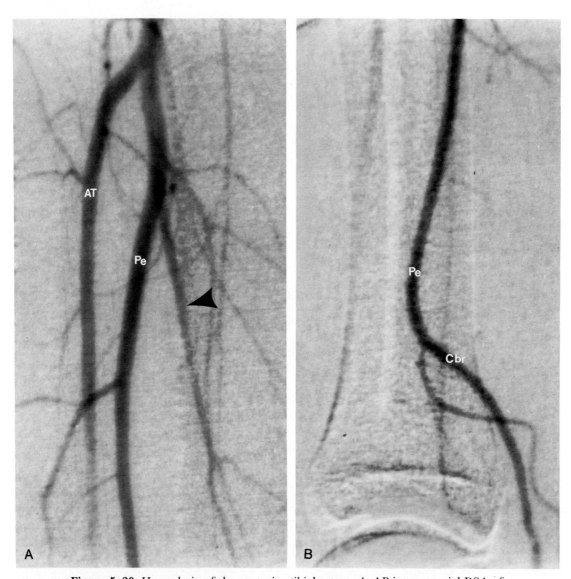

Figure 5–20. Hypoplasia of the posterior tibial artery. *A,* AP intra-arterial DSA of the proximal tibioperoneal region shows a hypoplastic posterior tibial artery *(black arrowhead)*. *B,* Lateral view of the distal lower extremity at the level of the ankle joint shows a large communicating branch of the peroneal artery continuing as the posterior tibial artery at the ankle.

AT   Anterior tibial
Cbr Communicating branch of peroneal
Pe   Peroneal

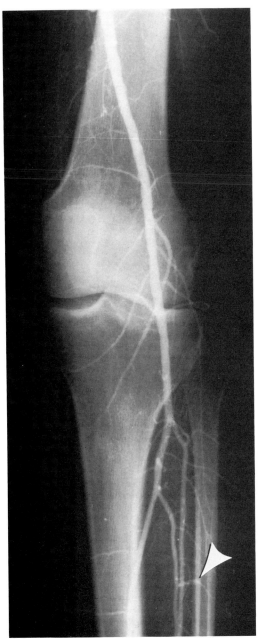

Figure 5–21. Nutrient artery of the fibula *(arrowhead)* arising from the proximal peroneal artery.

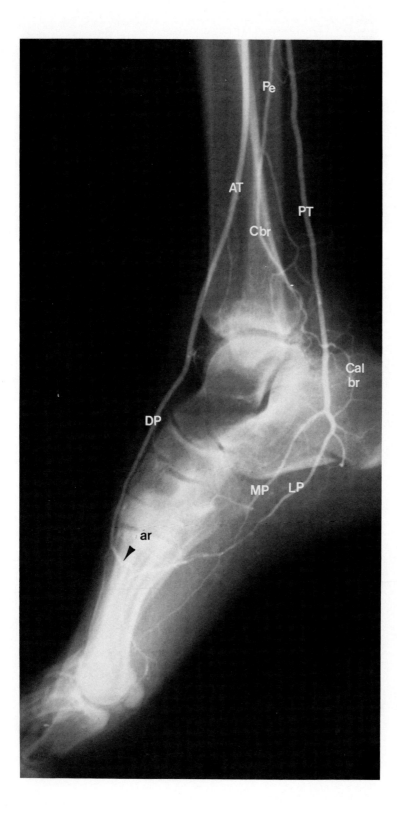

Figure 5–22. Normal arteriogram of the distal leg and foot.

ar	Arcuate
AT	Anterior tibial
Cal br	Calcaneal branches of peroneal artery
Cbr	Communicating branch of peroneal
DP	Dorsalis pedis
LP	Lateral plantar
MP	Medial plantar
Pe	Peroneal
PT	Posterior tibial

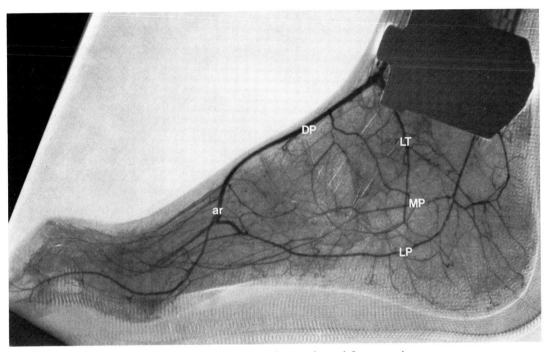

Figure 5–23. Subtraction film from a lateral foot arteriogram.

ar   Arcuate artery
DP   Dorsalis pedis
LP   Lateral plantar branch of the posterior tibial
LT   Lateral tarsal
MP   Medial plantar branch of the posterior tibial

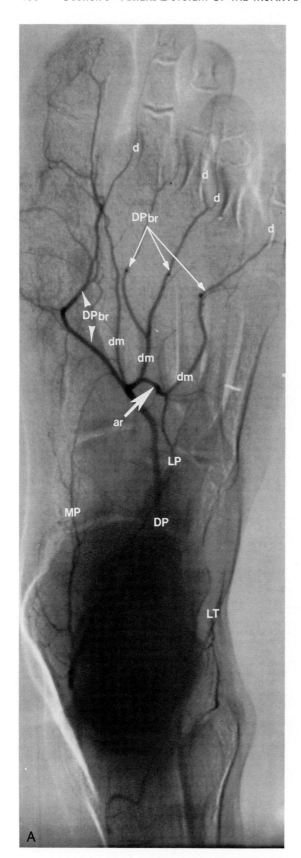

Figure 5–24. *A*, AP and *B*, lateral subtraction films from a foot arteriogram.

ar	Arcuate
d	Digital
dm	Dorsal metatarsal
DP	Dorsalis pedis
DPbr	Deep plantar branch
LP	Lateral plantar
LT	Lateral tarsal
MP	Medial plantar

Illustration continued on opposite page.

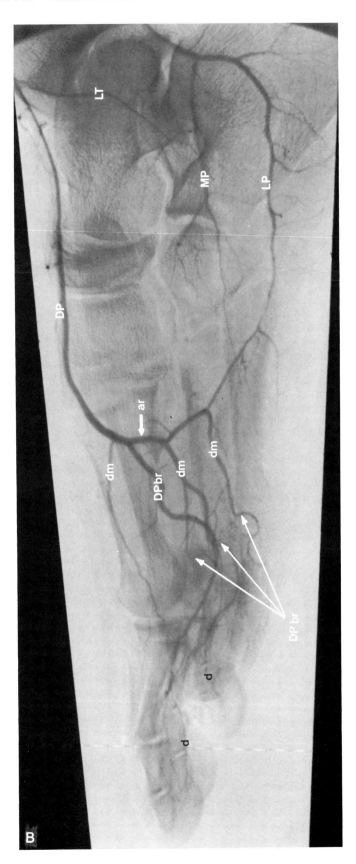

Figure 5–24. *Continued.*

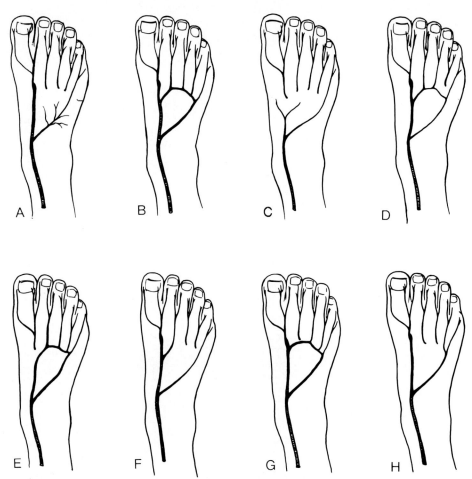

Figure 5–25. Diagram illustrating variant anatomy of dorsal arteries of the foot, indicating dorsal or plantar contribution to dorsal metatarsal arteries. (Redrawn after Lippert H and Pabst R: Arterial Variations in Man. Classification and Frequency. Munich, JF Bergmann Verlag, 1985.)

A   Dorsal metatarsal artery to the first digit originates from the dorsalis pedis artery, and the remainder are supplied from the plantar vessels (approximately 40 per cent of individuals).

B   Arcuate artery gives off all dorsal metatarsal arteries (approximately 20 per cent of individuals).

C   All dorsal metatarsal arteries are supplied by the plantar arch via the perforating branches, with only insignificant vascular contribution from the dorsalis pedis artery (approximately 10 per cent of individuals).

D   All dorsal metatarsal arteries except one (fourth) arise from the dorsalis pedis artery (approximately 6 per cent of individuals).

E   Only the first dorsal metatarsal artery receives vascular supply from the plantar arch (approximately 5 per cent of individuals).

F   Two dorsal metatarsal arteries arise from the dorsalis pedis artery, and two receive vascular supply from the plantar arch (approximately 5 per cent of individuals).

G   The second dorsal metatarsal artery receives vascular supply from the plantar arch (approximately 4 per cent of individuals).

H   The third and fourth metatarsal arteries receive vascular supply from the plantar arch (approximately 3 per cent of individuals).

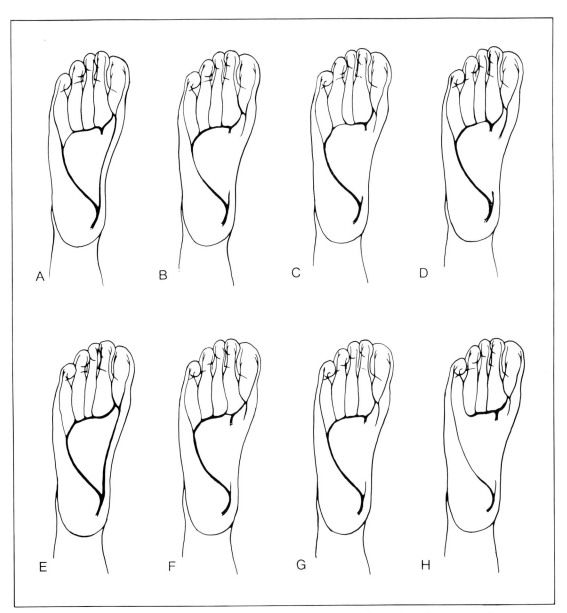

Figure 5–26. Variant anatomy of the plantar arch and branches. (Redrawn after Lippert H and Pabst R: Arterial Variations in Man. Classification and Frequency. Munich, JF Bergmann Verlag, 1985.)

A   Deep plantar branch of dorsalis pedis artery provides all four plantar metatarsal arteries (approximately 27 per cent).
B   Deep plantar arch supplies all plantar metatarsals and lateral branch to fifth digit (approximately 26 per cent).
C   Deep plantar branch provides the first three plantar metatarsal arteries (approximately 20 per cent).
D   Deep plantar branch provides the first and second metatarsal arteries (13 per cent).
E   All plantar metatarsal arteries arise from the lateral plantar branch of the posterior tibial artery (7 per cent).
F   First plantar metatarsal artery arises from the deep plantar branch (6 per cent).
G   Deep plantar and lateral plantar arteries are equally strong (approximately 1 per cent of individuals).
H   The plantar arch is incomplete. All plantar metatarsal arteries originate from the deep plantar branch of the dorsalis pedis artery (1 per cent).

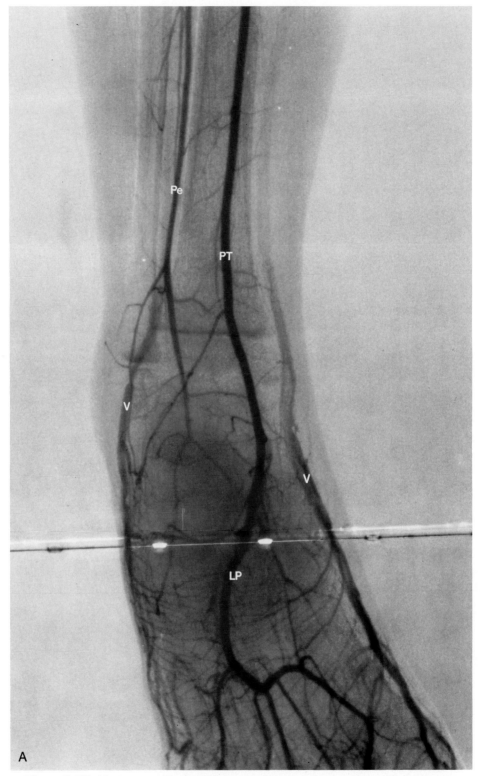

Figure 5–27. Absent anterior tibial artery. *A*, Anteroposterior view; *B*, lateral view.

Illustration and legend continued on opposite page.

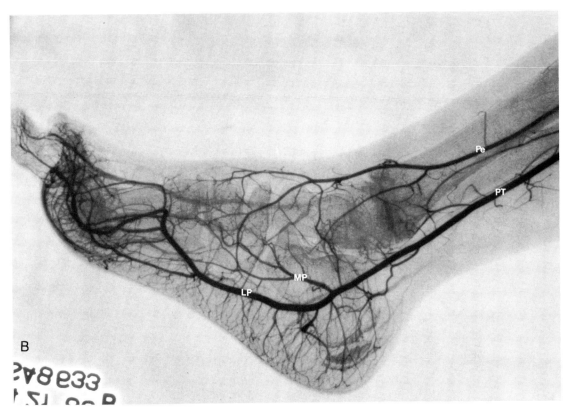

Figure 5–27. *Note:* All plantar metatarsal arteries originate from the lateral plantar branch. Venous opacification is from use of an intra-arterial vasodilator.

LP	Lateral plantar
MP	Medial plantar
Pe	Peroneal
PT	Posterior tibial
V	Veins

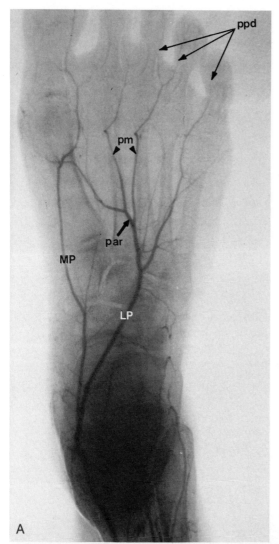

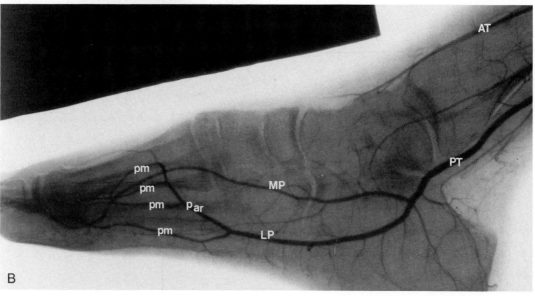

Figure 5–28. Hypoplasia of the distal anterior tibial artery. *A,* Anteroposterior view; *B,* lateral view. There is a large medial plantar artery that gives rise to the first plantar metatarsal artery.

AT	Anterior tibial
LP	Lateral plantar
MP	Medial plantar
par	Plantar arch
pm	Plantar metatarsal
ppd	Plantar proper digital
PT	Posterior tibial

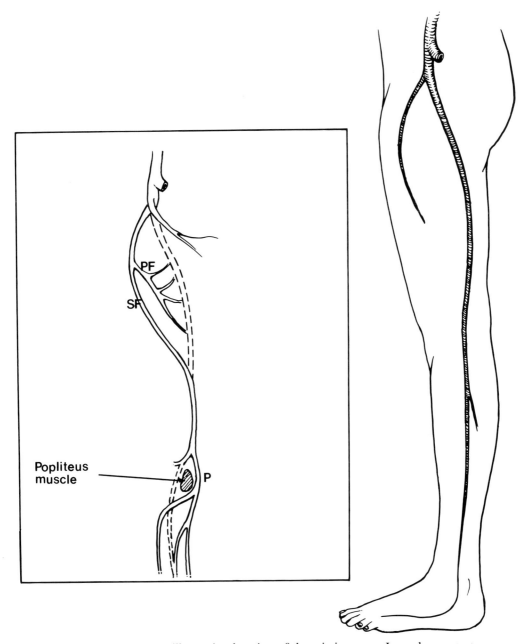

Figure 5–29. Diagram illustrating location of the sciatic artery. Inset demonstrates the normal vascular anatomy in the adult. The dashed lines represent the axial artery segments that have regressed.

P	Popliteal
PF	Profunda femoris
SF	Superficial femoral

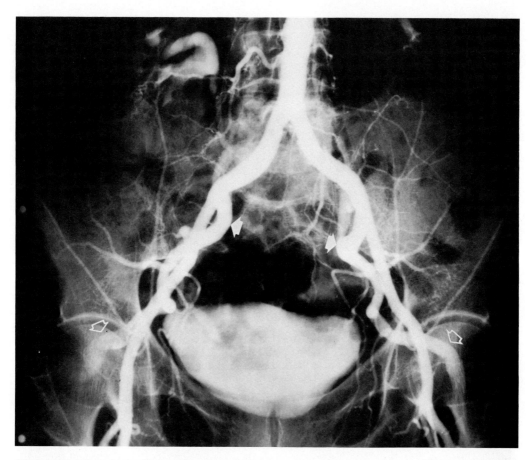

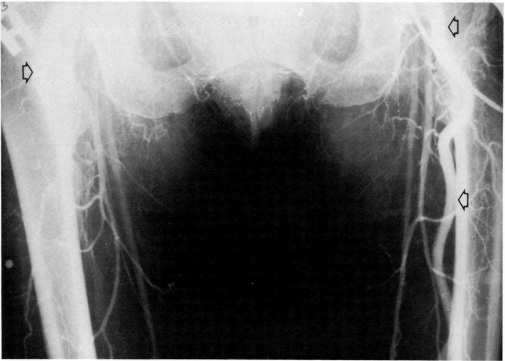

Figure 5–30. *Illustration continued on opposite page.*

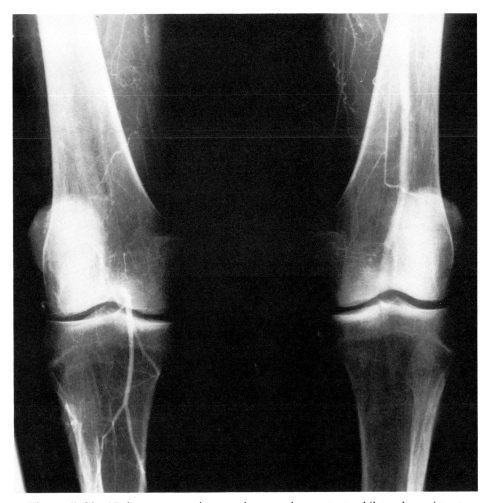

Figure 5–30. AP lower extremity arteriogram demonstrates bilateral persistent sciatic arteries *(open arrows)*. Closed arrows point to the large internal iliac arteries. *Note:* Bilateral superficial femoral arteries are also present with occlusion of the right sciatic artery and popliteal artery reconstitution. (Courtesy of Dr. J. Nepper-Rasmussen. Reproduced with permission from Ugeskrift For Laeger 149:710, 1987.)

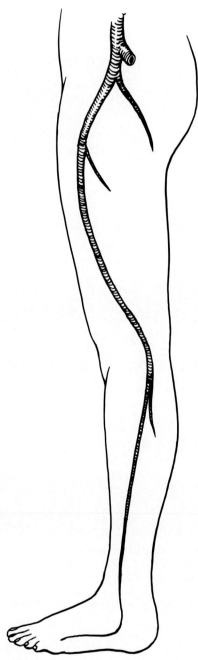

Figure 5–31. Diagram illustrating position of the persistent saphenous artery.

Section II

VENOUS SYSTEM OF THE TRUNK AND EXTREMITIES

Chapter Six

SUPERIOR VENA CAVA AND THORACIC VEINS

CAROLINE LUNDELL, M.D.
SAADOON KADIR, M.D.

SUPERIOR VENA CAVA (Figs. 6–1 to 6–3)

The superior vena cava is formed by the junction of the two brachiocephalic (innominate) veins at the lower margin of the first right costal cartilage. It is about 7 cm in length and 2 cm in width and contains no valves. It courses downward behind the first and second intercostal spaces to enter the superior posterior aspect of the right atrium at the level of the third costal cartilage. The lower half of the superior vena cava lies within the pericardium. Its major tributaries include the brachiocephalic, azygos, and small veins from the pericardium and mediastinum.

VARIANT ANATOMY OF THE SUPERIOR VENA CAVA
(Figs. 6–4 and 6–5)

A double superior vena cava is the most common variant. It is observed in 0.3 per cent of the general population and in 4.3 per cent of patients with congenital heart disease. This results from failure of the left brachiocephalic vein to form and persistence of the left anterior cardinal vein. The left superior vena cava drains into the right atrium via the coronary sinus.

A single left superior vena cava occurs if the right anterior cardinal vein regresses rather than the left anterior cardinal vein. In this case, the right-sided cranial drainage is directed to the left via the left brachiocepahlic vein. The single left superior vena cava also drains into the right atrium via the coronary sinus.

163

BRACHIOCEPHALIC (INNOMINATE) VEINS
(Figs. 6–1, 6–2, 6–5, 6–6, and 6–9)

The brachiocephalic veins are formed by the junction of the internal jugular and subclavian veins at the base of the neck and upper thorax. The right brachiocephalic vein is about 2.5 cm long and lies behind the sternal end of the clavicle and anterolateral to the brachiocephalic artery. The left brachiocephalic vein is about 6 cm long and begins behind the sternal end of the left clavicle. It lies anterior to the left subclavian, common carotid, and brachiocephalic arteries, superior to the aortic arch, and behind the upper half of the manubrium. It joins the right brachiocephalic vein behind the inferior margin of the first anterior rib to form the superior vena cava. Rarely, the brachiocephalic veins may open separately into the right atrium. Valves are not present in these veins.

Major tributaries include the following:

1. Vertebral veins
2. Internal thoracic (mammary) veins. These form a single trunk on each side at about the third costal cartilage. They drain the anterior intercostal and musculophrenic veins and lie medial to the internal thoracic (mammary) artery.
3. Inferior thyroid veins
4. First posterior intercostal veins (inconstant). On the left, this occasionally receives the bronchial and left pericardiophrenic veins.

In addition, the left brachiocephalic vein receives the following:

5. Superior intercostal vein. This is formed by the second, third, and occasionally the fourth posterior intercostal veins.
6. Thymic and pericardial veins occasionally.

The freely communicating thyroid venous plexus drains via the superior, middle, and inferior thyroid veins. The superior and usually middle thyroid veins drain into the internal jugular veins. The inferior thyroid veins drain into the brachiocephalic veins on each side close to the superior vena cava. Frequently, both inferior thyroid veins form a common trunk, which then enters the superior vena cava or left brachiocephalic vein. The inferior thyroid veins may also drain branches from the esophagus, trachea, and inferior larynx.

AZYGOS-HEMIAZYGOS VENOUS SYSTEMS (Figs. 6–8 to 6–11)

Most frequently, the azygos vein forms at the L_1–L_2 level and occasionally below the renal veins (lumbar azygos vein). At the T_{12} level it is joined by the right ascending lumbar and right subcostal (twelfth intercostal) veins. Rarely, the lumbar azygos vein is absent and the azygos vein forms at T_{12} from the right ascending lumbar and subcostal veins. It ascends in the posterior mediastinum anterior and usually slightly to the right of the midline. At the T_4 or T_5 level, it arches anteriorly to join the superior vena cava, just before the latter's entry into the pericardium.

Major tributaries to the azygos vein include the following:

1. Hemiazygos–accessory hemiazygos veins
2. Right superior intercostal vein (second to fourth intercostal veins)
3. Right posterior fifth to eleventh intercostal veins

In addition, the azygos veins also receive esophageal, mediastinal, pericardial, and right bronchial veins.

The hemiazygos vein also forms at the L_1–L_2 level. About the T_{12} level it is joined by the left subcostal and ascending lumbar veins. It ascends anterior to the spine and slightly to the left of the midline. At the T_8 level, it passes to the right behind the aorta, esophagus, and thoracic duct, to join the azygos vein. Major tributaries include the following:

1. Esophageal and mediastinal veins
2. Left bronchial veins (these may drain into left superior intercostal or accessory hemiazygos vein
3. Left eighth to twelfth posterior intercostal veins
4. Occasionally, upper lumbar veins.

In two thirds of cases, the hemiazygos vein communicates with the left renal vein.

The accessory hemiazygos vein is the most variable of the three veins comprising the azygos-hemiazygos system and also lies on the left side in the upper thorax. It is joined by the left fourth or fifth to seventh or eighth posterior intercostal veins and occasionally the left bronchial veins. It crosses to the right to join the azygos vein at the T_7 level. Occasionally, it joins the hemiazygos vein and may also drain into the left superior intercostal vein and subsequently into the brachiocephalic vein (Fig. 6–9).

VARIANT ANATOMY

In over 95 per cent of individuals, a right azygos and left hemiazygos vein are present. In 1 to 2 per cent of individuals, separate right and left azygos veins are present. In about 1 to 2 per cent of individuals, a single azygos vein located in the midline may be present (mostly without a hemiazygos vein), in which case both right and left intercostal veins drain directly into the azygos vein. In about 0.5 per cent of individuals, the azygos vein ascends more lateral than usual and drains into the superior vena cava at a higher level, resulting in the formation of an azygos lobe. Anastomoses between the azygos, hemiazygos, and accessory hemiazygos veins are variable (usually one to five or more). The azygos-hemiazygos venous system has numerous valves that are frequently incompletely formed. Rarely, the azygos vein is absent.

REFERENCES

1. Abrams HL: The vertebral and azygos venous systems and some variations in systemic venous return. Radiology 69:508–525, 1957.
2. Anderson RC, Adams P Jr, Burke B: Anomalous inferior vena cava with azygos continuation (infrahepatic interruption of the inferior vena cava). Report of 15 new cases. J Pediatr 59:370–383, 1961.
3. Campbell M, Deuchar DC: The left sided superior vena cava. Br Heart J 16:423–439, 1954.
4. Hatfield MK, Vyborny CJ, MacMahon H, et al: Congenital absence of the azygos vein: A cause for "aortic nipple" enlargement. AJR 149:273–274, 1987.
5. Haswell DM, Berrigan TJ Jr: Anomalous inferior vena cava with accessory hemiazygos continuation. Radiology 119:51–54, 1976.
6. Nandy K, Blair CB Jr: Double superior venae cavae completely paired azygos veins. Anat Rec 151:1–9, 1965.
7. Shumacker HB Jr, King H, Waldhausen JA: The persistent left superior vena cava. Surgical implications, with special reference to caval drainage into the left atrium. Ann Surg 165:797–805, 1967.

Figures 6–1 through 6–11 on following pages.

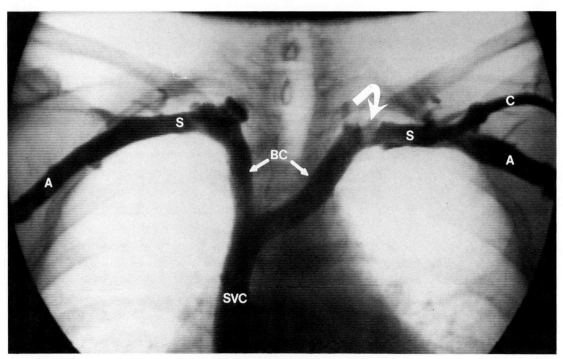

Figure 6–1. Bilateral upper extremity digital subtraction venogram. Curved arrow points to inflow of unopacified blood from the left internal jugular veins.

A	Axillary
BC	Brachiocephalic
C	Cephalic
S	Subclavian
SVC	Superior vena cava

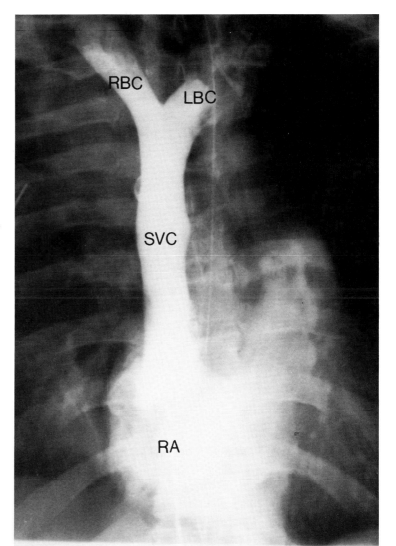

Figure 6–2. Anteroposterior superior vena cavagram.

LBC	Left brachiocephalic vein
RA	Right atrium
RBC	Right brachiocephalic vein
SVC	Superior vena cava

Figure 6–3. Digital subtraction left subclavian venogram. (Reproduced from Kadir S: Diagnostic Angiography. Philadelphia, WB Saunders Company, 1986.)

BC	Brachiocephalic vein
MPA	Main pulmonary artery
RA	Right atrium
RV	Right ventricle
S	Subclavian vein
SVC	Superior vena cava

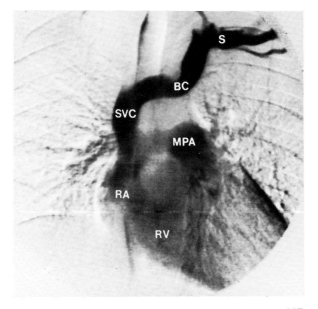

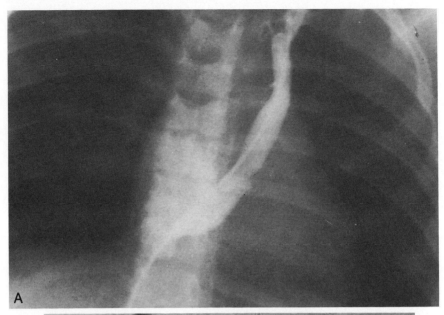

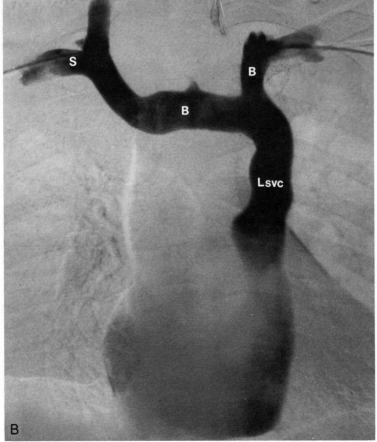

Figure 6–4. *Illustration continued on opposite page.*

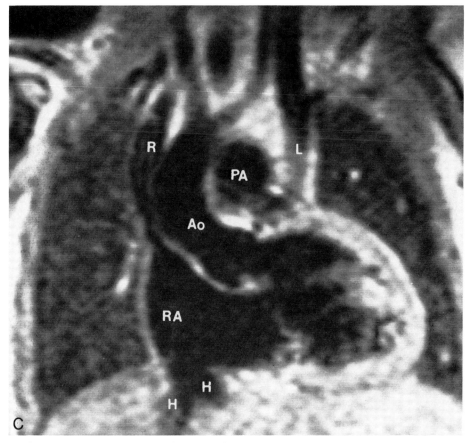

Figure 6–4. *A*, Angiogram shows a left superior vena cava. The catheter passage is via the right atrium and coronary sinus into the left SVC. *B*, Bilateral subclavian venograms show a left SVC. *C*, Coronal image from a magnetic resonance scan shows a duplicated SVC. (Courtesy of William Jones, M.D.).

Ao   Ascending aorta
H   Hepatic veins
L   Left SVC
PA   Main pulmonary artery
R   Right SVC
RA   Right atrium

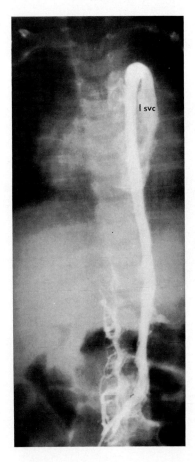

Figure 6–5. Absent inferior vena cava and hemiazygos continuation with drainage via the left superior vena cava (l svc). (From Kadir S: Diagnostic Angiography. Philadelphia, WB Saunders Company, 1986.)

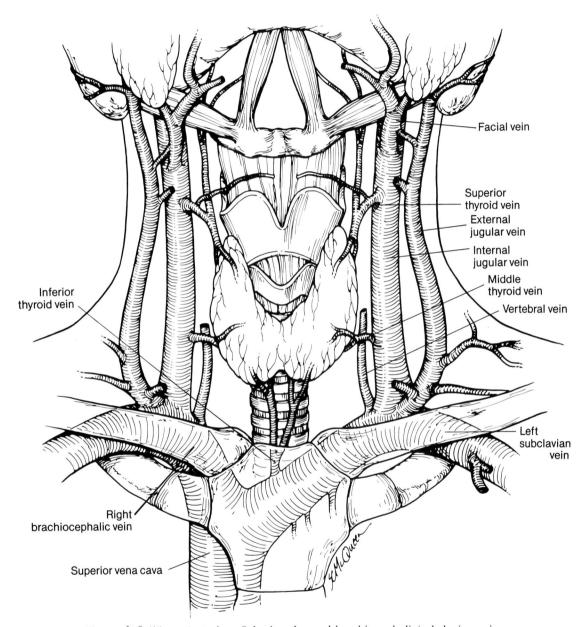

Figure 6–6. The tributaries of the jugular and brachiocephalic/subclavian veins.

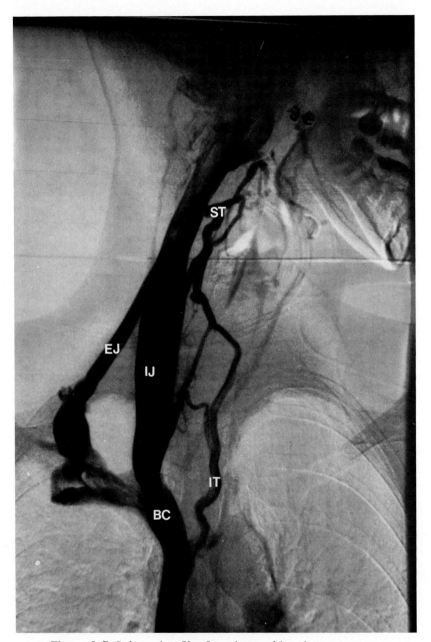

Figure 6–7. Subtraction film from internal jugular venogram.

BC   Brachiocephalic
EJ   External jugular
IJ   Internal jugular
IT   Inferior thyroid
ST   Superior thyroid

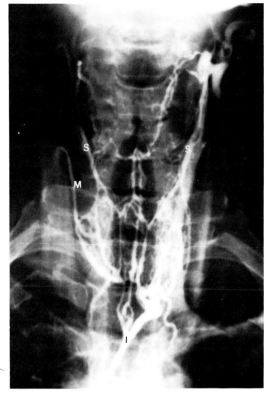

Figure 6–8. Retrograde inferior thyroid venogram demonstrating the thyroid venous plexus. (From Kadir S: Diagnostic Angiography. Philadelphia, WB Saunders Company, 1986. Courtesy of John Doppman, M.D.)

I   Inferior thyroid vein
M Middle thyroid vein
S   Superior thyroid vein

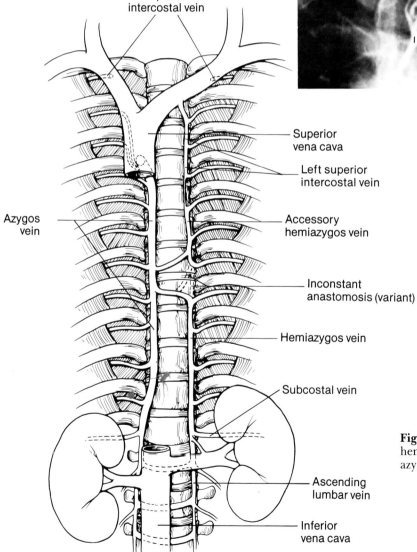

Figure 6–9. The azygos-hemiazygos-accessory hemiazygos venous system.

173

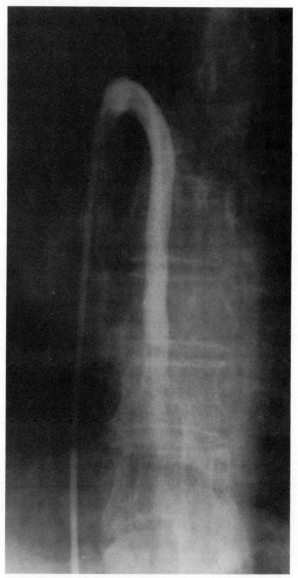

Figure 6–10. Azygos venogram. Contrast injection opacifies a normal-caliber azygos vein.

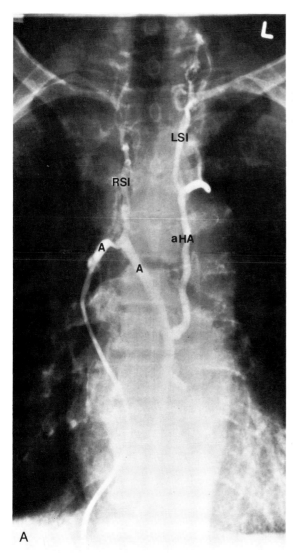

Figure 6–11. *A,* AP and *B,* lateral azygos venogram. Arrowheads point to contrast in superior vena cava.

A	Azygos
aHA	Accessory hemiazygos
IC	Intercostal vein
LBC	Left brachiocephalic vein
LSI	Left superior intercostal
RSI	Right superior intercostal

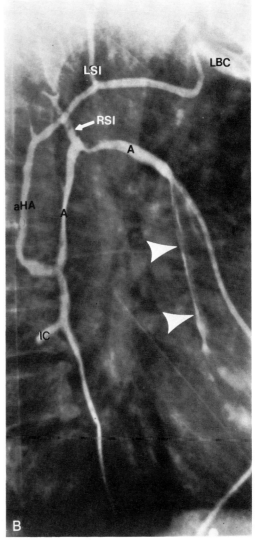

Chapter Seven

UPPER EXTREMITY VEINS

CAROLINE LUNDELL, M.D.
SAADOON KADIR, M.D.

HAND AND WRIST (Figs. 7–1 and 7–2)

The dorsal and palmar digital veins course along the sides of the fingers. The dorsal digital veins join to form three metacarpal veins that drain into the superficially located dorsal venous network in the hand. The dorsal digital veins from the radial aspect of the second finger and thumb and the ulnar side of the fifth finger also join this network. Drainage from this network along the lateral aspect is via the cephalic vein and medially via the basilic vein.

In the palm, both a superficial and a deep venous system are present. These are interconnected by means of intercapitular veins passing between the metacarpal heads. In the superficial system, the proper palmar digital veins join to form three or four common palmar digital veins, which subsequently form the superficial palmar venous arch. In the deep system, the proper palmar digital veins join to form three or four palmar metacarpal veins, which form the deep palmar venous arch. The deep palmar arch lies proximal to the superficial palmar arch, and both venous arches parallel the corresponding arterial arches. Veins from the deep and superficial palmar arches continue along each side of the hand and wrist to form the radial and ulnar veins. Small branches from the deep palmar arch and the proximal radial and ulnar veins at the wrist form a carpal venous network. Branches from this carpal venous network then join to form the anterior and posterior interosseous veins.

FOREARM AND UPPER ARM (Figs. 7–1 to 7–8)

Superficial Veins

The superficial system, which is the predominant venous system of the upper extremity, is composed of the (1) dorsal venous network of the hand,

177

(2) superficial veins of the palm, (3) median cubital and antebrachial veins, (4) basilic vein, and (5) cephalic vein. A great amount of variation is present in the superficial veins of the forearm. Either the cephalic or basilic vein can predominate or one may be absent.

Cephalic Vein

The cephalic vein originates from the dorsal venous network on the radial aspect of the distal forearm. It courses across the elbow joint and along the biceps brachii ventrolaterally. In the upper arm, it enters the infraclavicular fossa behind the pectoralis major muscle and passes through the clavipectoral fossa. It joins the superior aspect of the axillary vein just below the clavicle. Occasionally, a branch connects the cephalic vein to the external jugular vein. In addition, an accessory cephalic vein frequently connects the dorsal venous network in the hand to the cephalic vein at the mid-forearm. Occasionally, the accessory cephalic vein may originate in the mid-forearm.

Basilic Vein

The basilic vein begins from the dorsal venous network adjacent to the ulnar side of the forearm and courses along the dorsomedial (ulnar) aspect of the forearm. In the upper forearm it crosses over to the ventral surface in the antecubital region. In the upper arm, it lies medial to the biceps and passes through the deep fascia in the mid-upper arm. It then continues medial to the brachial artery to the inferior border of the teres major muscle where it joins the brachial veins to become the axillary vein.

Median Cubital Vein

The median cubital vein is a large but inconstant vein in the antecubital fossa which connects the cephalic and basilic veins. Occasionally, it provides the primary venous drainage for the cephalic vein.

Medial Antebrachial Vein

The medial antebrachial vein drains the superficial palmar venous plexus. It continues proximally along the ulnar aspect of the anterior forearm and terminates in the basilic or median cubital vein. Occasionally, it divides in the upper forearm, with one branch joining the cephalic vein and the other joining the basilic vein. It communicates with the deep veins of the forearm.

Deep Veins

The deep veins of the upper extremity are usually paired and follow their respective arteries and include the (1) deep palmar venous arch, (2) radial, ulnar, and interosseous veins in the forearm, (3) brachial veins, and (4) axillary vein. The deep veins of the forearm and upper arm are usually relatively small, since the superficial veins provide the predominant venous return of the upper extremities. Valves are more numerous in the deep venous system, and perforating veins connect the deep and superficial venous systems.

The radial and ulnar veins arise from the deep and superficial palmar venous arches. The radial veins are smaller than the ulnar veins. The anterior and posterior interosseous veins are formed by small veins of the carpal venous network at the wrist and course along the anterior and posterior surfaces of the interosseous membrane in the forearm. Close to the elbow, the ulnar veins receive both interosseous veins and also send a large branch to the median cubital vein.

The three pairs of deep veins of the forearm join anterior to the elbow to form the brachial veins. These are paired and lie on each side of the brachial artery. They join the basilic vein at the lower margin of the teres major muscle to form the axillary vein. The medial branch of the brachial vein may join the basilic vein prior to its becoming the axillary vein.

Axillary Vein

The axillary vein begins at the inferior border of the teres major at the junction of the basilic and brachial veins and ends at the outer border of the first rib, where it becomes the subclavian vein. The axillary vein lies medial and inferior to the axillary artery. The medial cord of the brachial plexus lies between the axillary artery and vein. Valves are usually present in the axillary vein just proximal to the junction with both brachial and cephalic veins.

Subclavian Vein

The subclavian vein is the continuation of the axillary vein and extends from the lateral border of the first rib to the sternal end of the clavicle, where it joins the internal jugular vein to form the brachiocephalic vein. The subclavian vein lies posterior and superior to the subclavian artery. The only major tributary to the subclavian vein is the external jugular vein. The dorsal scapular and occasionally the anterior jugular vein may join it. It often has valves about 2 cm proximal to its junction with the internal jugular vein.

REFERENCES

1. Rominger CJ: Normal axillary venogram. AJR 1958; 80:217–224.
2. Thomas ML, Andress MR: Axillary phlebography. Radiology 1971; 113:713–721.
3. Theron J, Djindjian R: Cervicovertebral phlebography using catheterization: A preliminary report. Radiology 1973; 108:325–331.

Figures 7–1 through 7–8 on following pages.

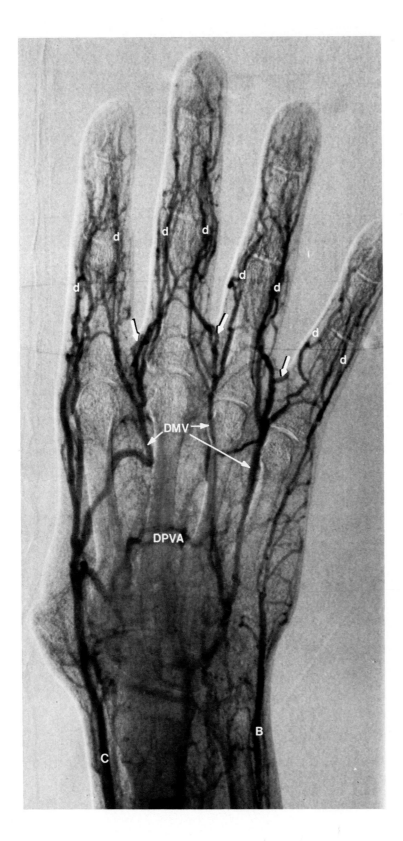

Figure 7–1. Hand veins seen on venous phase of brachial arteriogram. There is surgical absence of the thumb. Arrows point to the intercapitular veins.

B Basilic vein
C Cephalic vein
d Digital veins
DMV Dorsal metacarpal
   veins
DPVA Deep palmar
   venous arch

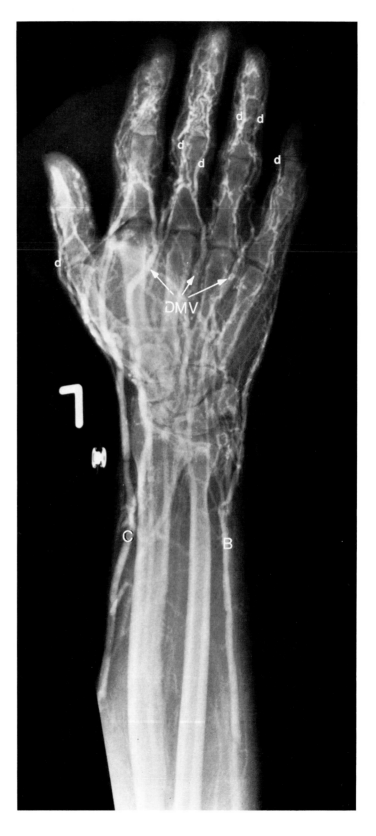

Figure 7–2.   Venous phase of brachial arteriogram showing the deep and superficial veins of the hand and forearm.

B   Basilic vein
C   Cephalic vein
d   Digital veins
DMV   Dorsal metacarpal
            veins

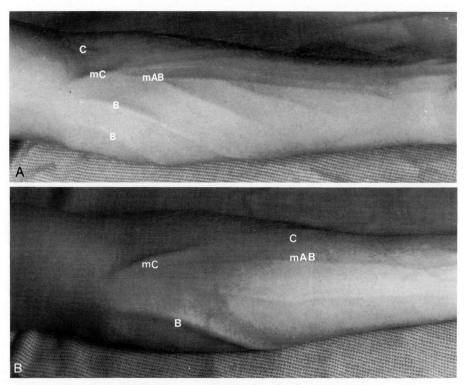

Figure 7–3. Photographs showing the forearm veins.

B	Basilic
C	Cephalic
mAB	Median antebrachial
mC	median cubital

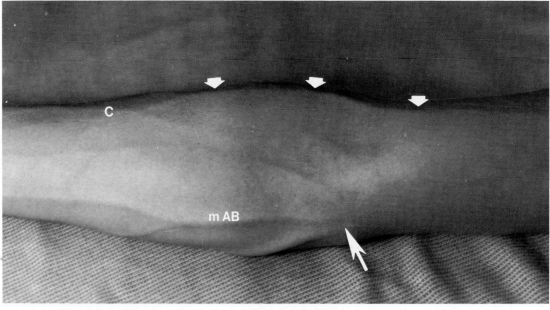

Figure 7–4. Photograph showing accessory cephalic vein *(short arrows)*. Long arrow points to basilic vein.

C	Cephalic
mAB	Median antebrachial

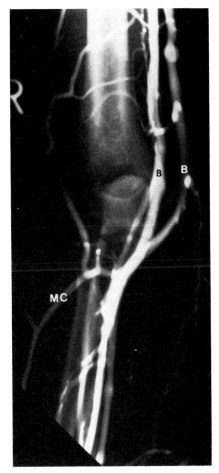

Figure 7–5. Upper forearm veins. The basilic vein is duplicated. (From Kadir S: Diagnostic Angiography. Philadelphia, WB Saunders Company, 1986.)

B	Basilic
MC	Median cubital

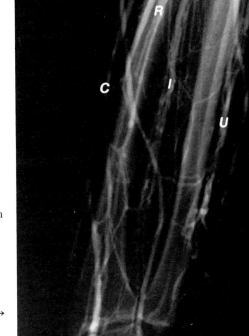

Figure 7–6. Forearm veins seen on closed system venography.

B	Basilic
C	Cephalic
I	Interosseus
R	Radial
U	Ulnar

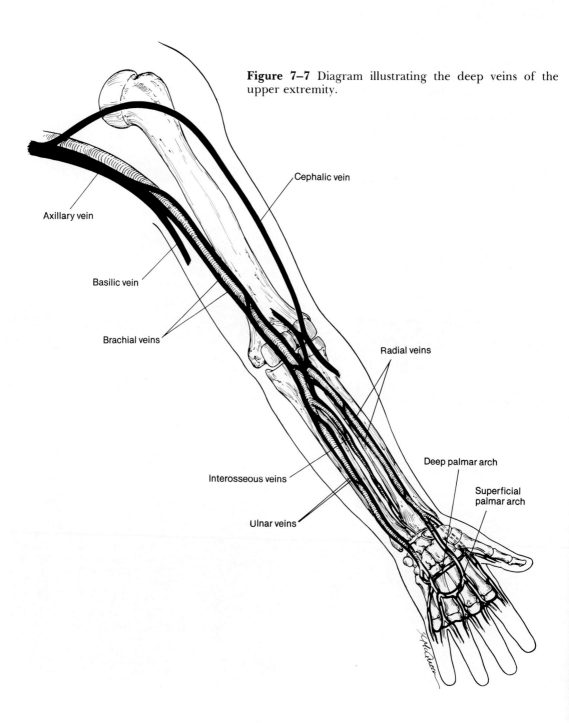

Figure 7–7 Diagram illustrating the deep veins of the upper extremity.

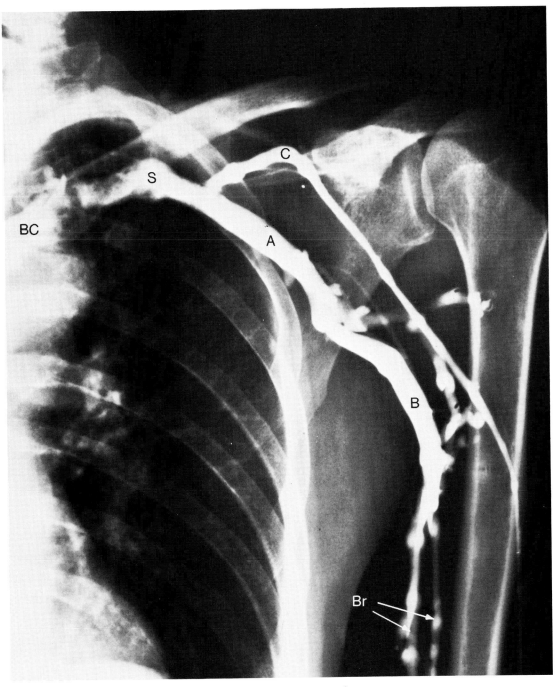

Figure 7–8. Upper arm veins.

A   Axillary
B   Basilic
BC Brachiocephalic
Br Brachial
C   Cephalic
S   Subclavian

Chapter Eight

INFERIOR VENA CAVA AND SPINAL VEINS

CAROLINE LUNDELL, M.D.
SAADOON KADIR, M.D.

EMBRYOLOGY (Fig. 8–1)

The retroperitoneal venous system develops from three paired fetal veins. The paired posterior cardinal (postcardinal) veins are the earliest veins to drain the caudal portion of the embryo at about four weeks. They drain predominantly the mesonephros initially and also the abdomen, pelvis, and lower limb buds. Two other paired veins develop and gradually replace the posterior cardinal veins. The subcardinal veins form at about the fifth week and parallel the posterior cardinal veins anteromedially. The subcardinal veins form multiple interconnections with the posterior cardinal veins and gradually assume the drainage of the mesonephros veins. A venous network develops between the two subcardinal veins called the subcardinal anastomosis or sinus. The subcardinal anastomosis receives drainage from both the posterior cardinal and subcardinal veins. The more caudal portions of both posterior cardinal veins then regress. At about the seventh week, the supracardinal veins develop posteromedial to the posterior cardinal veins and lateral to the subcardinal veins. The upper right subcardinal vein develops a connection with the capillaries of the primitive liver and also joins with the vitelline veins; it eventually enlarges and becomes the intrahepatic portion of the inferior vena cava. The suprahepatic portion of the inferior vena cava (segment between liver and right atrium) develops from the right vitelline vein. The prerenal portion of the inferior vena cava (segment between kidneys and liver) is derived from the subcardinal anastomosis. The renal segment of the inferior vena cava is formed by the subcardinal-supracardinal venous anastomosis. The postrenal segment of the inferior vena cava (segment below kidneys) is formed from the

TABLE 8–1. Embryology of the Retroperitoneal Veins

Veins	Time of Development and Location	Contribution
1. Posterior cardinal veins	(Develop at about 4 weeks)	Do not contribute to IVC formation. Failure to regress on right leads to retrocaval ureter.
2. Subcardinal veins	(Develop at about 5 weeks) Located ventral and medial to posterior cardinal veins	Form prerenal IVC. Establish three main communications: 1. Between left and right subcardinal vein; 2. With posterior cardinal veins; 3. With hepatic veins.
3. Supracardinal veins	(Develop at about 7 weeks) Dorsal and medial to posterior cardinal veins	Form the azygos and hemiazygos veins. Form the postrenal IVC.

lower portion of the right supracardinal vein. Table 8–1 summarizes the key development stages.

Absence of the right inferior vena cava results from failure of the right subcardinal vein to connect with the liver, in which case blood is shunted into the right supracardinal vein. Venous drainage from the lower body reaches the heart via the azygos vein and superior vena cava. This anomaly is frequently associated with congenital heart disease.

Above the subcardinal anastomosis, the left posterior cardinal and subcardinal veins regress except for the portions just above and below the renal vein which form the left adrenal and gonadal veins. Since these portions of the right subcardinal vein are retained, the right adrenal and gonadal veins arise from the inferior vena cava. If the left subcardinal vein fails to regress, a double inferior vena cava is formed.

The right supracardinal vein and proximal portion of the right posterior cardinal vein form the azygos veins. The left supracardinal and proximal portions of the posterior cardinal veins form the hemiazygos, accessory hemiazygos, and left superior intercostal veins. The remainder of the left supracardinal vein regresses.

The lower limb buds initially drain into the posterior cardinal veins and later into the iliac veins. A transverse connection develops between the right and left iliac veins; this becomes the left common iliac vein. With further development, venous drainage from the lower extremities gradually shifts from the posterior cardinal veins into the right supracardinal vein.

INFERIOR VENA CAVA (Figs. 8–2 and 8–3)

The inferior vena cava is formed at the L_5 level by the junction of the common iliac veins and drains the lower half of the body. In the lower abdomen, it courses upward retroperitoneally just anterior to the right side of the spine and psoas muscle. In the upper abdomen, the inferior vena cava lies posterior to the duodenum, pancreas, lesser sac, and liver and just anterior to the crus of the right hemidiaphragm. In its intrahepatic portion, the inferior vena cava lies in a groove along the posterior surface of the caudate lobe. It enters the thorax through the tendinous portion of the diaphragm, then courses slightly anterior and medial for about 2.5 cm. The inferior vena cava then passes through the serous pericardium to enter the inferior aspect of the right atrium at approximately the T_9 level. The inferior vena cava is very distensible, with an average diameter of 2.5 cm and is valveless, although a semilunar valve is present on the left anteriorly at the orifice of the inferior vena cava into the right atrium (Eustachius valve), which is rudimentary in the adult but functional in the fetus. In addition to the common iliac veins, major tributaries to the inferior vena cava include the ascending lumbar, renal, adrenal, gonadal, inferior phrenic, and hepatic veins.

The ascending lumbar veins join the common iliac veins and connect with the iliolumbar and lumbar veins. The ascending lumbar veins course posterior to the psoas and anterior to the transverse processes. Superiorly, these join the subcostal veins about the T_{12} level to form the azygos vein on the right and hemiazygos on the left. Four lumbar veins are present bilaterally which course transversely anterior to the roots of the transverse processes of the first four lumbar vertebrae. The lumbar veins drain the vertebral plexuses. The first and second lumbar veins may terminate in the inferior vena cava, ascending lumbar, or azygos veins. The third and fourth lumbar veins course anterolateral to the vertebral bodies and terminate in the posterior inferior vena cava.

VARIANT ANATOMY OF THE INFERIOR VENA CAVA
(Figs. 8–4 to 8–6)

Persistence of both right and left supracardinal veins results in a double postrenal inferior vena cava. This occurs in about 2 per cent of individuals. In this instance, the left inferior vena cava drains into the left renal vein. Persistence of the lower left supracardinal vein (rather than the right supracardinal vein) results in a left-sided inferior vena cava. This is observed in 0.5 per cent of individuals. In this case, the left-sided inferior vena cava joins the left renal vein, then crosses the aorta anteriorly to the right to join the normal prerenal portion of the inferior vena cava. Occasionally, the left inferior vena cava crosses behind the aorta.

Absence of the hepatic segment of the inferior vena cava is due to failure of the right subcardinal vein branches to join the veins of the primitive liver. In this case, the postrenal segment of the inferior vena cava joins the azygos-hemiazygos veins to drain into the superior vena cava (absent prerenal segment of the inferior vena cava with azygos continuation). The hepatic veins drain directly into the right atrium.

VERTEBRAL VENOUS PLEXUS (Figs 8–7 to 8–9)

The vertebral venous plexus is divided into internal and external spinal canal venous components. These veins are valveless, and interconnections throughout the vertebral venous plexus are abundant. Both internal and external venous plexuses drain into the intervertebral veins, which exit from the neural foramina bilaterally to join the lateral sacral, ascending lumbar, posterior intercostal, and cervical vertebral veins.

The internal vertebral venous plexus lies in the spinal canal between the dura and vertebrae and is composed of six longitudinal veins, two paired veins anteriorly, and two single veins posteriorly. This plexus receives the basivertebral vein and small tributaries from the spinal canal. At each vertebral level, the anterior and posterior internal (epidural) veins are connected by transverse veins that join the intervertebral veins laterally at the neural foramina.

The anterior external vertebral plexus courses anterior to the vertebral body to drain small branches of the basivertebral vein, then joins the intervertebral veins laterally. The posterior external vertebral plexus lies along the posterior surface of the spinous and transverse processes and articular facets. It then joins the posterior internal vertebral venous plexus to drain into the intervertebral veins.

REFERENCES

1. Anderson RC, Heilig W, Novick R, et al: Anomalous inferior vena cava with azygos drainage: So called absence of the inferior vena cava. Am Heart J 49:318–322, 1955.
2. Edwards EA: Clinical anatomy of lesser variations of the inferior vena cava and a proposal for classifying the anomalies of the vessel. Angiology 2:85–99, 1951.
3. Gryska PF, Earthrowl FH: Left sided inferior vena cava. Arch Surg 94:363–364, 1967.
4. Hirsch DM, Chan K-F: Bilateral inferior vena cava. JAMA 185:729–730, 1963.
5. Mayo J, Gray R, St Louis E, et al: Anomalies of the inferior vena cava. AJR 140:339–345, 1983.
6. Milloy FJ, Anson BJ, Cauldwell EW: Variations in the inferior caval veins and in their renal and lumbar communications. Surg Gynecol Obstet 115:131–142, 1962.
7 Senecail B, Lefevre C, Person H, et al: Radiologic anatomy of duplication of the inferior vena cava: a trap in abdominal imaging. A report of 8 cases. Surg Radiol Anat 9:151–157, 1987.

Figures 8–1 through 8–9 on following pages.

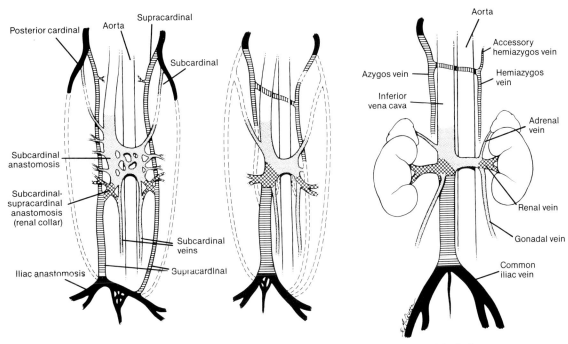

Figure 8–1. Development of renal, adrenal, and gonadal veins and inferior vena cava.

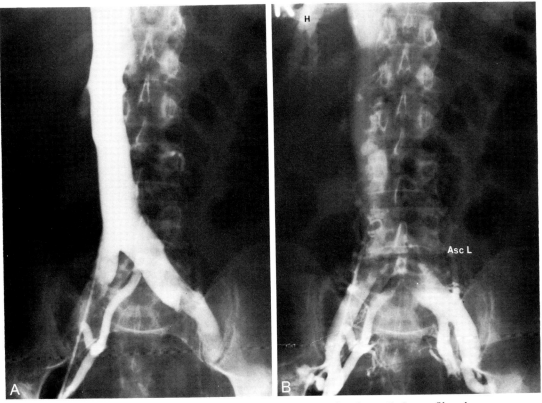

Figure 8–2. Normal inferior vena cavagram. *A*, Early phase. *B*, Later film shows reflux of contrast medium into pelvic and hepatic (H) veins. Asc L = Ascending lumbar vein.

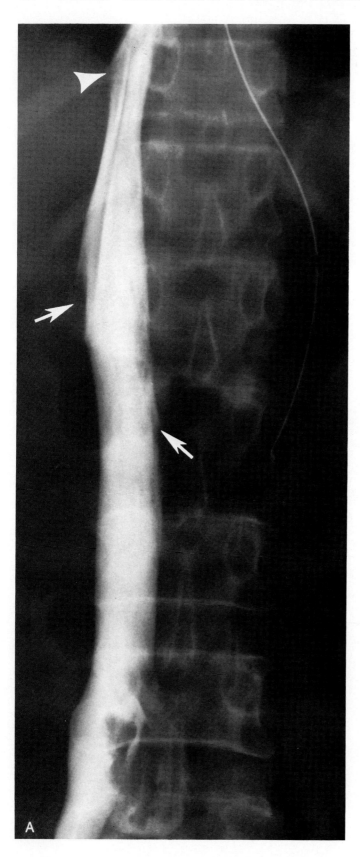

Figure 8–3. *A,* Anteroposterior and *B,* lateral views of the inferior vena cava. Arrows indicate renal vein inflow. Arrowhead indicates hepatic vein inflow.

Illustration continued on opposite page.

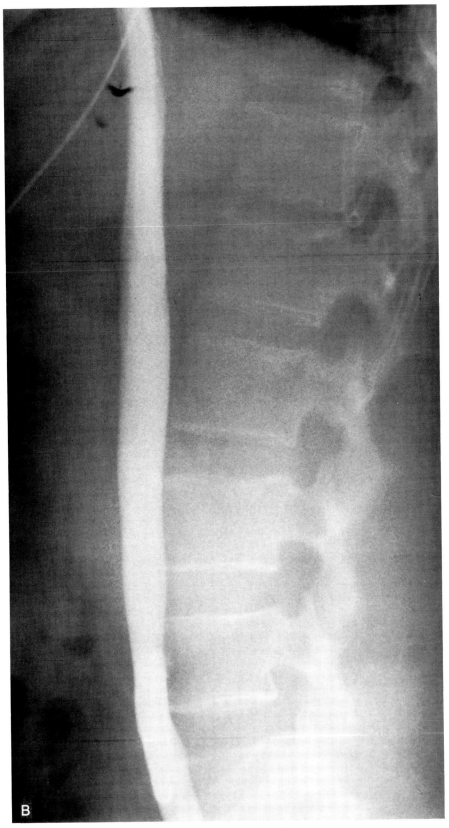

Figure 8–3. *Continued.*

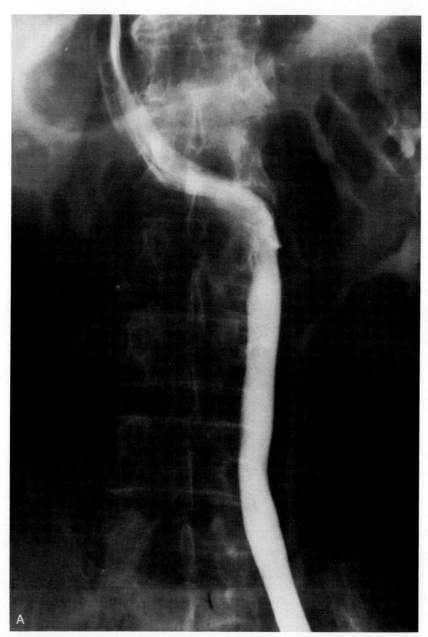

Figure 8–4. Left inferior vena cava. *A,* The inferior vena cava joins the left renal vein and crosses over to the right to continue as a right prerenal vena cava. *B,* AP and *C,* lateral views from a left-sided inferior vena cavagram show that it crosses to the right in front of the abdominal aorta. Arrowheads point to catheter in aorta.

Illustration continued on opposite page.

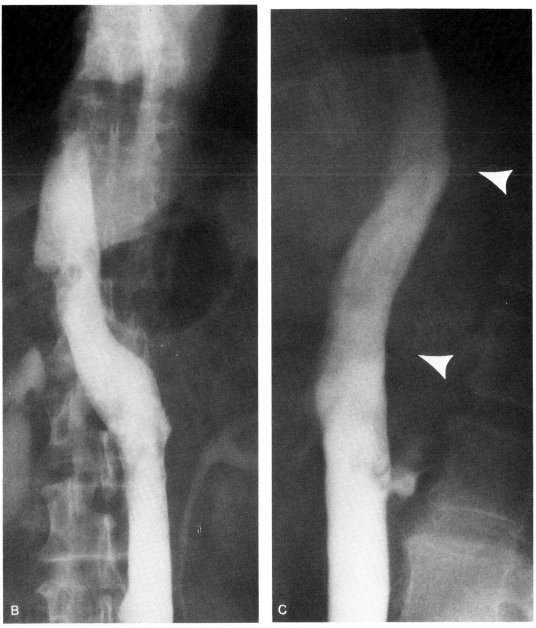

Figure 8–4. *Continued.*

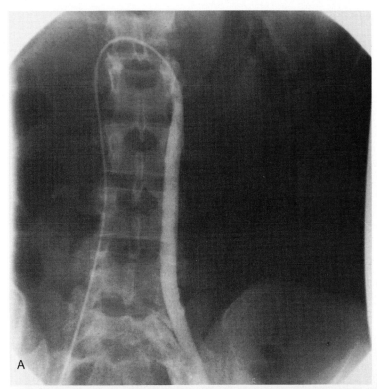

Figure 8–5. Duplicated inferior vena cava. *A,* Catheter has been introduced for contrast injection into left inferior vena cava via the right inferior vena cava. *B,* Coronal image from a magnetic resonance scan from another person shows duplication of the infrarenal (postrenal) vena cava. The left vena cava crosses behind the aorta. (*B* courtesy of William Jones, M.D.)

A   Abdominal aorta
L   Left inferior vena cava
R   Right inferior vena cava

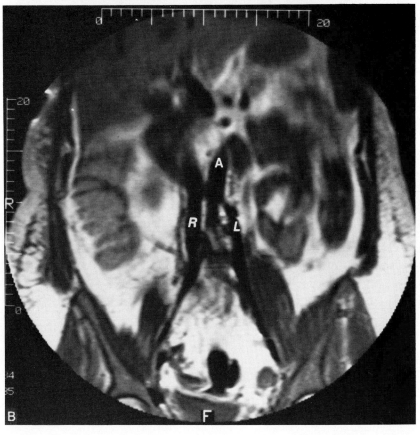

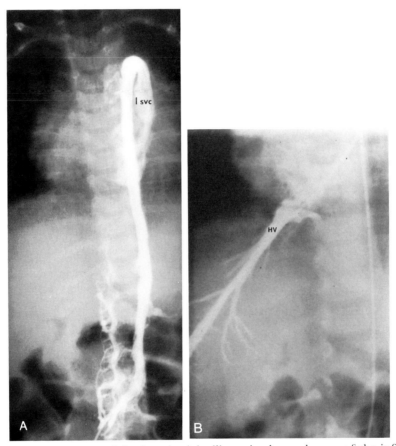

Figure 8–6. *A*, Contrast injection via right iliac vein shows absence of the inferior vena cava with hemiazygos continuation. *B*, Hepatic venogram in the same patient shows drainage directly into the right atrium.

HV   Hepatic vein
lsvc   Left superior vena cava

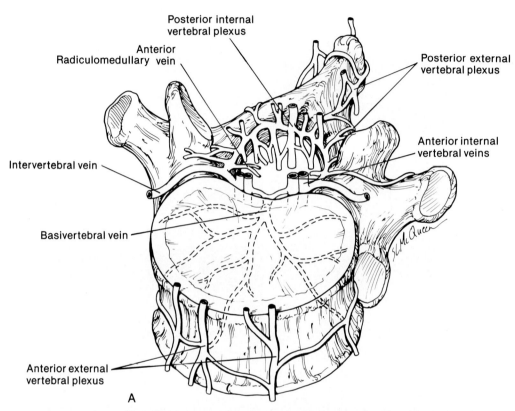

Figure 8–7. Epidural and paravertebral veins. *A,* Diagram showing internal and external vertebral veins. *B,* Axial and *C,* frontal vein showing the epidural and paravertebral veins. (*B* and *C,* from Kadir S.: Diagnostic Angiography. Philadelphia, WB Saunders Company, 1986.)

aivv   Anterior internal vertebral veins
bvv   Basivertebral vein
icv   Infrapedicular communicating vein
iv   Intervertebral vein
pivv   Posterior internal vertebral veins
pv   Paravertebral vein
rmv   Radiculomedullary vein
scv   Suprapedicular communicating vein
sv   Segmental vein

Illustration continued on opposite page.

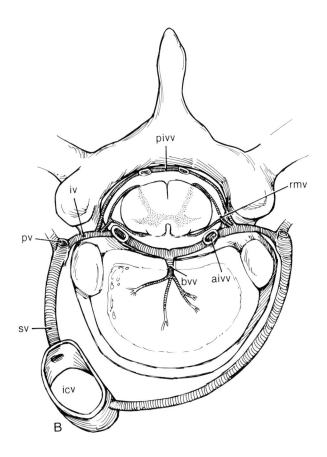

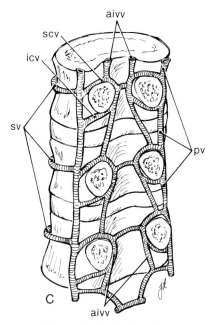

Figure 8–7. *Continued.*

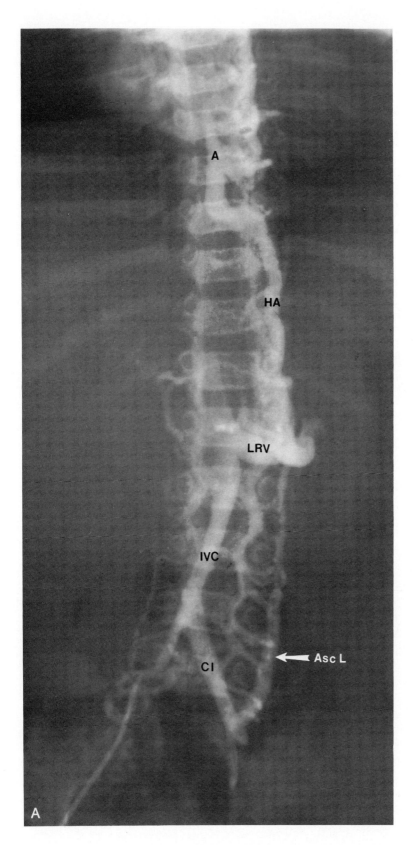

Figure 8–8. *A*, Anteroposterior and *B*, lateral inferior vena cavagram in a child shows the paravertebral veins (in the lumbar region). The vertebral veins are opacified on the AP image as a result of caval compression in the supine position by a large abdominal mass.

A   Azygos
AscL   Ascending lumbar
CI   Common iliac
HA   Hemiazygos vein
IVC   Inferior vena cava
LRV   Left renal

Illustration continued on opposite page.

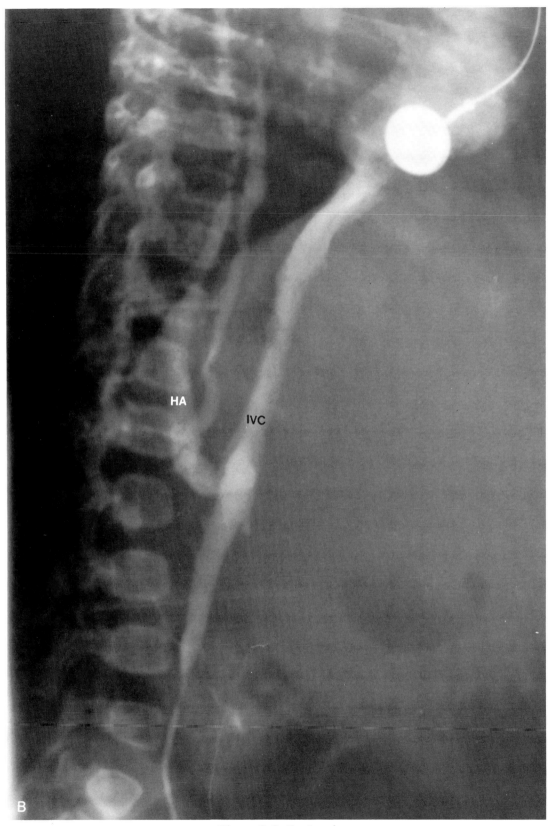

Figure 8–8. *Continued.*

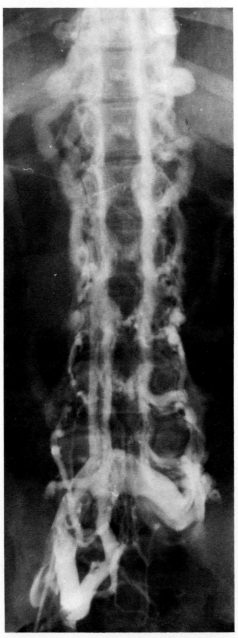

Figure 8–9. Anteroposterior inferior vena cavagram shows a dilated vertebral venous plexus.

Chapter Nine

LOWER EXTREMITIES AND PELVIS

CAROLINE LUNDELL, M.D.
SAADOON KADIR, M.D.

The veins of the lower extremities are divided into superficial, deep, and perforating veins. The superficial veins are located in the subcutaneous tissues superficial to the fascia. The deep veins accompany the arteries and lie deep to the fascia and muscles. The perforating veins penetrate the deep fascia to connect the superficial and deep venous systems. Venous flow is normally from superficial to deep veins and is directed by bicuspid valves, which are present in all three venous groups. Valves are more numerous in the deep venous system and in the distal veins. Valves are more numerous in the lower than in the upper extremities.

VEINS OF THE FOOT

Superficial Veins (Fig. 9–1)

The dorsal digital veins join to form three or four dorsal metatarsal veins that overlie the base of the toes. These then unite to form the dorsal venous arch, which gives rise to the medial and lateral marginal veins that lie along each side of the foot. These continue up the leg as the greater and lesser saphenous veins. An additional network of superficial veins is present proximal to the dorsal venous arch. This network communicates with the deep veins of the foot as well as the medial and lateral marginal veins and the veins along the anterior leg.

The superficial veins in the sole of the foot form a plantar cutaneous venous arch that extends along the base of the toes and joins the medial and lateral marginal veins. In addition, there is a plantar cutaneous venous network that lies proximal to this plantar cutaneous venous arch. This communicates with the deep plantar veins and the plantar cutaneous venous arch and drains predominantly into the medial and lateral marginal veins.

Deep Veins (Fig. 9–2)

The plantar digital veins also form three or four plantar metatarsal veins that join to form the deep plantar venous arch. This parallels the deep plantar arterial arch. The deep plantar venous arch, which is the largest vein in the foot, divides into medial and lateral plantar veins. The latter accompany the corresponding arteries and join behind the medial malleolus to form the posterior tibial veins.

The deep veins of the foot communicate with the dorsal veins at several points: (1) plantar digital veins with dorsal digital veins, (2) plantar metatarsal veins via perforating veins, and (3) medial and lateral plantar veins with greater and lesser saphenous veins.

VEINS OF CALF

In the calf, the three main deep venous trunks follow their respective arteries. These veins are usually paired but are occasionally single and may interconnect (see Figure 9–4). They join in the upper one third of the calf along with the calf muscular veins to form the popliteal vein.

Tibial and Peroneal Veins (Figs. 9–3 and 9–4)

The posterior tibial veins originate as a direct continuation of the medial and lateral plantar veins. They ascend in the fascial plane between the superficial and deep muscles of the posterior compartment (predominantly soleus), which they drain. The posterior tibial veins are joined by the peroneal veins in the proximal one third of the calf prior to entering the popliteal vein. The peroneal veins originate from multiple tributaries at the ankle and course just posterior to the interosseous membrane to drain the muscles of the lateral and posterior compartments.

The anterior tibial veins are a direct continuation of the dorsal venous arch. They course along the anterior aspect of the interosseous membrane. The anterior tibial veins leave the anterior compartment through the interosseous membrane just inferior to the fibular head to join the posterior tibial vein in the posterior compartment, to form the popliteal vein.

The muscular veins of the calf include the soleus and gastrocnemius veins. The soleus veins may be present as multiple pairs and join either the posterior tibial veins or the peroneal veins below the popliteal fossa. The gastrocnemius veins are more variable and usually consist of two pairs of large medial veins and two smaller lateral veins that drain into the popliteal veins above the knee.

Popliteal Vein (Figs. 9–5 and 9–6)

This vein is formed at the lower border of the popliteus muscle by confluence of the anterior and posterior tibial veins. In the lower part of the popliteal fossa, it lies medial to the popliteal artery. As it passes between the gastrocnemius muscle it lies posterior to the artery. Further proximal it lies posterolateral to the artery. The popliteal vein has three or four valves.

FEMORAL VEINS (Figs. 9–7 and 9–8)

The superficial femoral vein begins at the adductor hiatus as a continuation of the popliteal vein. The common femoral vein is formed in the proximal thigh just below the inguinal ligament by the junction of the superficial and deep femoral veins. The common femoral vein is 4 to 10 cm in length and continues as the external iliac vein above the inguinal ligament. The superficial femoral vein courses posterolateral to the superficial femoral artery in the lower adductor canal and medial to the superficial femoral artery in the upper adductor canal. It is most often single but may be paired or partially duplicated in 25 per cent of individuals. The only major tributary of the superficial femoral vein is the deep femoral vein. Major tributaries of the common femoral vein include the greater saphenous vein and the lateral and medial circumflex femoral veins in 86 per cent of individuals. The femoral vein has several valves. The most constant sites are the superficial femoral vein just below the deep femoral vein insertion and the common femoral vein just below the inguinal ligament.

The deep femoral vein (profunda femoris) lies in the proximal two thirds of the thigh and originates from muscular tributaries in the posterior thigh. It courses anterior to the deep femoral artery and terminates in the superficial femoral vein. In about 50 per cent, the deep femoral vein has a large connection inferiorly with the popliteal vein or superficial femoral vein at the adductor canal. Major tributaries of the deep femoral vein include perforating veins of the posterior thigh and occasionally the medial and lateral circumflex femoral veins.

ILIAC VEINS (Figs. 9–1, 9–9 to 9–11)

The external iliac vein begins at the inguinal ligament as the superior continuation of the common femoral vein. Anterior to the sacroiliac joint it is joined by the internal iliac vein to form the common iliac vein. On the right side, the distal external iliac vein lies medial to the external iliac artery, then passes behind it as it ascends. On the left side, the external iliac vein lies medial to the external iliac artery. Major tributaries of the external iliac vein include the inferior epigastric, deep circumflex iliac, and pubic veins. The inferior epigastric vein drains part of the anterior abdominal wall and joins the external iliac vein about 1 cm above the inguinal ligament. Superiorly, it communicates with the superior epigastric vein. The deep circumflex iliac vein joins the external iliac vein about 2 cm above the inguinal ligament. The pubic vein connects the external iliac and obturator veins.

Internal Iliac (Hypogastric) Veins (Figs. 9–9 and 9–12)

The internal iliac vein is formed by the junction of its tributaries near the upper part of the sciatic foramen. The internal iliac vein lies posterior and slightly medial to the internal iliac artery and joins the external iliac vein at the pelvic brim anterior to the sacroiliac joint. It drains the pelvic organs, the majority of the pelvic wall muscles, and the perineum.

Tributaries to the internal iliac vein follow their respective arteries (except for the iliolumbar vein) and consist of three major groups: (1) veins arising external to the pelvis (superior and inferior gluteal, internal pudendal, and obturator veins), (2) posterior pelvic veins, and (3) internal pelvic veins that drain the pelvic viscera (inferior and middle hemorrhoidal, vesical, prostatic, uterine, and vaginal veins).

Veins Arising External to the Pelvis

The superior and inferior gluteal veins drain the buttocks and upper posterior thigh, respectively, and enter the pelvis inferior to the sciatic foramen. The inferior gluteal vein communicates with superficial veins via the buttocks by numerous perforating veins to provide collateral flow between the femoral and internal iliac veins. The internal pudendal veins begin in the prostatic venous plexus in the male and the uterovaginal plexus in the female and form a single vein on each side which joins the internal iliac or inferior hemorrhoidal veins. It receives tributaries from the penis, scrotum or labia, and inferior hemorrhoidal veins. The obturator vein begins in the proximal adductor region of the thigh and passes through the obturator foramen into the pelvis to join the internal iliac vein. Occasionally, the obturator vein is replaced by an enlarged pubic vein, which joins the external iliac vein.

Posterior Pelvic Veins

In the posterior pelvis, the lateral sacral veins interconnect via the sacral venous plexus on the anterior surface of the sacrum. These communicate with the paravertebral veins.

Internal Pelvic Veins

The hemorrhoidal venous plexus drains via superior, middle, and inferior hemorrhoidal veins. The superior hemorrhoidal vein drains into the inferior mesenteric vein. The middle hemorrhoidal vein varies significantly in size and joins the internal iliac vein. The inferior hemorrhoidal vein joins either the internal iliac vein or the internal pudendal vein. The hemorrhoidal venous plexus also communicates with the vesical plexus in the male and the uterovaginal plexus in the female.

The vesical plexus surrounds the inferior aspect of the bladder and base of prostate (or vagina) and connects with the prostatic or vaginal venous plexuses. The bladder is drained by superior, middle, and inferior vesical veins, which join to form a single trunk on each side before entering into the internal iliac vein.

The superficial dorsal veins of the penis and clitoris drain into the external pudendal veins. The uterine plexus lies in the broad ligaments and joins the ovarian and vaginal venous plexuses; it drains by two uterine veins on each side, which join the internal iliac vein. The vaginal plexus is located posterior to the vagina and communicates with the uterine, vesical, and hemorrhoidal plexuses; it drains via single vaginal veins on each side into the internal iliac vein.

SAPHENOUS VEINS (Figs. 9–1 and 9–13)

The greater (long) and lesser (short) saphenous veins are direct continuations of the medial and lateral marginal veins of the foot, respectively, and are the major superficial veins of the legs. Both veins have numerous valves. A valve is located close to the junction of the greater saphenous vein with the femoral vein. A valve is also present at the junction of the lesser saphenous vein with the popliteal vein.

Greater Saphenous Vein

The greater saphenous vein is the longest vein in the body. It courses anterior to the medial malleolus and posteromedial to the medial femoral condyle and drains anteriorly into the common femoral vein about 3 cm below the inguinal ligament. It has numerous connections to other superficial veins and to a lesser extent to the deep veins. It usually has three large tributaries: (1) at the ankle, it is joined by perforating veins from the posterior tibial veins; (2) at the calf, it communicates with the lesser saphenous vein; and (3) just below the knee, it has two or three large tributaries. Multiple (often three) arcades connect the greater and lesser saphenous veins.

Accessory Saphenous Veins

The lateral accessory saphenous vein, which drains the anterior and lateral aspect of the thigh, joins the greater saphenous vein in the upper thigh. The large accessory saphenous vein (also called medial accessory saphenous vein), which is formed by numerous tributaries from the posterior and medial thigh, joins both the greater and lesser saphenous veins. The anterior femoral cutaneous vein is an important tributary that drains the anterior thigh and joins the saphenous vein in the upper thigh.

Three veins join the greater saphenous vein just prior to its entrance through the saphenous opening: the superficial epigastric, superficial circumflex iliac, and superficial external pudendal veins. The superficial epigastric vein drains the lower abdominal wall and connects superiorly with veins draining the thoracic wall via the thoracoepigastric vein. It terminates in the greater saphenous vein, usually lateral to the accessory saphenous veins. The superficial circumflex iliac vein also drains the anterior abdominal wall and upper and lateral parts of the thigh and terminates in the greater (60 per cent) or lateral accessory (40 per cent) saphenous veins. The superficial external pudendal vein drains the upper medial thigh, lower medial inguinal region, and scrotum or labia majora. It terminates in the greater (90 per cent) or accessory saphenous vein (10 per cent).

The thoracoepigastric vein represents an important collateral pathway for the inferior vena cava. It lies in the anterolateral portion of the trunk and communicates with the superficial epigastric vein and subsequently the common femoral vein below and the lateral thoracic and subsequently the axillary veins above.

Lesser Saphenous Vein (Fig. 9–14)

The lesser saphenous vein begins posterior to the lateral malleolus and ascends in the middle of the back of the calf to join the popliteal vein about 3 to 7.5 cm above the level of the knee joint. In the lower part of the popliteal fossa, it passes between the two heads of the gastrocnemius muscle. Less frequently, the lesser saphenous vein may terminate in the greater saphenous vein in the proximal thigh or bifurcate, with its branches joining the greater saphenous, popliteal, or deep posterior calf veins. It receives numerous cutaneous branches from the posterior aspect of the leg. Occasionally, a large branch joins the medial accessory saphenous vein.

PERFORATING VEINS (VENAE COMITANTES)
(Figs. 9–13 to 9–15)

The perforating veins connect the deep (subfascial) and superficial (epifascial) veins in the leg and foot and by means of valves function to prevent backward flow from deep to superficial veins. In the foot, they connect the superficial dorsal and plantar venous arches. In the ankle and calf, the perforating veins connect the greater saphenous and the deep veins. Boyd's vein is a well-known perforating vein that connects the posterior tibial deep veins to the gastrocnemius veins. In the thigh, perforating veins connect the greater saphenous vein or one of its branches to the superficial femoral vein at the adductor hiatus.

REFERENCES

1. Almen T, Nylander G: Serial phlebography of the normal lower leg during muscular contraction and relaxation. Acta Radiol 57:264–272, 1962.
2. Greitz T: Phlebography of the normal leg. Acta Radiol 44:1–20, 1955.
3. Haage H: Zur Darstellung der V. saphena magna. Fortschr Rontgenstr 124:480–482, 1976.
4. Helander CG, Lindbom A: Retrograde pelvic venography. Acta Radiol 51:401–414, 1959.
5. Jacobsen BH: The venous drainage of the foot. Surg Gynecol Obstet 131:22–24, 1970.
6. Kuster G, Lofgren EP, Hollinshead WH: Anatomy of the veins of the foot. Surg Gynecol Obstet 127:817–823, 1968.
7. Ternberg JL, Butcher HR Jr: Evaluation of retrograde pelvic venography. Arch Surg 91:607–609, 1965.
8. Thomas ML: Phlebography. Arch Surg 104:145–151, 1972.
9. Thomas ML, Fletcher EWL: The techniques of pelvic phlebography. Clin Radiol 18:399–402, 1967.

Figures 9–1 through 9–15 on following pages.

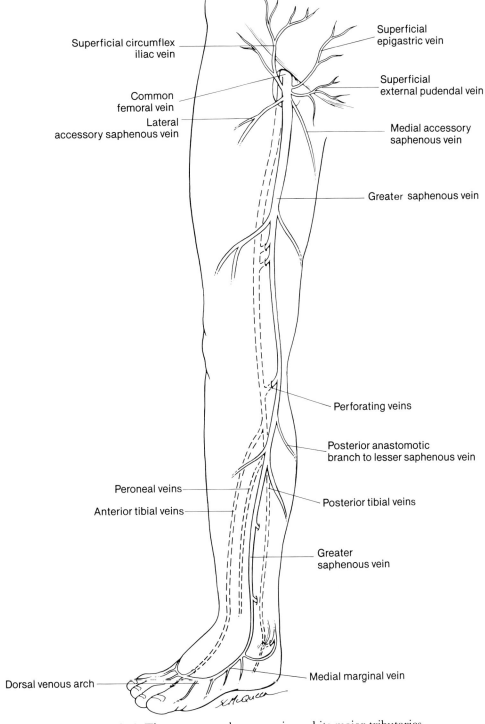

Figure 9–1. The greater saphenous vein and its major tributaries.

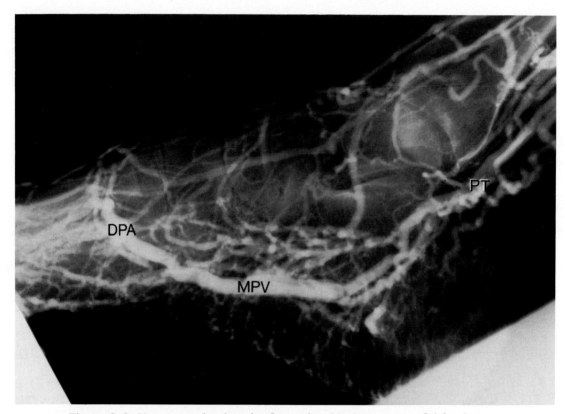

Figure 9–2. Venogram showing the foot veins. Numerous superficial veins are opacified.

DPA   Deep plantar venous arch
MPV   Medial plantar vein
PT   Posterior tibial vein

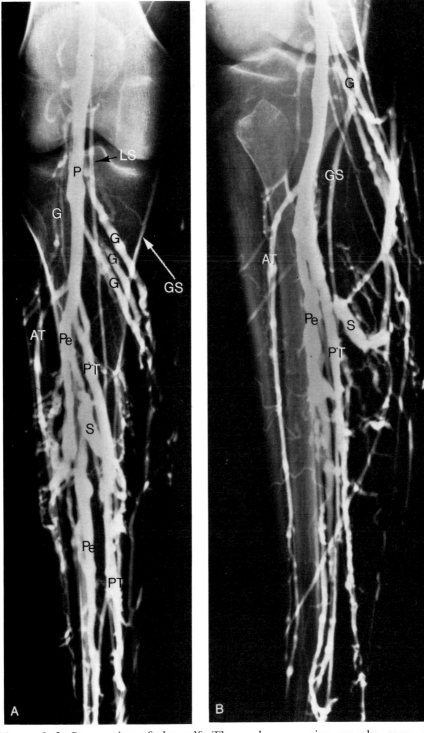

Figure 9–3. Deep veins of the calf. The saphenous veins are also seen. *A*, Anteroposterior and *B*, lateral projections. (From Kadir S: Diagnostic Angiography. Philadelphia, WB Saunders Company, 1986.)

AT	Anterior tibial	P	Popliteal
G	Gastrocnemius	Pe	Peroneal
GS	Greater saphenous	PT	Posterior tibial
LS	Lesser saphenous	S	Soleal

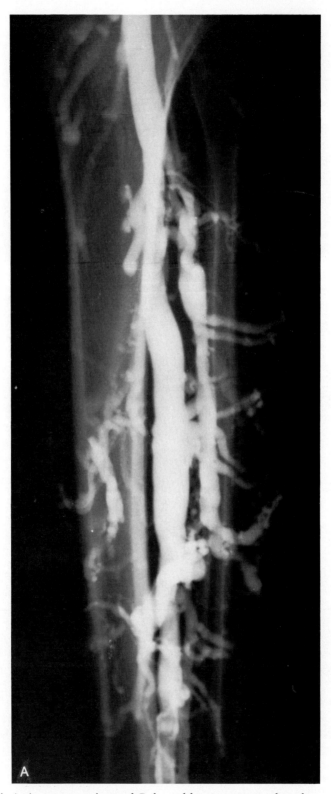

Figure 9–4. *A,* Anteroposterior and *B,* lateral leg venograms show large peroneal veins. Anterior tibial veins do not opacify and the posterior tibial veins are absent.

Illustration continued on opposite page.

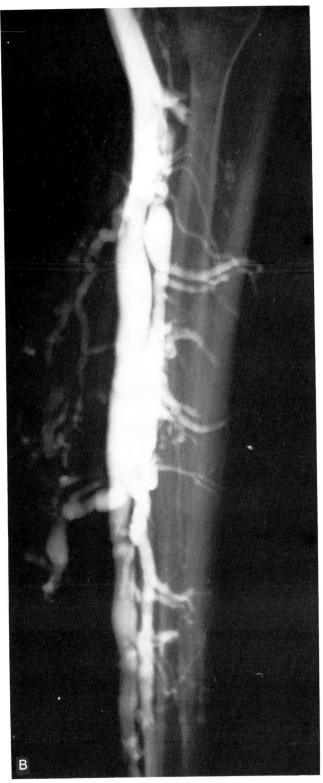

Figure 9–4. *Continued.*

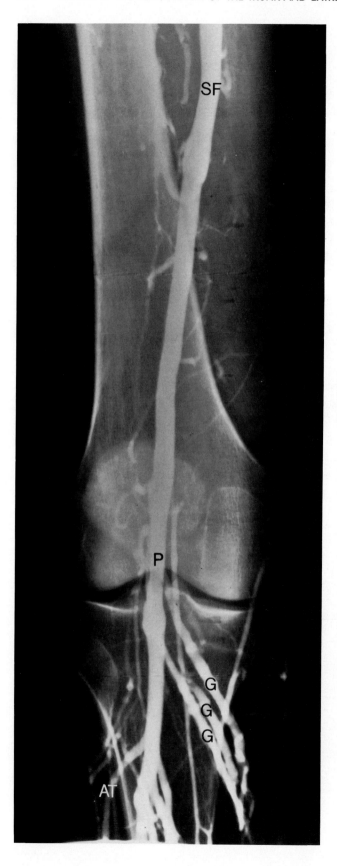

Figure 9–5. Anteroposterior popliteal venogram. (From Kadir S: Diagnostic Angiography. Philadelphia, WB Saunders Company, 1986.)

AT   Anterior tibial veins
G   Gastrocnemius veins
P   Popliteal vein
SF   Superficial femoral vein

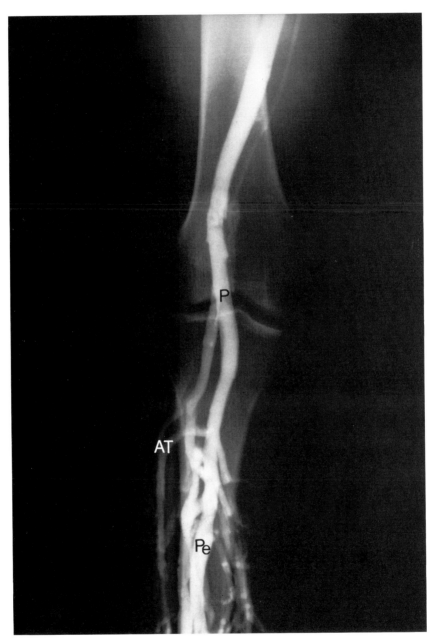

Figure 9–6. Partial duplication of popliteal vein.

AT Anterior tibial
P   Popliteal
Pe Peroneal

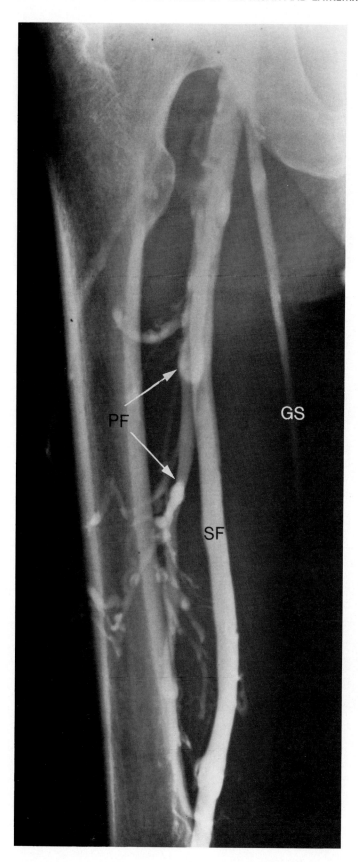

Figure 9–7. Femoral veins. (From Kadir S: Diagnostic Angiography. Philadelphia, WB Saunders Company, 1986.)

GS Greater saphenous vein
PF Profunda (deep) femoris vein
SF Superficial femoral vein

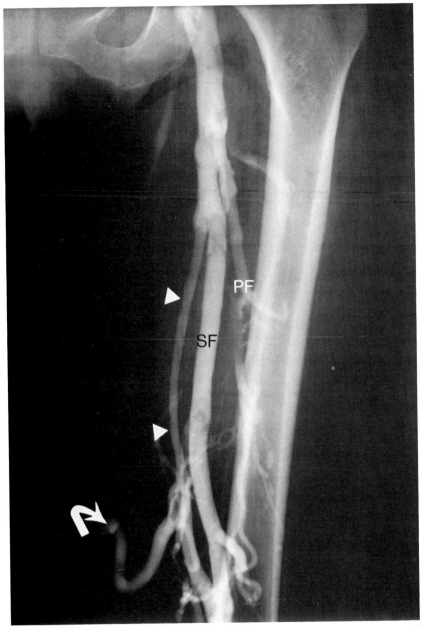

Figure 9–8. Duplicated superficial femoral vein. Arrowheads point to smaller second channel. Curved arrow points to large incompetent perforating vein.

PF   Profunda femoris vein
SF   Superficial femoral vein

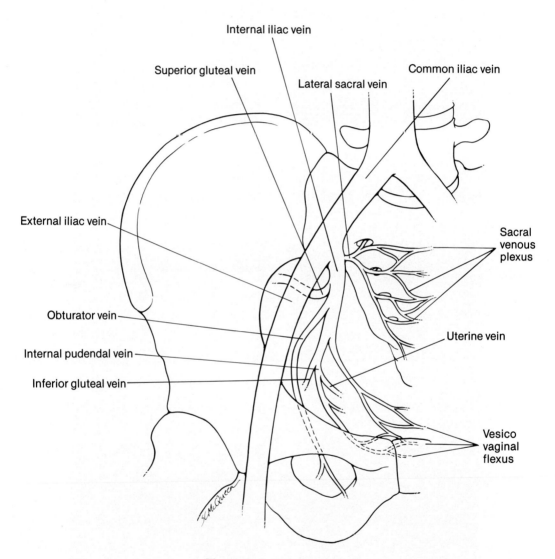

Figure 9–9. The iliac veins.

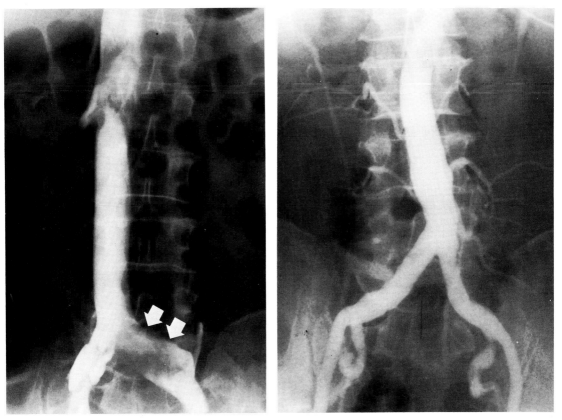

Figure 9–10. Common iliac compression from abdominal aorta and iliac arteries. *Left,* Inferior vena cavagrams show compression of the left common iliac vein *(arrows)* by the distal aorta and proximal iliac arteries *(right).* (From Kadir S: Diagnostic Angiography. Philadelphia, WB Saunders Company, 1986.)

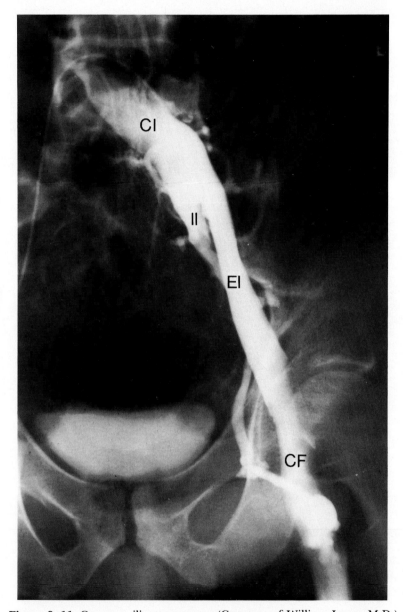

Figure 9–11. Common iliac venogram. (Courtesy of William Jones, M.D.)

CF	Common femoral vein
CI	Common iliac vein
EI	External iliac vein
II	Internal iliac vein

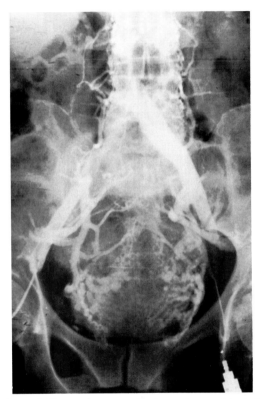

Figure 9–12. Bilateral iliac venogram in a patient with inferior vena caval obstruction shows dilated vesical and uterine veins. (From Kadir S: Diagnostic Angiography. Philadelphia, WB Saunders Company, 1986.)

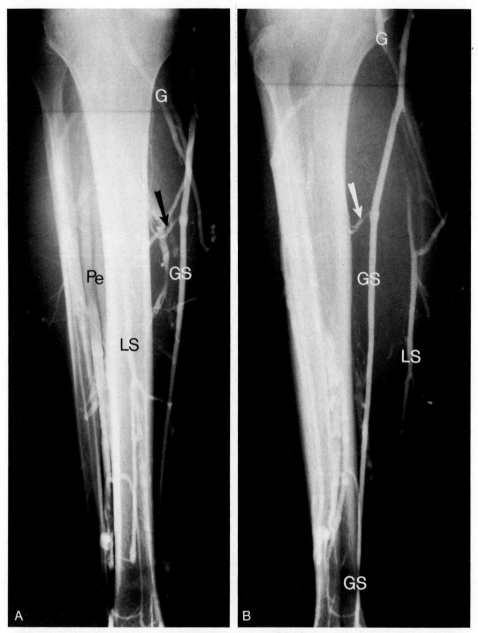

Figure 9–13. Venograms showing the lesser and greater saphenous veins. *A,* AP and *B,* lateral views of the lower leg. Arrow points to perforating veins. *C* and *D,* Radiograph with higher positioning showing the lesser and greater saphenous veins.

G   Gastrocnemius veins
GS   Greater saphenous vein
LS   Lesser saphenous vein
Pe   Peroneal vein
SF   Superficial femoral vein

Illustration continued on opposite page.

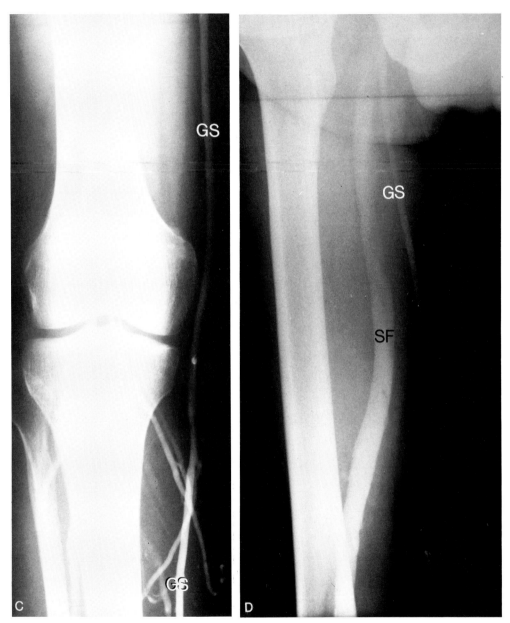

Figure 9–13. *Continued.*

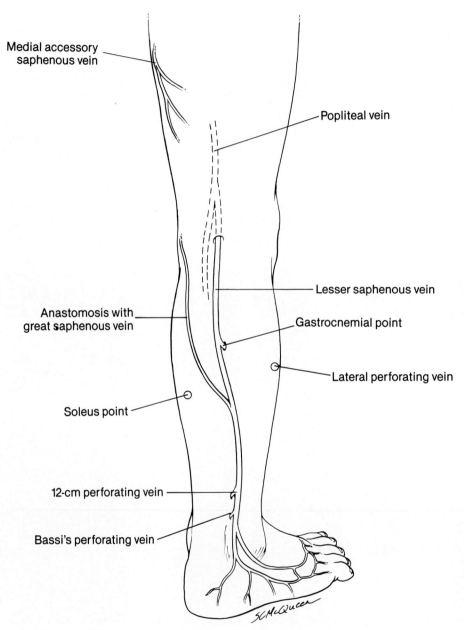

Figure 9–14. The lesser saphenous vein and site of major perforating veins.

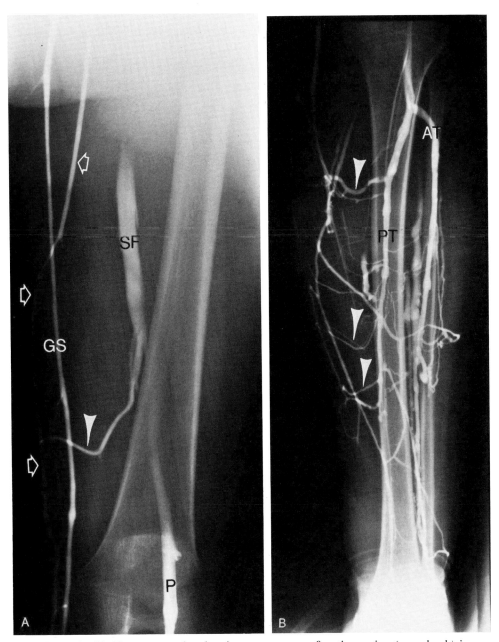

Figure 9–15. Venograms showing incompetent perforating veins *(arrowheads)* in calf *(A)* and thigh *(B)*. Open arrows in *A* indicate medial accessory saphenous vein. (From Kadir S: Diagnostic Angiography. Philadelphia, WB Saunders Company, 1986.)

AT   Anterior tibial
GS   Greater saphenous
P   Popliteal
PT   Posterior tibial
SF   Superficial femoral

Chapter Ten

PULMONARY ARTERIAL AND VENOUS ANATOMY

SAADOON KADIR, M.D.

EMBRYOLOGY (see Fig. 2–1, page 25)

The pulmonary arteries are derived from the sixth embryonal arches. The ventral portion of the left arch becomes a part of the main and left pulmonary arteries, with the dorsal segment persisting as the ductus arteriosus. On the right side, the sixth arch persists as the proximal right pulmonary artery (RPA).

PULMONARY ARTERIES (Fig. 10–1)

The main pulmonary artery (MPA) lies intrapericardial, has a straight anteroposterior (AP) course, and is best seen on the lateral or craniocaudad angulated AP beam arteriogram. At the level of the fifth thoracic vertebra, it divides into the left and right pulmonary arteries.

Pulmonary artery branches generally follow the segmental bronchi. However, variations in the number of vessels supplying a pulmonary segment are common, with additional accessory branches occurring frequently.

Right Pulmonary Artery (Figs. 10–2 to 10–8)

The RPA is longer than the left and has a slightly inferior sloping course to the right hilus, lying behind the ascending aorta, superior vena cava, and right upper lobe pulmonary vein and anterior to the right mainstem bronchus and esophagus. At the hilus of the lung, it divides into a superior (ascending branch) and an inferior trunk (descending branch, interlobar artery). The former supplies the upper lobe, and the latter trunk supplies the middle and lower lobes.

Right Upper Lobe

The ascending branch divides into three segmental arteries: apical, posterior, and anterior. The apical and posterior segmental arteries frequently arise together. The posterior and anterior segmental arteries immediately divide into ascending and descending subsegmental branches. In approximately 90 per cent of individuals, the upper lobe receives one or more accessory branches from the proximal descending right pulmonary artery (Figs. 10–2 and 10–3). Most frequently (approximately 70 per cent), these branches supply the posterior segment but may also supply the anterior segment. Occasionally, the entire apical/posterior segments may be supplied by such a vessel (Fig. 10–6).

In approximately 20 per cent of individuals, the ascending branch ends in a true trifurcation (apical, posterior, and anterior segmental arteries), or there may be two large ascending branches supplying the upper lobe (approximately 15 per cent) (Fig. 10–7). The distribution of the upper lobe arteries is not strictly segmental, as crossover supply to other segments occurs, most commonly between the apical and posterior segments. On the AP arteriogram, the upper lobe vessels show a constant relationship from medial to lateral: apical, posterior, and anterior segmental arteries.

Middle Lobe

The middle lobe arteries originate from the anteromedial aspect of the descending right pulmonary artery. On the AP arteriogram, the medial segmental artery overlies the basal segmental arteries, and the lateral segmental artery projects lateral and craniad to the anterior basal artery, which lies below the minor fissure. Both vessels are often difficult to identify on the same projection. The middle lobe is supplied by a single vessel in 50 per cent of individuals. In the remainder, there are two or more separate branches from the descending branch of the pulmonary artery to each segment of the middle lobe. Either of these segmental arteries may arise together (common origin) with a lower lobe segmental artery.

Right Lower Lobe

The superior segment is supplied by a single artery (80 per cent) and occasionally by two or three branches arising from the descending RPA close to and opposite the origin of the middle lobe arteries (Fig. 10–2 and 10–3). On the AP arteriogram this vessel usually lies between the anterior segmental (upper lobe) and the lateral segmental (middle lobe) arteries.

The descending RPA gives off, in sequence, the medial basal and anterior basal segmental arteries and subsequently divides into the terminal branches: lateral and posterior basal segmental arteries. Occasionally, the medial basal artery is duplicated or may be absent. This branching order is observed in approximately 50 per cent of individuals. In the remainder, the branching is random. In addition, subsegmental branches arise directly from the descending RPA.

On the AP arteriogram the basal segmental arteries show a more or less constant location irrespective of the order in which the branches arise. From medial to lateral these are:

Medial basal: Commonly overlies the right atrium
Posterior basal: Most dependent branch
Lateral basal: Together with the posterior basal, constitutes the terminal branch of the RPA
Anterior basal: Extends laterally to the costophrenic sulcus

Left Pulmonary Artery (Figs. 10–9 to 10–12)

The left pulmonary artery (LPA) is shorter and represents the continuation of the MPA. On the AP arteriogram this vessel appears foreshortened and is best evaluated in the left anterior oblique projection. From its proximal segment, it provides branches to the upper lobe and the lingula and continues inferiorly to supply the lower lobe segmental branches.

Left Upper Lobe and Lingula (Fig. 10–12)

The formation of a common trunk similar to the right upper lobe PA occurs infrequently (approximately 18 per cent) on the left side. The upper lobe branches arise in more or less random order, frequently forming small trunks of two or more branches. In all, three to seven branches may originate from the proximal LPA to supply the upper lobe and lingula. On the average there are five separate upper lobe arteries. The lingular arteries arise from the left interlobar artery in around 90 per cent. In the remainder they arise together with the other upper lobe vessels. On arteriography, the location of the left upper lobe vessels is similar to that of the right upper lobe. From medial to lateral—apical-posterior, anterior, and lingular branches project below the anterior segmental artery.

Left Lower Lobe (Fig. 10–11)

At or distal to the origin of the lingular artery(ies) the descending LPA gives off the superior segmental artery. Occasionally, this vessel originates above the lingular artery and frequently there are two or more separate vessels. The descending LPA then divides into the lower lobe branches. Frequently, the division is into two major trunks: anterior-lateral basal and posterior basal artery. In other cases, the anterior and medial segmental arteries form a common trunk (approximately 50 per cent) (see Fig. 10–9*B*). A true medial basal segmental artery is not identifiable on all normal left pulmonary arteriograms.

On the AP arteriogram, the location of these vessels is similar to that of the right lower lobe, i.e., from medial to lateral:

Medial basal: Identified only inconstantly
Posterior basal: Most medial and frequently the largest and lowest reaching branch
Lateral basal:
Anterior basal: Extends laterally toward the costophrenic sulcus

PULMONARY VEINS (Figs. 10–13 and 10–16)

The right lung is drained by superior and inferior pulmonary veins. The superior pulmonary vein is usually formed by the junction of four veins: the apical, anterior, and posterior segmental veins and the middle lobe vein comprising lateral and medial segmental veins. Occasionally, the middle lobe veins empty directly into the left atrium or drain via the inferior pulmonary vein. The inferior pulmonary vein is formed by the junction of the superior and common basal pulmonary vein. The latter has two tributaries, the superior and inferior basal pulmonary veins.

The left lung is also drained by two sets of pulmonary veins. The upper vein is formed by the confluence of three veins—apical-posterior (apical and posterior segmental veins), anterior segmental, and lingular veins. The latter has two tributaries, the superior and inferior lingular veins. The left inferior pulmonary vein is formed by two veins, the superior and common basal pulmonary veins. The latter is also formed by the junction of the superior and inferior basal pulmonary veins.

The superior and inferior pulmonary veins drain separately into the left atrium but may form a confluence on one or both sides. Occasionally, the middle lobe or other segmental veins may drain into the left atrium independently. Rarely, the left and right superior or inferior pulmonary veins have a common opening in the left atrium.

REFERENCES

1. Aviado DM: The lung circulation. New York, Pergamon Press, 1965.
2. Boyden EA: Segmental anatomy of the lungs. New York, McGraw-Hill, 1955.
3. Boyden EA, Hamre CJ: An analysis of variations in the bronchovascular patterns of the middle lobe in fifty dissected and twenty injected lungs. J Thorac Surg 21:172–188, 1951.
4. Elliott FM, Reid L: Some new facts about the pulmonary artery and its branching pattern. Clin Radiol 16:193–198, 1965.
5. Herrnheiser G, Kubat A: Systematische anatomie der lungen gefässe. Z Anat Entwickelungsgesch 105:570–653, 1936.
6. Jefferson KE: The normal pulmonary angiogram and some changes seen in chronic nonspecific lung disease. Proc Roy Soc Med 58:677–681, 1965.
7. Nagaishi C: Functional anatomy and histology of the lung. Baltimore, University Park Press, 1972.

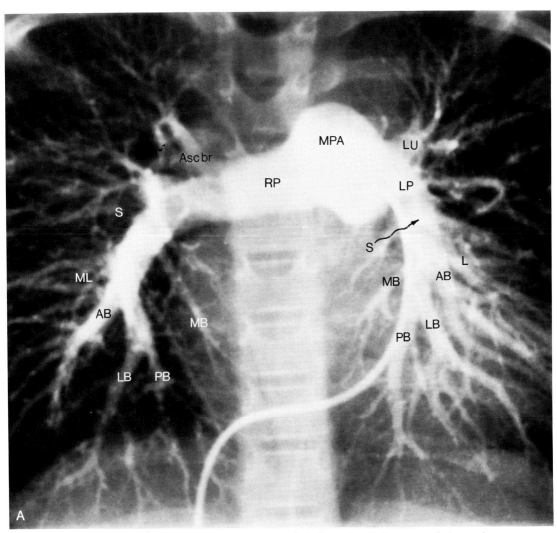

Figure 10–1. *A* and *B*, Anteroposterior and *C*, lateral arteriograms of the main pulmonary artery from different individuals. Arrows point to pulmonary valve. In *C*, the left pulmonary artery branches are labeled.

AB	Anterior basal
Asc br	Ascending branch of right pulmonary artery
L	Lingular arteries
LB	Lateral basal segmental artery
LP	Left pulmonary artery
LU	Upper lobe branches of left pulmonary artery
MB	Medial basal segmental artery
ML	Middle lobe arteries
MPA	Main pulmonary artery
PB	Posterior basal segmental artery
RP	Right pulmonary artery
S	Superior segmental artery

Illustration continued on following page.

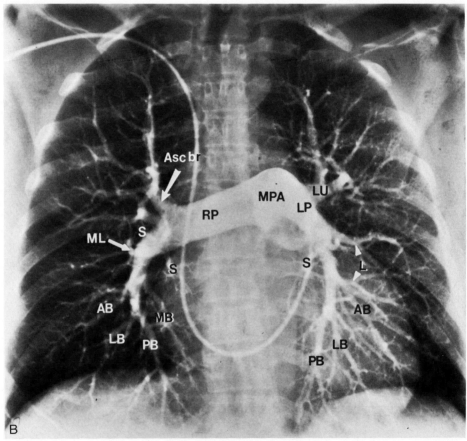

Figure 10–1. *Continued.*

Illustration continued on following page.

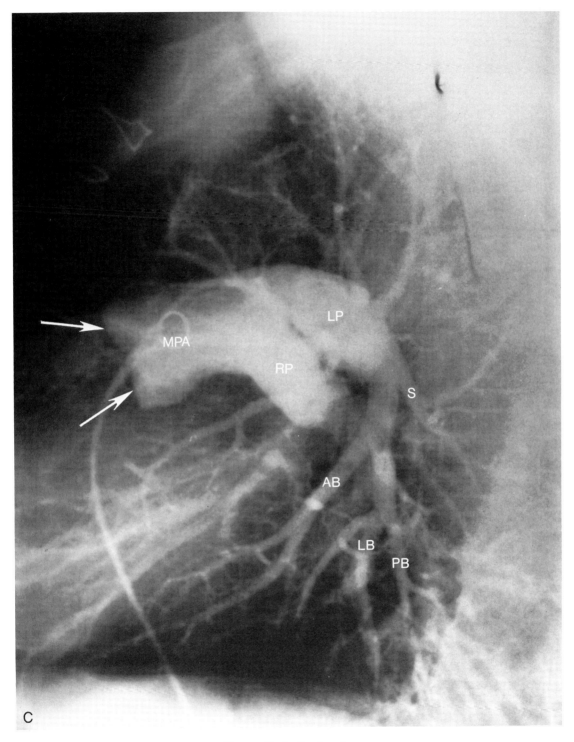

Figure 10–1. *Continued.*

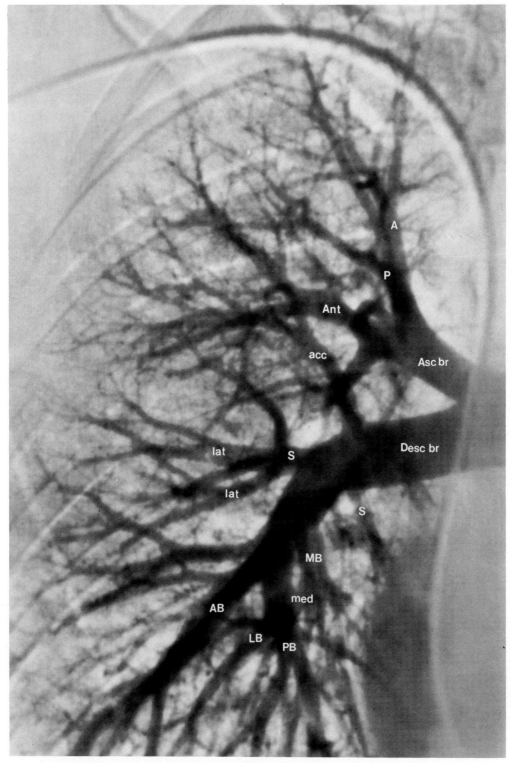

Figure 10–2. Subtraction film from an anteroposterior right pulmonary arteriogram. *Note:* The proximal superior segmental right lower lobe and lateral segmental right middle lobe vessels are superimposed. Multiple subsegmental arteries have independent origins from the pulmonary artery.

Legend continued on opposite page.

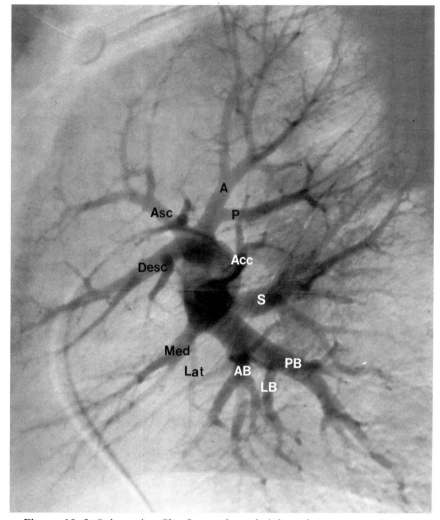

Figure 10–3. Subtraction film from a lateral right pulmonary arteriogram.

A	Apical segmental artery of right upper lobe
AB	Anterior basal segmental artery
Acc	Accessory branch to right upper lobe
Asc	Ascending branch anterior segment right upper lobe artery
Desc	Desending branch anterior segment right upper lobe artery
Lat	Lateral segmental branches of middle lobe artery
LB	Lateral basal segmental artery
Med	Medial segmental middle lobe branch
P	Posterior segmental artery of right upper lobe
PB	Posterior basal segmental artery
S	Superior segmental artery of right lower lobe

Figure 10–2. *Continued.*

A	Apical segmental artery of right upper lobe		lat	Lateral segmental artery of middle lobe
AB	Anterior basal segmental artery		LB	Lateral basal segmental artery
acc	Accessory branch to right upper lobe		MB	Medial basal segmental artery
Ant	Anterior segmental artery of right upper lobe		med	Medial segmental artery of middle lobe
Asc br	Ascending branch of right pulmonary artery		P	Posterior segmental artery of right upper lobe
Desc br	Descending branch of right pulmonary artery		PB	Posterior basal segmental artery
			S	Superior segmental artery of right lower lobe

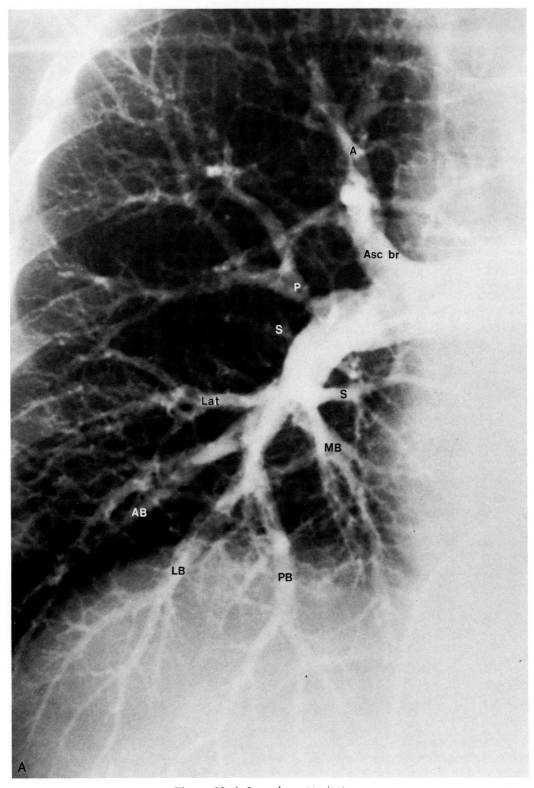

Figure 10–4. *Legend on opposite page.*

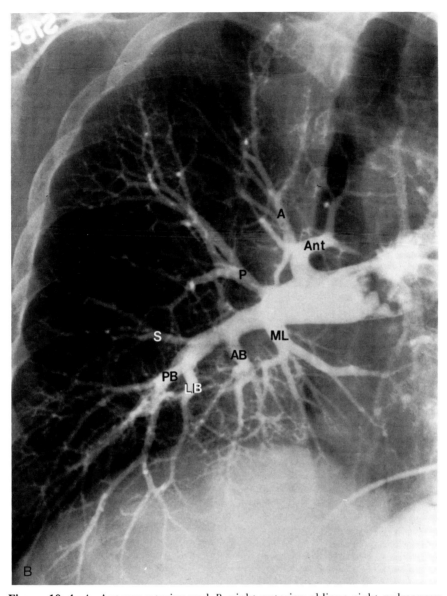

Figure 10–4. *A*, Anteroposterior and *B*, right anterior oblique right pulmonary arteriogram. The posterior segment of the right upper lobe is supplied by an accessory vessel from the interlobar pulmonary artery.

A	Apical segmental artery of right upper lobe
AB	Anterior basal segmental artery
Ant	Anterior segmental artery of right upper lobe
Asc br	Ascending branch of right pulmonary artery
Lat	Lateral segmental middle lobe artery
LB	Lateral basal segmental artery
MB	Medial basal segmental artery
ML	Middle lobe arteries
P	Posterior segmental artery of right upper lobe
PB	Posterior basal segmental artery
S	Superior segmental artery of right lower lobe

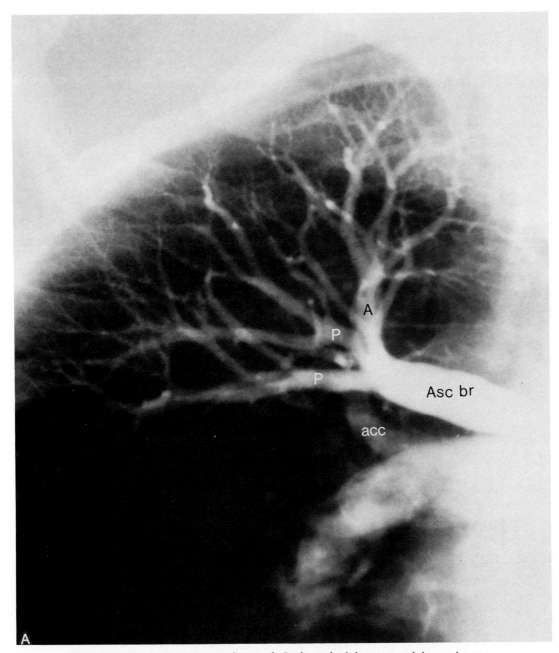

Figure 10–5. *A,* Anteroposterior and *B,* lateral right upper lobe pulmonary arteriograms. The ascending branch of the pulmonary artery supplies only the apical and posterior segments. The anterior segment is supplied by an accessory artery off the interlobar artery.

A	Apical segmental arteries
acc	Accessory branch to anterior segment
Asc br	Ascending branch of right pulmonary artery
P	Posterior segmental arteries

Illustration continued on opposite page.

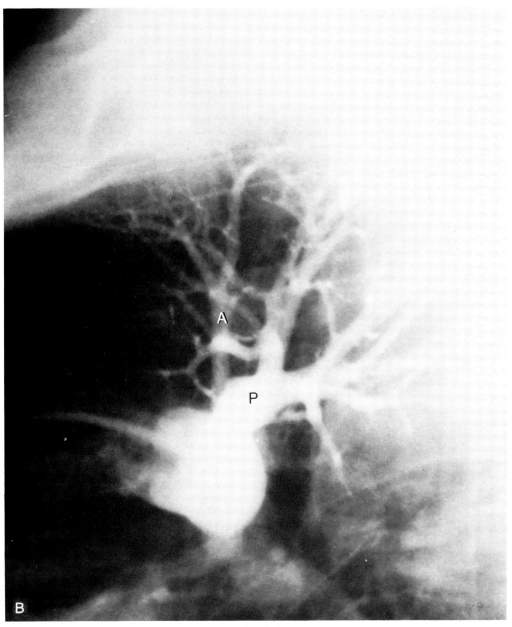

Figure 10–5. *Continued.*

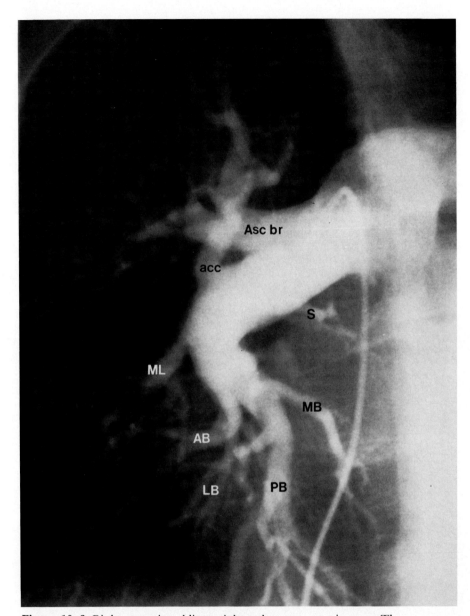

Figure 10–6. Right posterior oblique right pulmonary arteriogram. The accessory branch supplies the posterior as well as the apical segmental arteries.

AB	Anterior basal segmental artery
acc	Accessory right upper lobe artery
Asc br	Ascending branch of right pulmonary
LB	Lateral basal segmental artery
MB	Medial basal segmental artery
ML	Middle lobe artery
PB	Posterior basal segmental artery
S	Superior segmental artery of right lower lobe

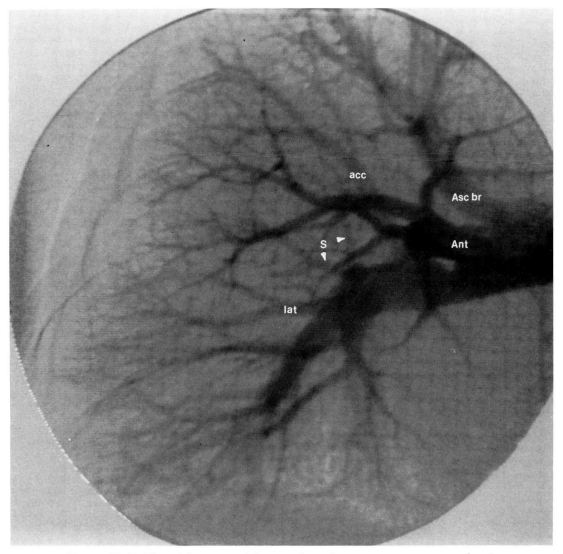

Figure 10–7. The right upper lobe arteries arise as two separate trunks. In addition, there is an accessory upper lobe branch from the interlobar artery.

acc	Accessory right upper lobe artery
Ant	Anterior segmental artery
Asc br	Ascending branch of right pulmonary artery
lat	Lateral segmental middle lobe artery
S	Superior segmental right lower lobe artery

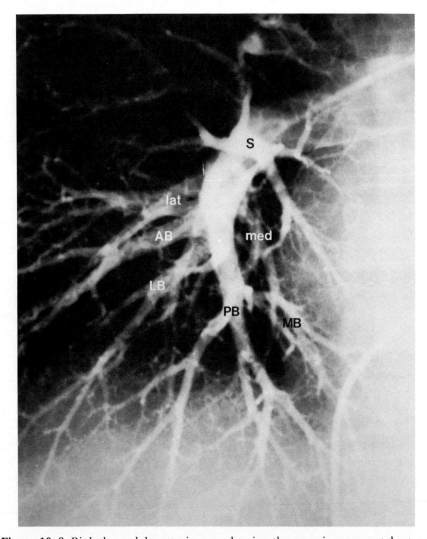

Figure 10–8. Right lower lobe arteriogram showing the superior segmental artery.

AB	Anterior basal segmental artery
LB	Lateral basal segmental artery
lat	Lateral segmental artery of middle lobe
MB	Medial basal segmental artery
med	Medial segmental artery of middle lobe
PB	Posterior basal segmental artery
S	Superior segmental artery

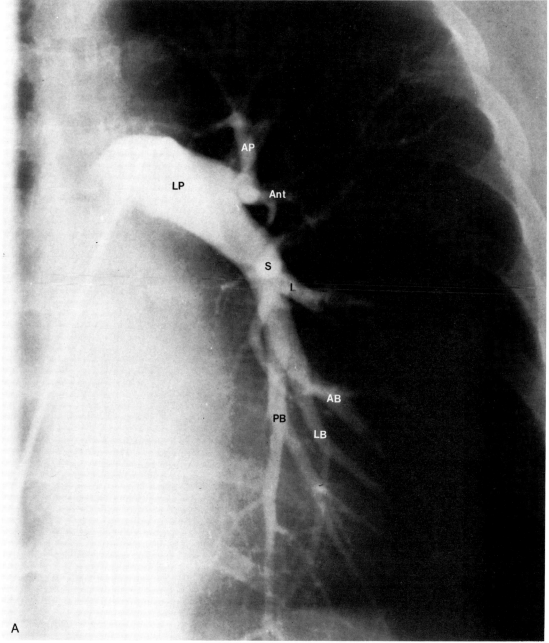

Figure 10–9. *A* and *B*, Anteroposterior and *C*, lateral left pulmonary arteriograms. In *B* the superior lingular artery and superior segmented left lower lobe arteries are superimposed. In addition, the lateral and posterior basal arteries are also superimposed.

A	Apical segmental artery of left upper lobe
AB	Anterior basal segmental artery
Ant	Anterior segmental branch of left upper lobe
AP	Apical posterior segmental branch
L	Lingular arteries
LB	Lateral basal segmental artery
LP	Left pulmonary artery
MB	Medial basal segmental artery
P	Posterior segmental artery
PB	Posterior basal segmental artery
S	Superior segmental artery of left lower lobe

Illustration continued on following page.

243

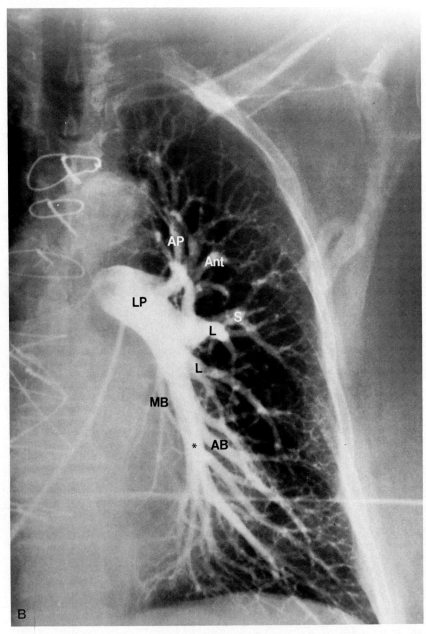

Figure 10–9. *Continued.*

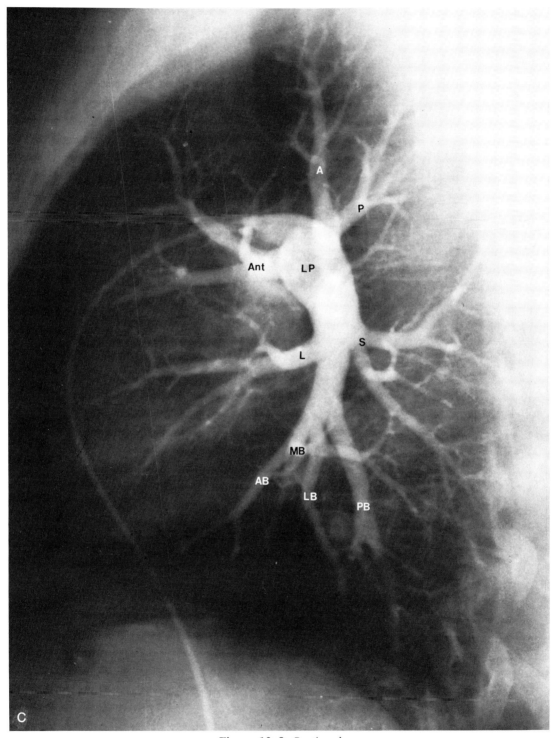

Figure 10–9. *Continued.*

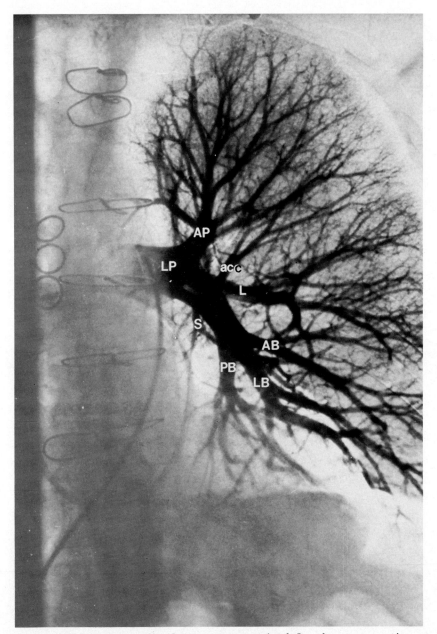

Figure 10–10. Subtraction film from anteroposterior left pulmonary arteriogram demonstrates the smaller peripheral pulmonary artery branches.

AB	Anterior basal segmental artery
acc	Accessory upper lobe artery
AP	Apical posterior segmental arteries
L	Lingular arteries
LB	Lateral basal segmental artery
LP	Left pulmonary artery
PB	Posterior basal segmental artery
S	Superior segmental artery

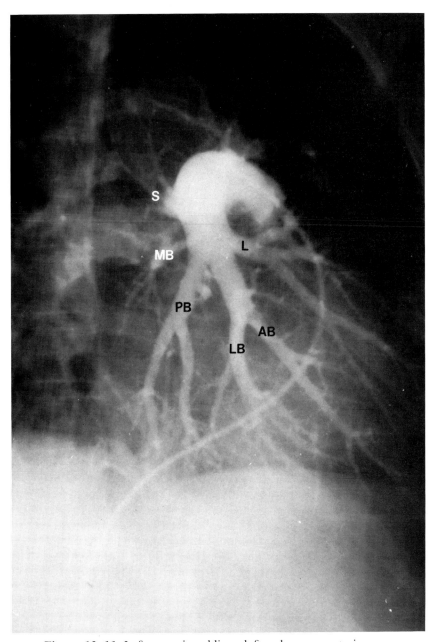

Figure 10–11. Left posterior oblique left pulmonary arteriogram.

AB	Anterior basal segmental artery
L	Lingual arteries
LB	Lateral basal segmental artery
MB	Medial basal segmental artery
PB	Posterior basal segmental artery
S	Superior segmental artery of left lower lobe

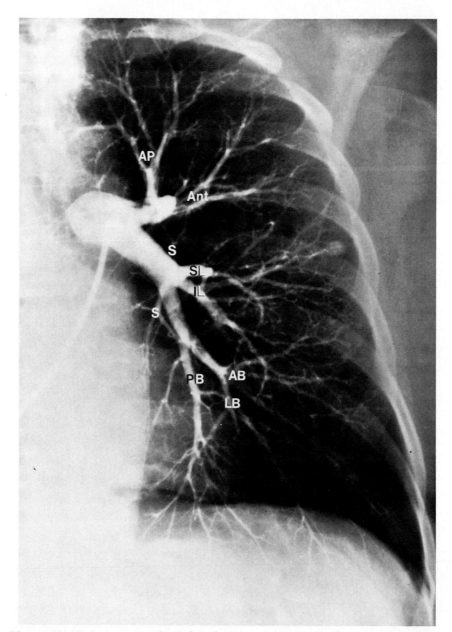

Figure 10–12. Anteroposterior left pulmonary arteriogram shows a single upper lobe trunk.

AB	Anterior basal segmental artery
Ant	Anterior segmental branch left upper lobe
AP	Apical posterior segmental branch
IL	Inferior lingular artery
LB	Lateral basal segmental artery
PB	Posterior basal segmental artery
S	Superior segmental artery
SL	Superior lingular artery

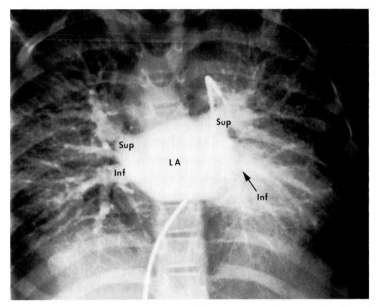

Figure 10–13. Venous phase of main pulmonary arteriogram showing the pulmonary veins and left atrium. (From Kadir S: Diagnostic Angiography. Philadelphia, WB Saunders Company, 1986.)

Inf	Inferior pulmonary vein
LA	Left atrium
Sup	Superior pulmonary vein

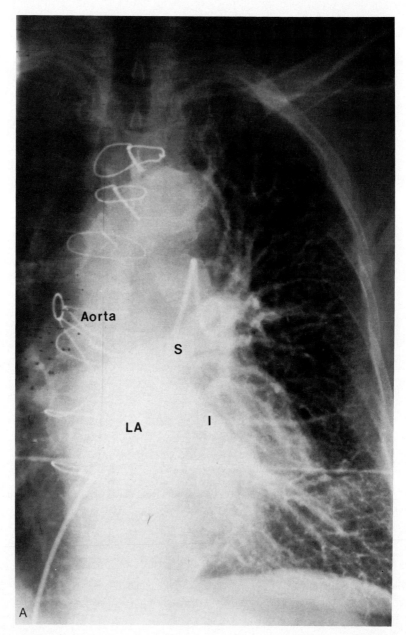

Figure 10–14. Levophase of pulmonary arteriogram. *A,* Anterior and *B,* lateral left pulmonary arteriogram shows the pulmonary veins, left atrium, left ventricle, and ascending aorta.

I	Inferior pulmonary veins
LA	Left atrium
LV	Left ventricle
S	Superior pulmonary vein

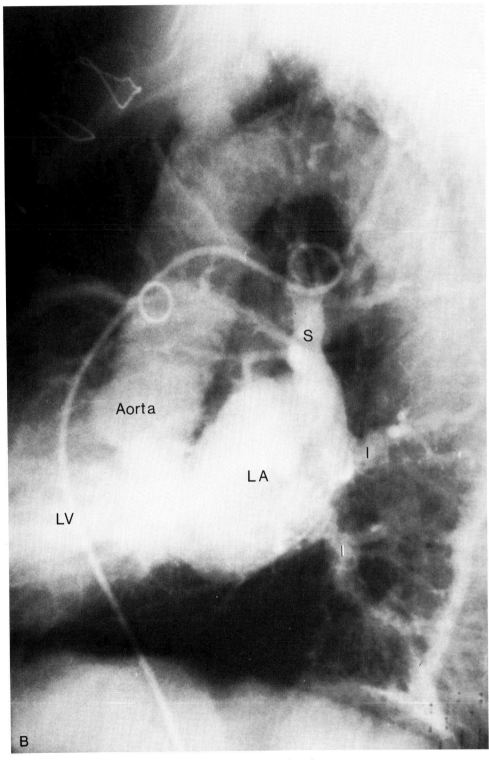

Figure 10–14. *Continued.*

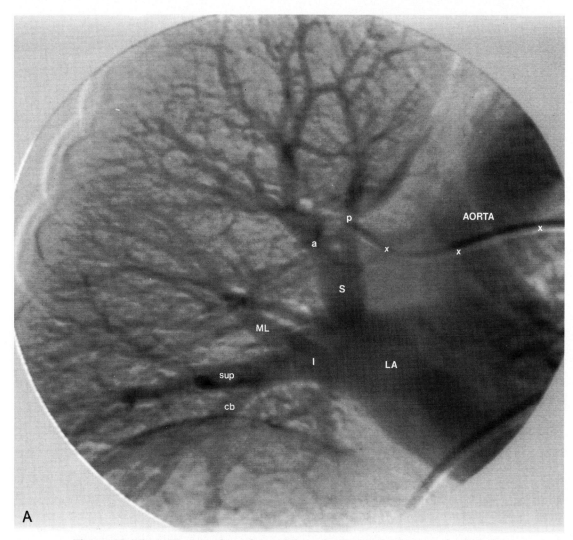

Figure 10–15. *A,* Venous phase from right pulmonary arteriogram showing the pulmonary veins. The middle lobe veins drain into the inferior pulmonary vein. *B,* Venous phase from another individual. The middle lobe vein joins the superior pulmonary vein.

a	Apical segmental vein
cb	Common basal pulmonary vein
I	Inferior pulmonary vein
LA	Left atrium
ML	Middle lobe vein
p	Posterior segmental vein
S	Superior pulmonary vein
sup	Superior basal pulmonary vein
xx	Catheter in right pulmonary artery

Illustration continued on opposite page.

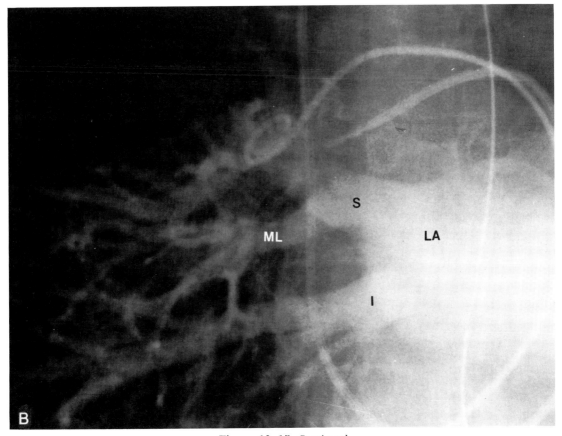

Figure 10–15. *Continued.*

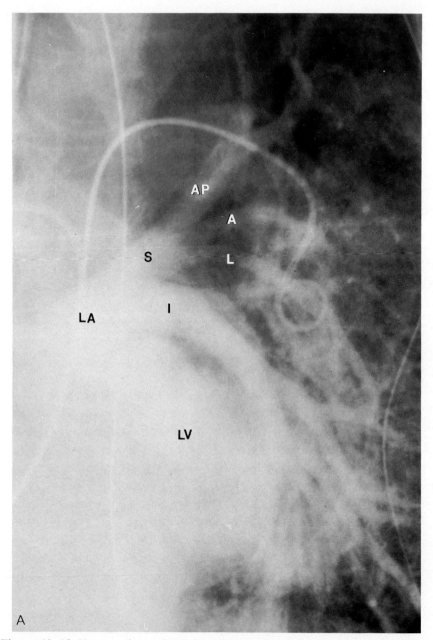

Figure 10–16. Venous phase of *A*, left and *B*, right pulmonary arteriogram shows a confluence of both upper and lower lobe veins with a single opening in the left atrium for each side.

A   Anterior segmental vein
AP Apical posterior segmental vein
I   Inferior pulmonary veins
L   Lingular veins
LA Left atrium
LV Left ventricle
S   Superior pulmonary veins

Illustration continued on opposite page.

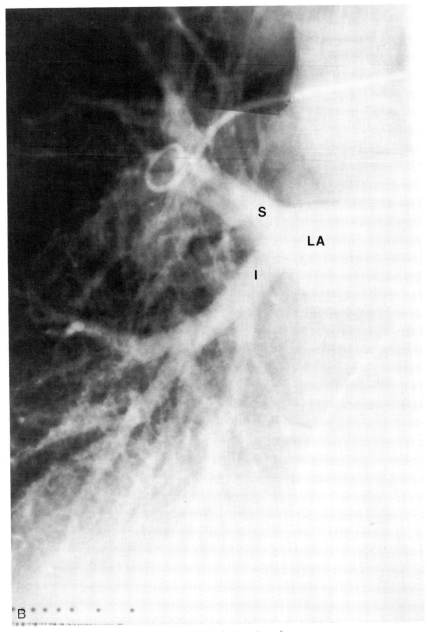

Figure 10–16. *Continued.*

ARTERIAL AND VENOUS ANATOMY OF THE REPRODUCTIVE ORGANS

Chapter Eleven

GONADAL VESSELS

SAADOON KADIR, M.D.

GONADAL ARTERIES (Figs. 11–1 to 11–5)

Embryologically, the gonadal arteries represent persistence of the lateral splanchnic branches of the aorta. In 80 per cent of individuals there is a single gonadal artery on each side. A common trunk of left and right gonadal arteries is rare. In the remainder, there are multiple gonadal arteries, more commonly on the left side. Occasionally there is a bifid origin. In this case one or both limbs may arise from the aorta or renal artery.

In the majority (greater than 70 per cent) of individuals, the gonadal arteries originate from the ventral surface of the abdominal aorta a few centimeters below the origin of the renal arteries. Less commonly, these originate at a higher level, frequently from the aorta at the level of the renal arteries or higher (Figs. 11–3 and 11–4). In about 20 per cent of individuals, a gonadal artery originates from a renal artery and rarely from the adrenal, lumbar, or iliac arteries.

Gonadal arteries arising from the suprarenal aorta usually form a sling around the renal vein. This has been implicated as a cause of varicocele. Their course is typically horizontal initially before turning downward. This permits differentiation from the lumbar arteries. The right gonadal artery lies anterior (ventral) to the inferior vena cava. If the origin is high, the course is posterior to the inferior vena cava and anterior to the right renal vein (Fig. 11–3).

The testicular artery has a laterally oriented course until it enters the inguinal canal (Fig. 11–5). The ovarian artery, which is usually quite tortuous distally, takes a medial course at the pelvic brim, crossing the iliac vessels as it lies in the suspensory ligament of the ovary. It gives off ovarian, ureteric, and tubal branches. It also provides an anastomotic branch to the uterine artery and another branch to the skin of the labia and inguinal area.

259

Proximally, the gonadal arteries provide branches to the ureter, perirenal and periureteric fat, and retroperitoneal lymph nodes and occasionally a branch to the adrenal gland. On aortography, the gonadal arteries are visualized in less than one third of individuals. Occasionally, they are enlarged and serve as collaterals for aortic occlusion (Fig. 11–5). The diameter of the normal gonadal artery is usually less than 1 mm.

GONADAL VEINS (Figs. 11–6 to 11–15)

The deep veins from the testicle and epididymis form the pampiniform plexus, which is drained by three or four veins via the internal and external spermatic and ductus deferens veins. The spermatic veins pass through the inguinal canal, where they intercommunicate. The external spermatic vein drains into the femoral vein via the inferior epigastric vein, and the internal spermatic vein follows the testicular artery to the renal vein. The ductus deferens vein drains into the internal iliac vein via the vesical veins.

The internal spermatic veins (three to five in number) unite to form two or three veins in the inguinal canal, and more centrally these frequently unite to form a single channel. (Fig. 11–9). However, there is considerable variation in the number of channels comprising the testicular (internal spermatic) veins and their anastomoses with other retroperitoneal veins. Frequently a single vein is present initially which breaks up into two or three frequently communicating parallel channels. On the left side, such multiple parallel channels occur in 50 per cent and on the right in around 40 per cent of individuals. Multiple parallel channels are less common in the ovarian veins.

The ovarian veins form a plexus near the ovary and uterus. Two veins emerge from this plexus and lie next to the ovarian artery (Fig. 11–8). They communicate freely with the uterine venous plexus. The central course and variations of the testicular and ovarian veins are similar, and they are discussed together as "gonadal veins." Peculiarities of each system are addressed separately.

The left gonadal vein joins the left renal vein at right angles, close to its junction with the inferior vena cava (IVC) but lateral to the junction of the adrenal vein and superior mesenteric artery crossing. In less than 1 per cent of individuals, the left gonadal vein joins the IVC. In the presence of a circumaortic renal vein, the gonadal vein may join either limb (pre- or retroaortic) (Fig. 11–15; also see Fig. 15–27*B*). Frequently, smaller tributaries join the other limb. In the presence of IVC duplication, the left gonadal vein joins the left IVC. The right gonadal vein joins the IVC slightly below the junction of the right renal vein and the IVC in approximately 60 per cent (occasionally as low as L_3–L_4). It joins the IVC at the renal vein–IVC junction in approximately 30 per cent of individuals and intrarenal branches in the remainder. Occasionally, the orifice of the right gonadal vein in the IVC is to the left of the midline.

Most frequently, there is a single large vein entering the renal vein or IVC. On the left side, in 30 per cent of individuals small accessory or two equal-sized channels may drain separately into the main renal vein, or one channel enters the intrarenal branches, inferior vena cava below the junction of the left renal vein, lumbar, or other retroperitoneal veins or may reunite with the main channel and drain into the left renal vein (Figs. 11–10 to 11–12). On the right side, accessory channels may drain into the renal vein or the inferior vena cava below the junction of the right renal vein and IVC in about 25 per cent of individuals.

The gonadal veins communicate with other retroperitoneal veins at the level of the iliac crest, with paravertebral, lumbar, and colic veins and with capsular renal and ureteric veins (Fig. 11–13). Trans-scrotal communications have been demonstrated in 3 to 5 per cent of individuals. These communications are important in the management of varicocele and infertility. Persistence of these communications may be responsible for recurrent varicoceles after embolization and surgical ligation.

Valves are present in 80 to 90 per cent of all gonadal veins (Figs. 11–13 and 11–14). The typical location of such valves is at the orifice or 1 to 4 cm below. In addition, one or more valves may be present in the mid-portion of these veins on the right in 90 per cent of individuals and on the left in around 60 per cent. Typically, a valve is present in the retroperitoneal collateral at the level of the iliac crest approximately 1 to 2 cm proximal to its junction with the gonadal vein. On retrograde renal venography, reflux of contrast medium into the gonadal vein may be demonstrated only in the presence of total valvar incompetence. If the valve is partially competent (as may be the case in the presence of a small to medium-sized varicocele), contrast may not reflux beyond the valve.

REFERENCES

1. Ahlberg NE, Bartley O, Chidekel N, et al: Phlebography in varicocele scroti. Acta Radiol [Diagn] 4:517–528, 1966.
2. Borell U, Fernström I: The adnexal branches of the uterine artery. An arteriographic study in human subjects. Acta Radiol 40:561–582, 1953.
3. Borell U, Fernström I: The ovarian artery. An arteriographic study in human subjects. Acta Radiol 42:253–265, 1954.
4. Comhaire F, Kunnen M, Nahoum C: Radiological anatomy of the internal spermatic vein(s) in 200 retrograde venograms. Int J Androl 4:379–387, 1981.
5. Coolsaet BLRA: The varicocele syndrome: Venography determining the optimal level for surgical management. J Urol 124:833–839, 1980.
6. Gaudin J, Lefeure C, Person H, et al: The venous hilum of the testis and epididymis: Anatomic aspect. Surg Radiol Anat 10:233–242, 1988.
7. Kurrat HJ, Hesse M: Doppelbildung der Arteria testicularis sinistra mit Ursprungs und Verlaufsvarianten—Eine entwicklungsgeschichtliche Betrachtung. Anat Anz 145:303–307, 1979.
8. Merklin RJ, Michels NA: The variant renal and suprarenal blood supply with data on the inferior phrenic ureteral and gonadal arteries. A statistical analysis based on 185 dissections and review of the literature. J Inter Coll Surg 29:41–76, 1958.
9. Murray RR, Mitchell SE, Kadir S, et al: Comparison of recurrent varicocele anatomy following surgery and percutaneous balloon occlusion. J Urol 135:286–289, 1986.
10. Nordmark L: Angiography of the testicular artery. Acta Radiol [Diagn] 18:25–32, 1977.
11. Notkovich H: Variations of the testicular and ovarian arteries in relation to the renal pedicle. Surg Gynecol Obstet 103:487–495, 1956.
12. Shinohara H, Nakatani T, Fukuo Y, et al: Case with a high positioned origin of the testicular artery. Anat Rec 226:264–266, 1990.
13. Sigmund G, Gall H, Bahren W: Stop-type and shunt-type varicoceles: Venographic findings. Radiology 163:105–110, 1987.

Figures 11–1 through 11–15 on following pages.

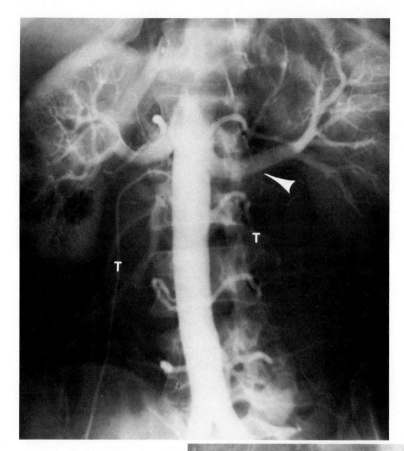

Figure 11–1. Testicular arteries (T). The left originates from the renal artery *(arrowhead)* and the right from the aorta.

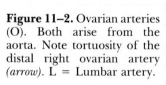

Figure 11–2. Ovarian arteries (O). Both arise from the aorta. Note tortuosity of the distal right ovarian artery *(arrow)*. L = Lumbar artery.

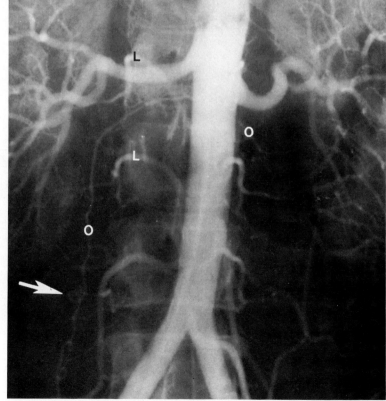

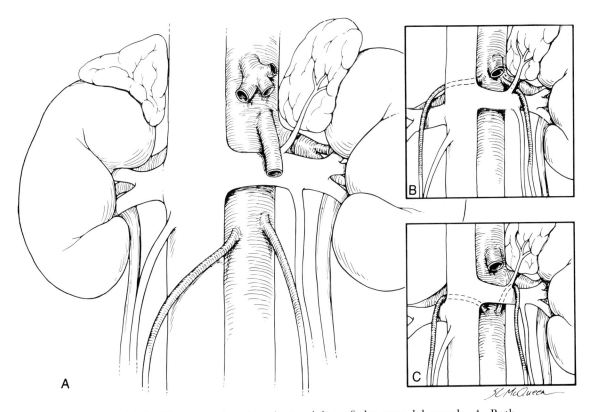

Figure 11–3. The normal and variant origins of the gonadal vessels. *A*, Both gonadal arteries originate from the ventral surface of the aorta. The vein joins the cava on the right and the renal vein on the left. *B*, Origin of gonadal arteries at the level of the renal arteries. The right gonadal artery lies posterior to the inferior vena cava and anterior to the renal vein. The left crosses the renal vein anteriorly. *C*, Infrarenal origin of gonadal arteries with a variant course. The right gonadal artery is retrocaval and anterior to the renal vein. The left artery also ascends initially to swing over the left renal vein.

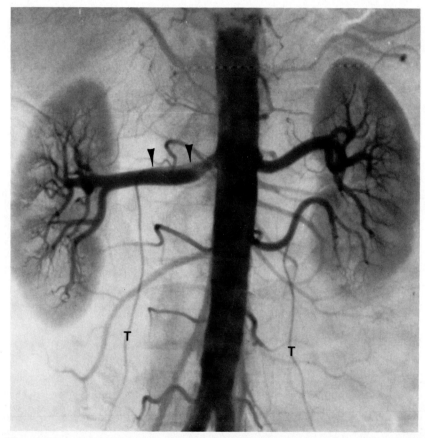

Figure 11–4. Retrocaval course of the right testicular artery *(arrowheads)* arising at the level of the renal artery. The left testicular artery (T) arises from the aberrant left renal artery.

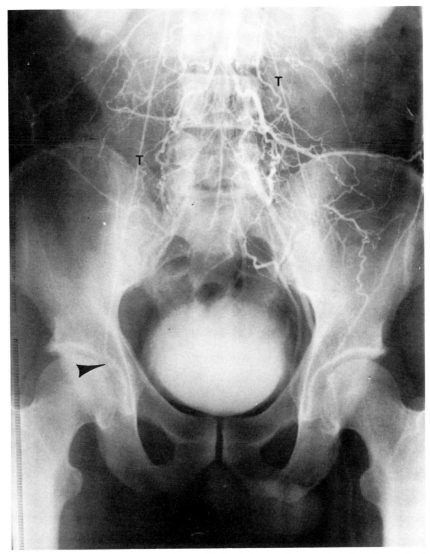

Figure 11–5. Aortogram in a patient with Leriche syndrome, showing the testicular arteries (T). Arrowhead points to where the right testicular artery enters the inguinal canal.

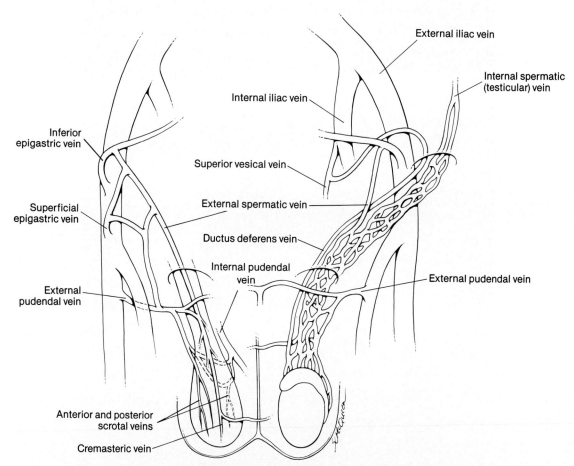

Figure 11–6. Diagram illustrating deep (left) and superficial (right) testicular venous drainage and potential collateral pathways.

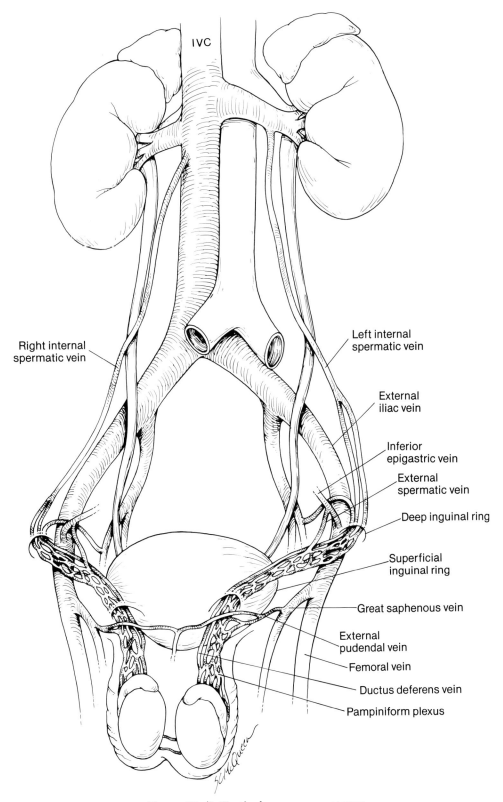

Figure 11–7. Testicular venous anatomy.

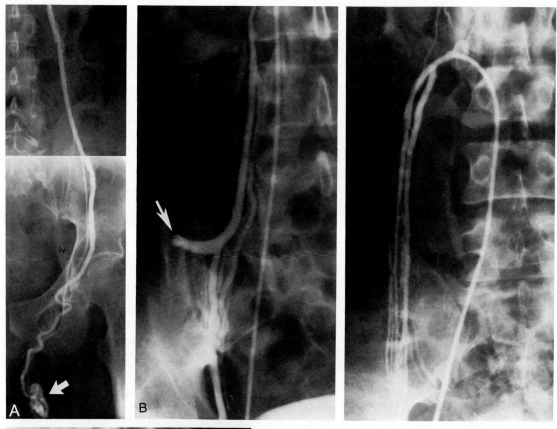

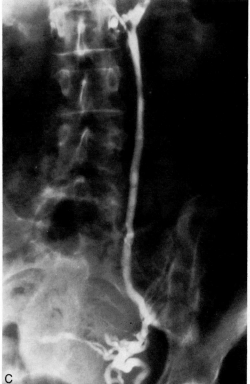

Figure 11–8. *A*, Retrograde left testicular venogram shows a varicocele *(arrow)*. There is opacification of the external iliac vein (iv). *B*, Retrograde right testicular venograms from two different individuals showing multiple channels. Arrow points to a venous valve in a large retroperitoneal communicating vein. *C*, Retrograde left ovarian venogram via cubital vein approach. *D*, Right ovarian venogram from another patient. There is opacification of the ovarian and uterine venous plexus and the internal iliac vein via the uterine vein.

II	Internal iliac
O	Ovarian
U	Uterine
xxx	Catheter

Illustration continued on opposite page.

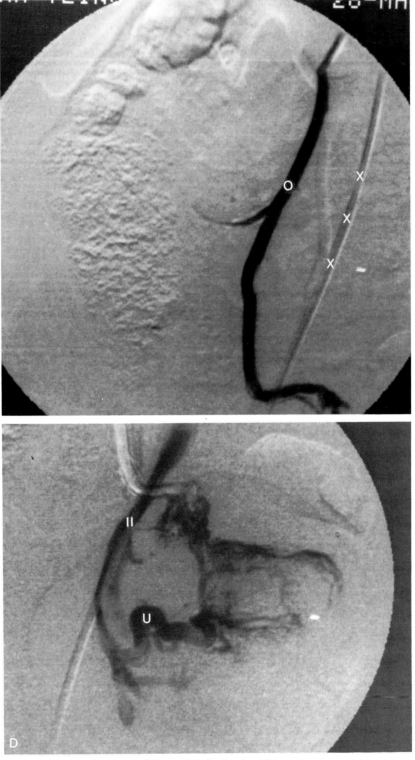

Figure 11–8. *Continued.*

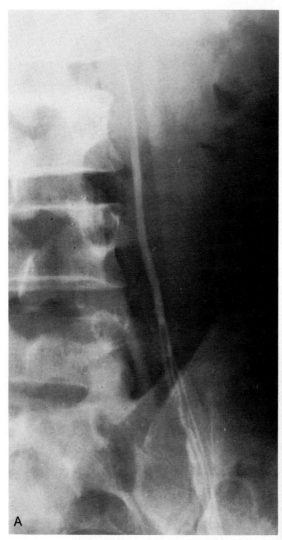

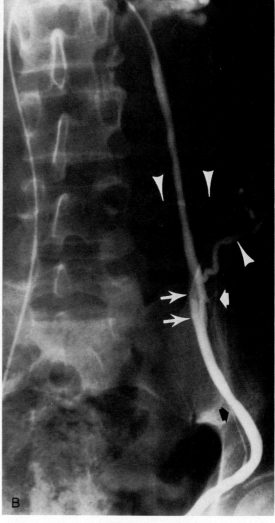

Figure 11–9. *A,* Multiple channels unite to form a single gonadal vein. *B,* Small parallel vein *(small wide arrows)* and segmental duplication *(large arrows)* of the left gonadal vein. Arrowheads point to communication between gonadal and paravertebral veins and vena cava.

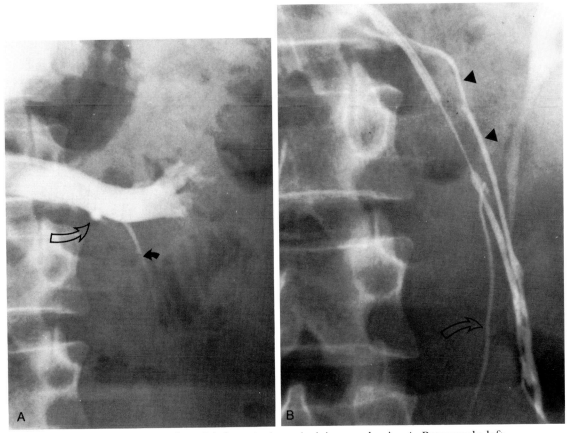

Figure 11–10. Duplicated left testicular vein joins renal vein. *A*, Retrograde left renal venogram opacifies the proximal segment of a laterally located smaller testicular vein *(solid arrow)* and a valve *(open arrow)* at the orifice of another medially located channel. *B*, Catheterization of the medially located orifice using a coaxial system. Both channels opacify on contrast injection. Arrowheads point to the lateral channel. Open arrow points to a collateral to the paravertebral veins.

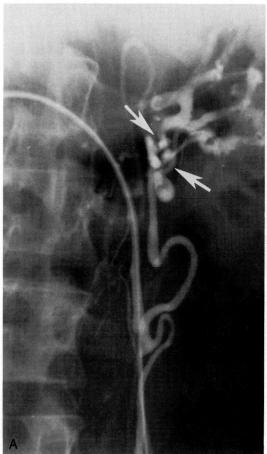

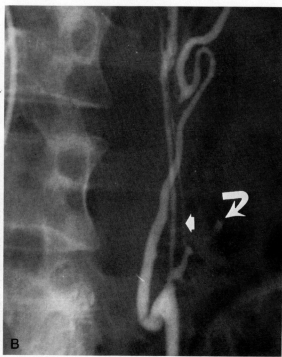

Figure 11–11. Duplicated left testicular vein with one channel joining an intrarenal vein. *A,* Left testicular venogram opacifies a tortuous channel joining an intrarenal vein *(arrows). B,* Radiograph with lower positioning shows a small, third channel *(straight short arrow).* Curved arrow points to the communication with the colic veins.

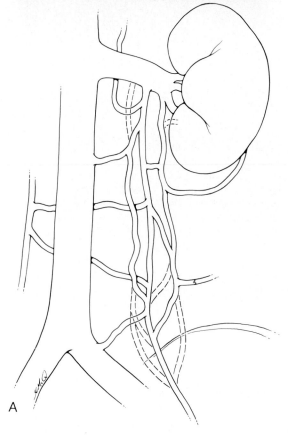

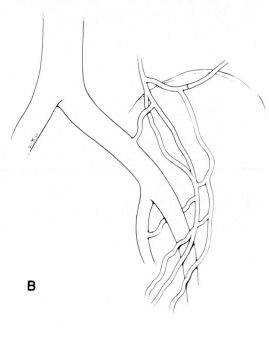

Figure 11–12. Different collateral pathways for gonadal venous drainage.

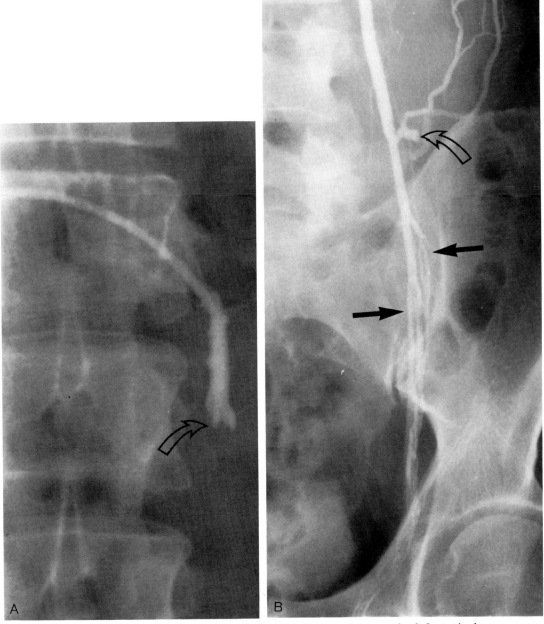

Figure 11–13. Competent testicular vein valve. *A,* Retrograde left testicular venogram. The vein does not opacify beyond the valve *(arrow).* *B,* Contrast injection after selective catheterization using an open ended wire; multiple channels *(solid arrows)* are seen. In addition, there are several collaterals communicating with the retroperitoneal veins. Open arrow points to another valve in the vein communicating with the colic veins.

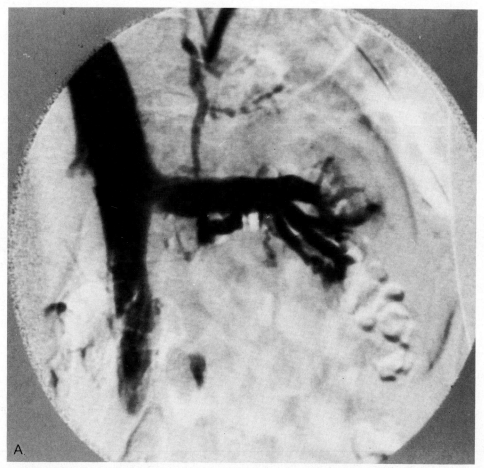

Figure 11–14. Nonvisualization of gonadal vein on retrograde renal venogram. A frequent pitfall of retrograde renal venography for demonstration of gonadal veins. *A,* There is good opacification of the renal vein but no gonadal vein is opacified. *B,* Selective catheterization and contrast injection demonstrate a large vein. There are several fine channels connecting with the renal capsular/pelvic veins *(arrows)*, main renal *(arrowhead)*, and other retroperitoneal veins.

Illustration continued on opposite page.

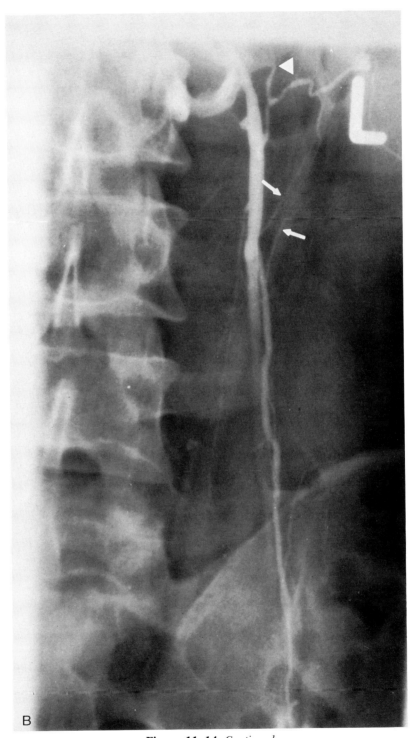

Figure 11–14. *Continued.*

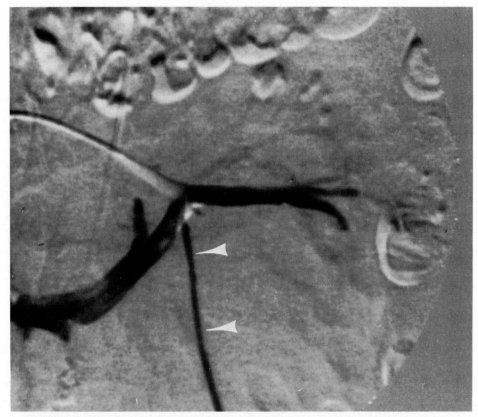

Figure 11–15. Gonadal vein *(arrowheads)* joining lower, posterior limb of a circum-aortic ring.

Chapter Twelve

PENILE AND UTERINE VESSELS

CHRISTIAN DELCOUR, M.D.,
SAADOON KADIR, M.D.

PENILE ARTERIES (Figs. 12–1 to 12–4)

The arterial supply to the penis is via the pudendal arteries. The internal pudendal artery is a branch of the anterior division of the internal iliac artery. In over 50 per cent of individuals, it arises together with the inferior gluteal artery. In another 15 per cent it forms a trunk with the obturator artery, and in the remainder it arises as an independent branch. After giving off the perineal artery to the perineum and scrotum at the urogenital diaphragm, it continues as the penile artery.

In the classic angiographic pattern, the penile artery gives off the following branches:

1. Artery of the bulb (bulbourethral artery): This is a short trunk that supplies the bulb and the corpus spongiosum. In the presence of vasodilatation of the penile arteries, this gives rise to an intense contrast stain in the proximal portion of the corpus spongiosum (Fig. 12–3). The corpus spongiosum is also supplied by a fine branch (spongiosal artery), which is not always opacified on arteriography. The urethral artery is also a fine caliber vessel that runs along the urethra and is frequently not demonstrated on angiography.

2. Cavernosal artery (also called the deep artery): This vessel enters the corpus cavernosum at the base of the penis and provides the helicine arteries that fill the sinusoidal spaces. Its intracavernosal distribution demonstrates significant variability.

3. The dorsal artery lies in the sulcus between the corpora cavernosa,

outside the latter, and continues to the glans. Distally, it anastomoses with the contralateral dorsal artery. It provides three to eight circumflex branches to the corpus spongiosum and anastomotic branches to the deep artery. The course of this vessel is best visualized if arteriography is performed during penile tumescence. In the flaccid state, the course is tortuous (Fig. 12–3). It supplies the glans and skin.

VARIANT ANATOMY (Figs. 12–5 to 12–7)

Numerous variations in the penile arterial supply are common. In addition, anastomoses are present with external pudendal, obturator, and hemorrhoidal arteries. The penile arteries may occasionally originate from the obturator or external pudendal arteries.

An accessory internal pudendal artery occurs in 6 to 10 per cent of individuals. This may arise from the anterior division of the internal iliac artery or from the superior vesical, obturator, or external iliac arteries. When present, this may be the main source of arterial supply to the corpora, providing the deep and dorsal arteries. In the latter case, the internal pudendal artery supplies the scrotum and perineal branches. Large, anastomotic channels exist between both sides in 15 per cent of individuals.

THE PROSTATE

The prostate gland receives its blood supply from branches of the internal pudendal artery, usually the inferior vesical or middle hemorrhoidal arteries. Venous drainage is via the prostaticovesical plexus into the internal iliac veins.

VENOUS ANATOMY (Figs. 12–8 to 12–12)

Venous drainage of the penis is via the superficial and deep dorsal veins, veins of the bulbus urethrae, and deep veins (venae profundae).

1. Superficial dorsal vein lies outside Buck's fascia and drains the skin and superficial structures into the external pudendal veins and then the greater saphenous vein (Fig. 12–11).

2. The deep dorsal vein lies adjacent to the dorsal artery between the corpora cavernosa, beneath Buck's fascia. This is the main drainage channel for the glans and corpus spongiosum and part of the corpora cavernosa. It drains into the prostaticovesical venous plexus and then the internal pudendal vein and internal iliac vein. Both deep and superficial venous systems have multiple anastomoses via the circumflex veins.

3. Veins of the bulbus drain the corpus spongiosum and are situated within it.

4. The deep veins (venae profundae penis) are the main drainage channels for the corpora cavernosa and drain into the prostaticovesical plexus and the internal pudendal veins. These are usually three or four in number.

5. Circumflex veins lie between the tunica albuginea and Buck's fascia and serve as communication between the deep and superficial dorsal veins. These drain the corpus spongiosum into the deep veins. The deep dorsal and circumflex veins have valves.

THE UTERINE ARTERIES AND VEINS (Figs. 12–13 to 12–15) (also see Figs. 4–12 and 4–18)

The uterine artery is a branch of the anterior division of the internal iliac artery. Figure 12–13 shows the anatomy of the uterine arteries. The end arteries in the uterine muscle are extremely tortuous and are also termed "helicine arteries." The branches of the uterine artery include the following:

1. Fundal branch to the fundus of the uterus. Occasionally this is a branch of the ovarian artery.
2. Cervicovaginal branches to the cervix and upper vagina. These anastomose with the vaginal artery and form the "azygos arteries" (two median, anteriorly and posteriorly located, parallel arteries).
3. Ovarian branch
4. Tubal branch
5. Small branch to the distal ureter

Venous drainage is via the uterine veins that drain into the internal iliac veins (see Fig. 11–8*D*).

REFERENCES

1. Bookstein JJ, Lang EV: Penile magnification pharmacoarteriography: Details of intrapenile arterial anatomy. AJR 148:883–888, 1987.
2. Bookstein JJ, Valij K, Parsons LC, et al: Pharmacoarteriography in the evaluation of impotence. J Urol 137:333–337, 1987.
3. Delcour C, Wespes E, Schulman CC, et al: Investigation of the venous system in impotence of vascular origin. Urol Radiol 6:190–193, 1984.
4. Delcour C, Wespes E, Vandenbosch G, et al: Impotence: Evaluation with cavernosography. Radiology 161:803–806, 1986.
5. Delcour C, Wespes E, Vandenbosch G, et al: Opacification of the glans penis during cavernosography. J Urol 139:732–733, 1988.
6. Delcour C, Vandenbosch G, Delatte P, et al: Penile arteriography: Technical advances. AJR 150:803–804, 1988.
7. Fernstrom I: Arteriography of the uterine artery. Acta Radiol, 1955.
8. Fernstrom I, Borell U: The adnexal branches of the uterine artery. Acta Radiol 40:561–582, 1953.
9. Fitzpatrick TJ: Venography of the deep dorsal venous and valvular system. J Urol 111:518–520, 1974.
10. Huguet JF, Clerissi J, Juhan C: Radiologic anatomy of pudendal artery. Eur J Radiol 1:278–284, 1981.
11. Juskiewenski S, Vaysse P, Moscovici J, Hammoudi S, Bouissou E: Study of the arterial blood supply to the penis. Anat Clin 4:101–107, 1982.
12. Michal V, Pospichal J: Phalloarteriography in the diagnosis of erectile impotence. World J Surg 2:233–248, 1977.
13. Reiss H: Role of spongiosography in study of penile veins. Urology 29:146–149, 1987.
14. Struyven J, Gregoir W, Giannakopoulos X, Wauters E: Selective pudendal arteriography. Eur Urol 5:233–242, 1979.
15. Tramier D, Argeme M, Huguet JF, Juhan C: Radiological anatomy of the internal pudendal artery (a. pudenda interna) in the male. Anat Clin 3:195–200, 1981.

Figures 12–1 through 12–15 on following pages.

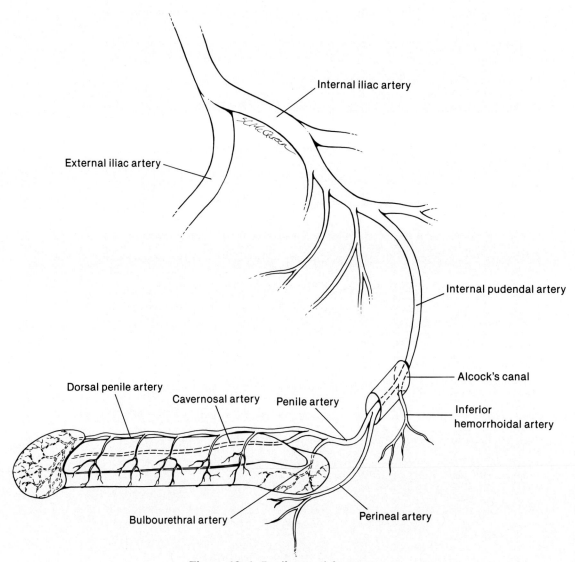

Figure 12–1. Penile arterial anatomy.

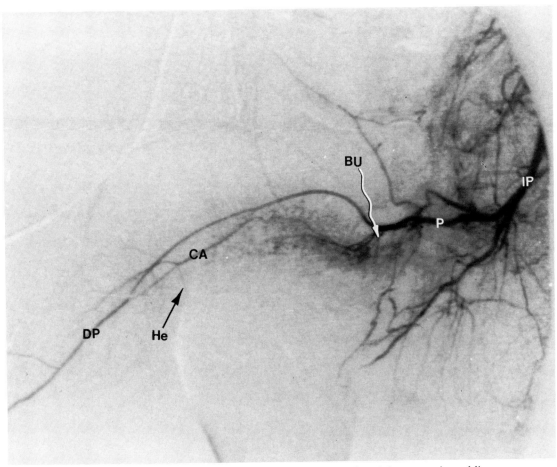

Figure 12–2. Left internal pudendal arteriogram in right posterior oblique projection showing the classic arterial anatomy of the penis.

BU Bulbourethral artery
CA Cavernosal artery
DP Dorsal penile artery
He Helicine arteries arising perpendicularly from the cavernosal artery
IP Internal pudendal artery
P   Penile artery

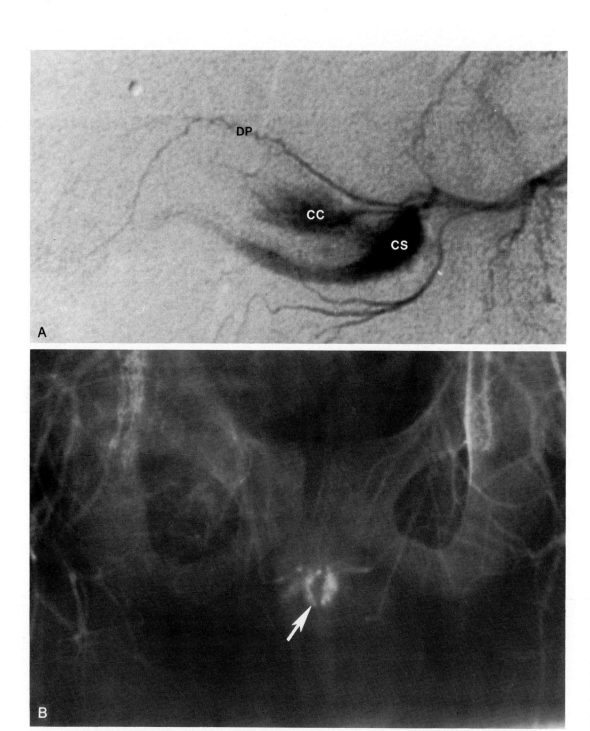

Figure 12–3. *A*, Left internal pudendal arteriogram showing intense blush in the corpus spongiosum (CS) and the proximal corpus cavernosum (CC). The dorsal penile artery (DP) is tortuous because the penis is in the flaccid state. *B*, AP pelvic arteriogram in a 15-year-old performed under general anesthesia shows an intense cavernosal blush *(arrow)*.

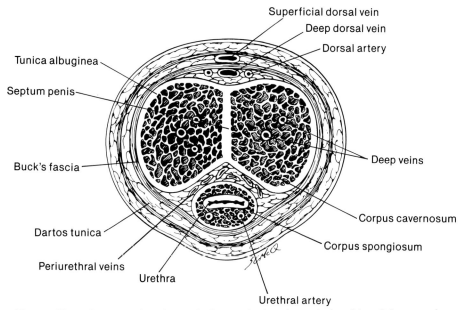

Figure 12–4. Cross-section through the penis showing relationship of the vascular structures.

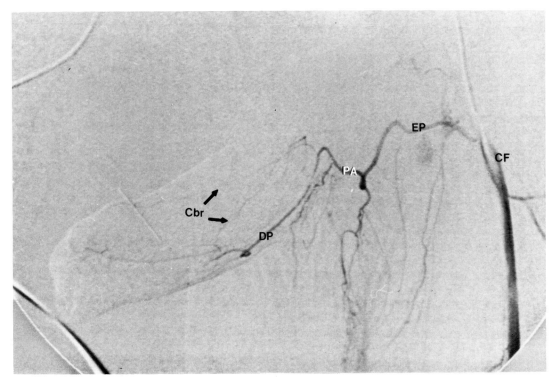

Figure 12–5. Variant arterial anatomy: The left penile artery originates from the external pudendal artery. The left dorsal penile artery and cavernosal branches are opacified.

Cbr	Cavernosal branches
CF	Common femoral artery
DP	Dorsal penile artery (left)
EP	External pudendal artery
PA	Penile artery (left)

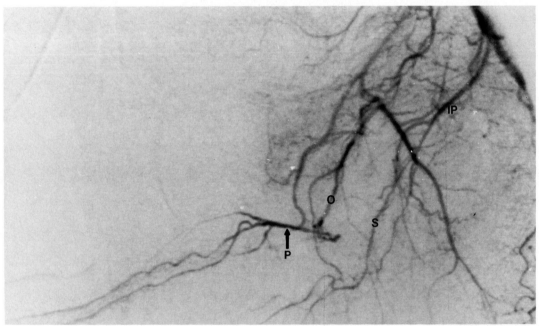

Figure 12–6. Variant arterial anatomy: The internal pudendal artery gives off only the scrotal artery. The penile artery is a continuation of the obturator artery.

IP	Internal pudendal artery
O	Obturator artery
P	Penile artery
S	Scrotal artery

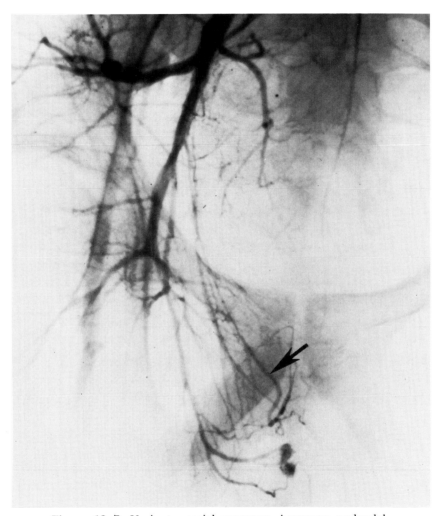

Figure 12–7. Variant arterial anatomy: Accessory pudendal artery *(arrow)*.

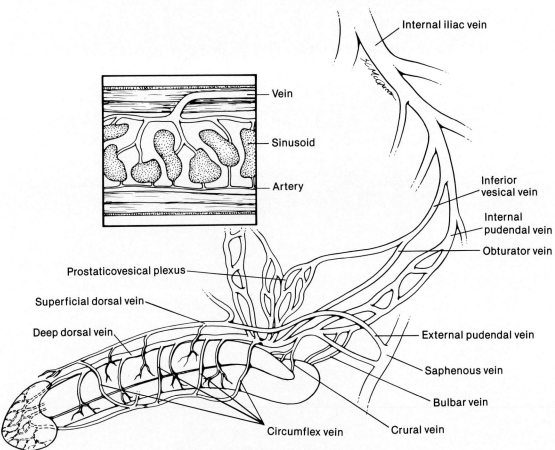

Figure 12–8. Normal venous anatomy.

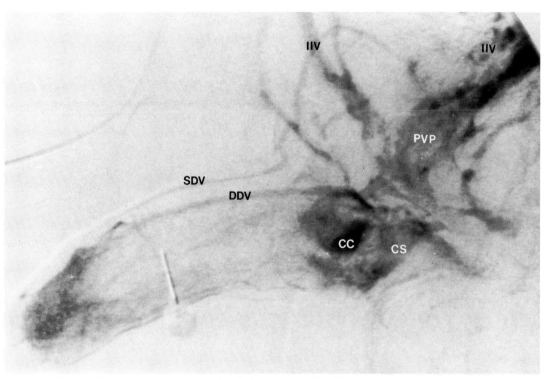

Figure 12–9. Venous phase of left internal pudendal arteriogram (same patient as in Figure 12–2). Drainage is mainly via the prostatic venous plexus.

CC	(Root of) corpus cavernosum
CS	(Root of) corpus spongiosum
DDV	Deep dorsal vein
IIV	Internal iliac veins
PVP	Prostatic venous plexus
SDV	Superficial dorsal vein

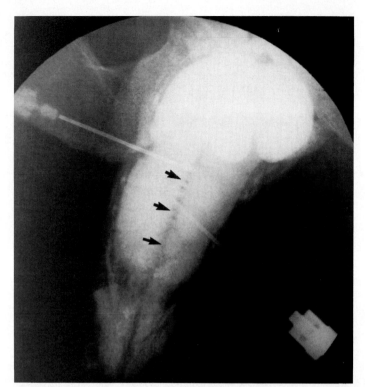

Figure 12–10. Cavernosogram shows a fenestrated septum *(arrows)*.

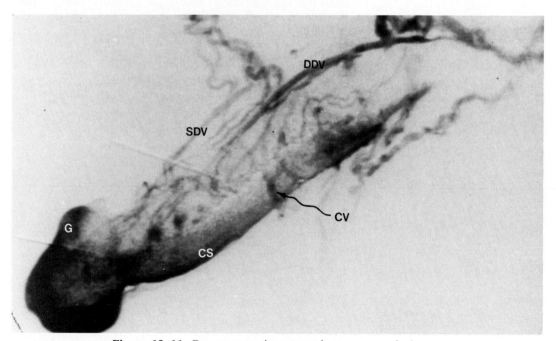

Figure 12–11. Corpus spongiosogram shows venous drainage.

CS   Corpus spongiosum
CV   Circumflex vein
DDV   Deep dorsal vein
G   Glans penis
SDV   Superficial dorsal vein

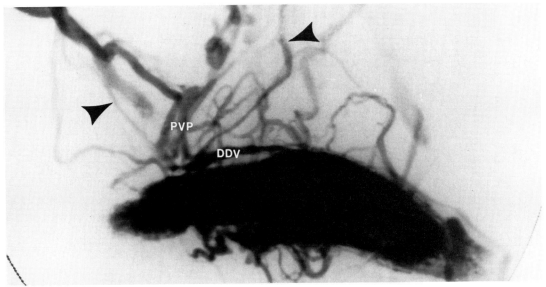

Figure 12–12. Digital cavernosogram without pharmacologic enhancement. Deep dorsal vein (DDV) drains primarily via the prostatic venous plexus (PVP) but also via the internal pudendal veins *(arrowheads)*.

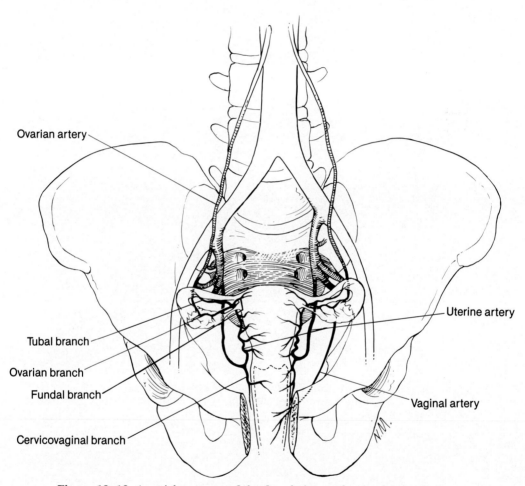

Ovarian artery

Tubal branch

Ovarian branch

Fundal branch

Cervicovaginal branch

Uterine artery

Vaginal artery

Figure 12–13. Arterial anatomy of the female internal reproductive organs.

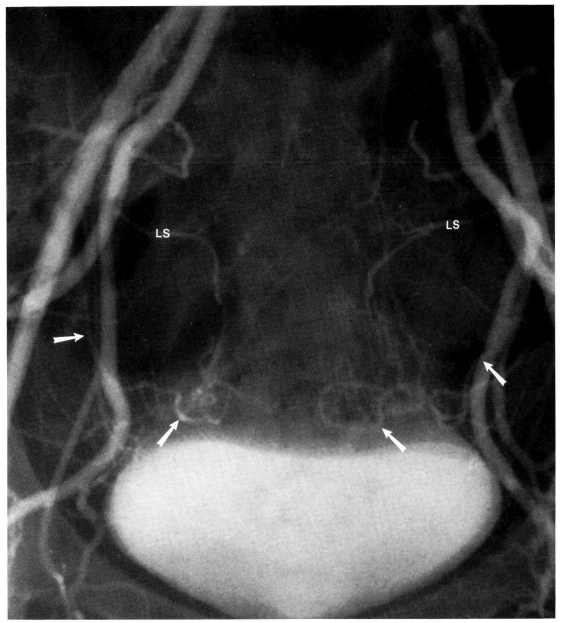

Figure 12–14. Anteroposterior pelvic arteriogram shows the uterine arteries *(arrows)*. LS = Lateral sacral arteries.

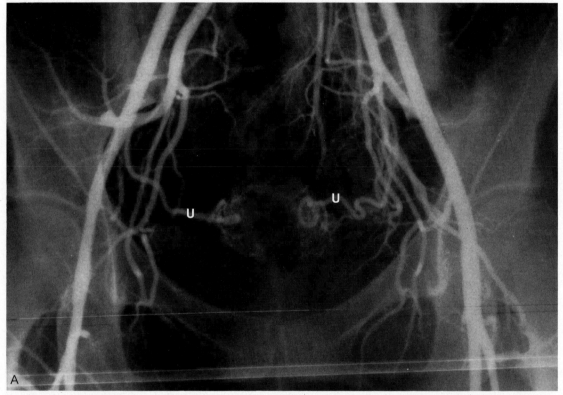

Figure 12–15. *A,* Early *B,* midcapillary, and *C,* late films from a pelvic arteriogram in a young woman, demonstrating the uterine vessels. Note typical, intense uterine parenchymal blush.

cv	Cervicovaginal branch
U	Uterine artery
V	Vaginal artery

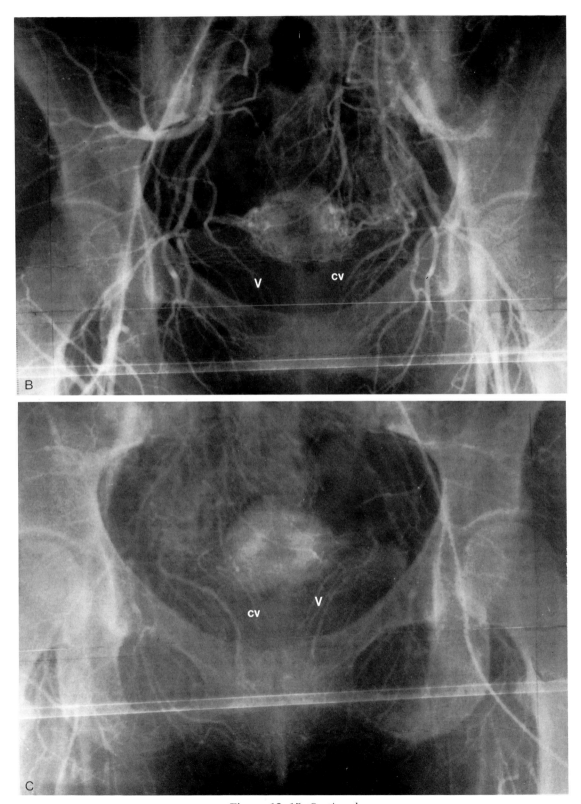

Figure 12–15. *Continued.*

ARTERIAL AND VENOUS SYSTEMS OF THE VISCERA

Chapter Thirteen

CELIAC, SUPERIOR, AND INFERIOR MESENTERIC ARTERIES

SAADOON KADIR, M.D.
CAROLINE LUNDELL, M.D.
MOHSIN SAEED, M.D.

EMBRYOLOGY (Fig. 13–1)

Both dorsal aortae provide ventral segmental (omphalomesenteric) arteries to the viscera. These give rise to the vitelline arteries. About the fourth week, fusion of the ventral roots and reduction in the number of segmental arteries leads to the formation of the three main ventrally oriented vessels: the celiac artery to the infradiaphragmatic portion of the foregut, the superior mesenteric to the midgut, and the inferior mesenteric artery to the hindgut. The celiac artery forms from the tenth cephalic root near the seventh cervical segment, then migrates caudally to the lower thoracic–upper lumbar level by about 7 weeks. The superior mesenteric artery forms from the thirteenth root near the T1–T3 segment and subsequently migrates caudally. The eleventh and twelfth roots regress. The inferior mesenteric artery originates from the twenty-first or twenty-second root.

The ventral segmental roots are connected longitudinally via a ventral anastomosis. Persistence of this ventral anastomosis between the superior mesenteric and celiac arteries and/or partial regression of another segment accounts for complete or partial replacement of the celiac artery branches to the superior mesenteric artery and vice versa. Persistence of the ventral anastomosis between the tenth and thirteenth vitelline arteries also gives rise to

297

TABLE 13–1. Celiac Artery: Normal and Variant Anatomy

Type	Incidence	Illustration
1. Classic anatomy: three branches		
Common hepatic, splenic, left gastric arteries	65–75%	Figs. 13–2 and 13–7
True trifurcation	25%	
2. Four branches: as above plus dorsal pancreatic or middle colic artery	5–10%	
3. Two branches		
Common hepatic and splenic arteries	2%	
Left gastric and splenic arteries	3%	
Left gastric and common hepatic arteries	<1%	
4. All branches arise independently	<1%	
5. Celiacomesenteric trunk	<1%	Fig. 13–6
6. Miscellaneous		
Common hepatic artery off superior mesenteric artery	2.5%	Fig. 13–9
Common hepatic artery off aorta	2%	Fig. 13–10
Splenic artery off superior mesenteric artery	<1%	

the persistent embryonic connection between the proximal celiac and superior mesenteric arteries, known as the arc of Bühler.

CELIAC ARTERY (Figs. 13–2 to 13–6 and 13–14; Table 13–1)

The celiac artery arises anteriorly from the abdominal aorta at the T12–L1 level. Its course is usually inferiorly directed but can be horizontal or craniad. Its length averages 1 to 2 cm prior to branching. The "classic" branching pattern is seen in 65 to 75 per cent of individuals in which it divides into the left gastric, common hepatic, and splenic arteries. In the remainder, one or more branches have a variant origin. The left gastric artery is usually the first branch. In 25 per cent there is a true trifurcation of all three branches. In less than 1 per cent, the celiac and superior mesenteric arteries form a common trunk.

HEPATIC ARTERIES (Figs. 13–7 to 13–15; Tables 13–1 to 13–3)

The common hepatic artery lies in the hepatoduodenal ligament to the left of the common bile duct and anterior to the portal vein. After the first major branch, the gastroduodenal artery, it continues as the proper hepatic artery. The intrahepatic distribution is segmental. Branches of the hepatic arteries maintain an anterior (to the portal vein) relationship. Anastomoses between the intrahepatic branches may occur to provide collateral flow.

In about 55 per cent, the "classic" hepatic arterial branching pattern is seen with the entire right, left, and middle hepatic arteries originating from the common hepatic artery off the celiac artery. Tables 13–1 to 13–3 list the variant anatomy.

The right hepatic artery crosses the hepatic duct posteriorly. In the liver substance, it divides into anterior and posterior segmental branches to the right lobe. The anterior segment frequently shows the typical caterpillar loop configuration and lies inferior to the posterior branch. The latter accompanies the posterior segmental bile duct and divides into superior and inferior branches.

TABLE 13–2. Hepatic Arteries: Normal and Variant Anatomy. Variations from the Classic Celiac Origin

Type	Incidence	Illustration
All hepatic branches off celiac artery	Approx. 75%	
Replaced or aberrant hepatic arteries	41%	
One vessel	31%	
Two or more vessels	10%	
Common hepatic artery		
Classic pattern: all hepatic branches off common hepatic	55%	Fig. 13–7
Common hepatic off superior mesenteric artery	2.5%	Fig. 13–9
Early division of common hepatic artery	Approx. 2%	Fig. 13–11
Common hepatic artery off aorta	2%	Fig. 13–10
Entire common hepatic off left gastric artery	<1%	
Aberrant right hepatic artery	24–26%	
Replaced: 17–18%		
Accessory: 7–8%		
Accessory right hepatic artery from gastroduodenal artery	2%	Fig. 13–12
Accessory right hepatic artery from superior mesenteric artery	4–6%	Fig. 13–13
Replaced right hepatic artery from superior mesenteric artery	10–12%	Fig. 13–9
Replaced right hepatic artery off aorta	<2%	Fig. 13–10
Aberrant left hepatic artery	23–25%	
Replaced: 15–18%		
Accessory: 7–8%		
Replaced left hepatic (off left gastric artery)	11–12%	Fig. 13–14
Replaced left hepatic off superior mesenteric artery (common hepatic off superior mesenteric artery)	2.5%	Fig. 13–9
Accessory left gastric off left hepatic artery	7%	
Accessory left hepatic off left gastric artery	11–12%	Fig. 13–14
Left gastric/left hepatic trunk from aorta	1–2%	Fig. 13–21
Middle hepatic artery		
From left hepatic artery	45%	Fig. 13–14
From right hepatic artery	45%	Fig. 13–10
From proper hepatic, gastroduodenal, right gastric or celiac artery	Approx. 10%	Fig. 13–14

It frequently provides a branch to the caudate lobe and the cystic and right gastric arteries. The left hepatic artery follows the left hepatic duct and divides into medial and lateral segmental branches (approximately 40 per cent). In approximately 25 per cent of cases, both branches have an independent origin from the common hepatic artery (Fig. 13–7D). In the remainder it divides into superior and inferior segmental branches (for the lateral segment), and one of these vessels gives off the medial segmental artery (middle hepatic artery) (35 per cent) (Fig. 13–9). In about 75 per cent, the left hepatic artery arises from the proper hepatic artery. In up to 12 per cent there is an accessory left hepatic artery off the left gastric artery (Fig. 13–14).

The middle hepatic artery supplies the medial segment of the left hepatic lobe and the quadrate lobe. It may also supply the caudate lobe and gallbladder.

TABLE 13–3. Hepatic Arteries: Variant Anatomy. Origin from Superior Mesenteric Artery

Type	Incidence
1. Overall incidence of hepatic branches from superior mesenteric artery	18–20%
2. Right hepatic artery from superior mesenteric artery	14–18%
Replaced right hepatic	10–12%
Accessory right hepatic	4–6%
3. Common hepatic artery from superior mesenteric artery	2.5%

The caudate lobe receives blood supply entirely from the right hepatic artery in approximately one third of individuals and in approximately 12 per cent entirely from the left hepatic artery. In 25 per cent of individuals there is a single caudate lobe branch. In the remainder there are two or three vessels supplying this portion of the liver.

CYSTIC AND BILIARY ARTERIES (Figs. 13–13 and 13–16; Table 13–4)

The cystic artery(ies) to the gallbladder lies posterior to the common hepatic duct. Table 13–4 lists the anatomic variations. At the gallbladder neck, it divides into superficial (to the anterior peritoneal) and deep (to the posterior nonperitoneal surface and gallbladder bed) branches. The deep cystic branch may arise separately from the right hepatic or less frequently from other vessels.

The arteries supplying the bile ducts are very small and frequently not demonstrated on angiography. The extrahepatic portion of the common duct is usually supplied by branches of the retroduodenal artery from the gastroduodenal artery. The intrahepatic biliary ducts are supplied from adjacent hepatic arterial branches.

RIGHT GASTRIC ARTERY (Figs. 13–9, 13–14, 13–17 and 13–18; Table 13–5)

The right gastric artery courses along the lesser curvature of the stomach and joins the posterior branches of the left gastric artery. It is 1 to 2 mm in diameter and supplies the pylorus and distal posterior aspect of the stomach. It is usually small and often not seen on nonselective angiography.

GASTRODUODENAL ARTERY (Figs. 13–3, 13–9, 13–18 and 13–19; Tables 13–5 and 13–7)

The gastroduodenal artery originates from the common hepatic artery in about 75 per cent of cases and arises almost always prior to the division of the hepatic artery into right and left branches. The variant anatomy is listed in Table 13–5.

TABLE 13–4. Cystic Arteries: Normal and Variant Anatomy

Type	Incidence	Illustration
1. Single artery	80%	Fig. 13–16
From right hepatic artery	Approx. 45%	
From accessory right hepatic off superior mesenteric artery	12%	
From distal common hepatic artery (bifurcation)	10%	
From left hepatic artery	Approx. 5%	
From proximal common hepatic artery	Approx. 2%	
From proper hepatic artery	2%	
From gastroduodenal artery	2%	
From celiac or superior mesenteric artery	<1%	
2. Two cystic arteries (separate origins)	19%	
Both from same branch or each from different branch		
Most commonly from right hepatic artery		
3. Three cystic arteries	<1%	

TABLE 13–5. Gastric Arteries: Normal and Variant Anatomy

Type	Incidence	Illustrations
Left gastric artery		
From celiac artery	90%	
Lienogastric trunk	Approx. 4%	
Directly off aorta	Approx. 3%	Fig. 13–21
Hepatogastric trunk	Approx. 2%	
Accessory branches from or to left hepatic artery distribution	23%	Figs. 13–14, 13–21
Gives off inferior phrenic artery	3–4%	Fig. 13–21
Right gastric artery		
From proper hepatic artery or proximally from a branch	40%	Fig. 13–9
From left or middle hepatic artery	40%	Fig. 13–7
From right hepatic artery	10%	
From gastroduodenal artery	8%	Fig. 13–17
From common hepatic artery	Approx. 2%	Fig. 13–7
Accessory left gastric branches		
From celiac artery	2%	
From splenic artery	6%	
Gastroepiploic arteries		
Complete gastroepiploic arcade	65%	
Incomplete or weak gastroepiploic arcade	35%	
Posterior gastric artery (ascending esophagogastric branch or accessory left gastric artery)	60%	Fig. 13–22
Gastroduodenal artery		
From a celiac artery branch	89%	
From common hepatic artery	75%	Fig. 13–7
From left hepatic artery	4%	
From right hepatic artery	6%	
From celiac artery directly	Rare	
From replaced or accessory hepatic arteries off superior mesenteric artery or aorta	11%	Fig. 13–9
From superior mesenteric artery	Approx. 4%	

The proximal gastroduodenal artery lies behind the first portion of the duodenum, anterior to the pancreas, and to the left of the common bile duct. Its major branches are the anterior and posterior superior pancreaticoduodenal arteries and the right gastroepiploic artery. Occasionally the right gastric and/or supraduodenal arteries originate from the gastroduodenal artery. Rarely, the jejunal branch may originate from the gastroduodenal artery (Fig. 13–7E).

The posterior superior pancreaticoduodenal artery arises 1 to 2 cm from the gastroduodenal artery origin and proximal to the anterior superior pancreaticoduodenal artery in 90 per cent of cases. It may also originate from the common, right hepatic, or superior mesenteric artery or may be absent. It supplies the posterior aspects of the pancreatic head and duodenum and the common bile duct. It is also called the retroduodenal artery.

The anterior superior pancreaticoduodenal artery arises from the distal gastroduodenal artery, behind the first part of the duodenum. It provides pyloric branches proximally and then courses to the anterior aspect of the pancreatic head. Both anterior and posterior superior pancreatioduodenal arteries anastomose with the corresponding inferior pancreaticoduodenal arteries to form the pancreaticoduodenal arcades, providing a major connection between the celiac and superior mesenteric arteries. Both arcades have numerous branches anastomosing with those of the dorsal and transverse pancreatic arteries.

The supraduodenal artery (1 to 2 mm in diameter) provides blood supply to the upper portion of the duodenum (anterior and posterior surfaces) and the pylorus. Its origin is variable. It may arise from the posterior superior pancreaticoduodenal, gastroduodenal, hepatic (right, middle, or proper), right gastric, or cystic arteries (Figs. 13–3*A*, 13–7, 13–14, 13–17, and 13–19). It communicates with the pancreaticoduodenal and right gastric branches. Occasionally, it is absent.

The right gastroepiploic artery is the terminal branch of the gastroduodenal artery. It courses along the greater curvature of the stomach and joins the left gastroepiploic artery from the splenic artery in around 90 per cent of cases, although this anastomosis is weak in 20 to 25 per cent of cases. The right gastroepiploic artery provides one or more branches to the pylorus and first portion of the duodenum and several branches to the greater curvature of the stomach. The proximal portion of the right gastroepiploic artery lies at some distance from the stomach wall.

The epiploic (omental) branches arise from the gastroepiploic arteries and descend in the greater omentum (Figs. 13–3, 13–7*B,* 13–9*B,* and 13–19). They are usually small branches and may join to form large epiploic arcades inferiorly. Branches from the epiploic arcade may join the middle and left colic, inferior pancreaticoduodenal, and transverse pancreatic arteries. The largest arcade, which parallels the gastroepiploic arteries, is called the arc of Barkow.

LEFT GASTRIC ARTERY (Figs. 13–15, 13–20, and 13–21; Tables 13–2 and 13–5)

The left gastric artery is usually the first and the smallest (4 to 5 mm in diameter) of the major branches of the celiac artery. It divides into anterior and posterior branches. The former further subdivides into two or three main branches. The posterior branch courses along the lesser curvature of the stomach to anastomose with the right gastric artery in most cases. It provides one to three branches to the distal esophagus and gastric cardia. Peripheral branches of the left gastric artery anastomose with short gastric arteries from the splenic artery, cardioesophageal branches of the left inferior phrenic artery, and esophageal artery branches. Accessory left gastric branches occur frequently, usually when the left gastric artery originates from the left hepatic artery. The variant anatomy is listed in Tables 13–2 and 13–5.

SPLENIC ARTERY (Figs. 13–2, 13–3, 13–7 to 13–9, 13–11, 13–16, 13–22 to 13–25; Table 13–6)

The splenic artery is usually the largest (6 to 10 mm in diameter) and most tortuous branch of the celiac artery, with an average length of 13 cm (8- to 32-

TABLE 13–6. Splenic Artery: Normal and Variant Anatomy

Type	Incidence	Illustrations
1. Early division	70%	
Division at splenic hilus	30%	Figs. 13–7, 13–11
2. Aberrant origin		
From superior mesenteric artery	<1%	Fig. 13–25
From right hepatic	<0.1%	Fig. 13–23
From aorta	<0.1%	
3. Location relative to pancreas		
Along upper border of pancreas	90%	
Behind pancreas	8%	
Intrapancreatic or prepancreatic	2%	

cm range). It courses superior and anterior to the splenic vein. Its major branches are pancreatic, posterior gastric, short gastric, and left gastroepiploic arteries.

The splenic artery divides into superior and inferior terminal branches. Each of these further subdivides into four to six segmental intrasplenic branches. The length of the terminal splenic branches varies greatly and is 1 to 12 cm (average 4 cm). The superior terminal branches are often much longer and usually provide the major splenic arterial supply. The inferior terminal branches are more variable and provide the left gastroepiploic artery. Both superior and inferior terminal branches supply polar arteries to the spleen.

A superior polar artery is seen in 65 per cent of cases and usually originates from the distal splenic artery near the hilum or less frequently from the superior terminal artery. The inferior polar artery is seen in 82 per cent of cases and usually arises from the left gastroepiploic artery or less often from the distal splenic or inferior terminal artery. Both polar arteries may give off small branches to supply adjacent viscera.

Between 4 and 10 short gastric arteries arise as small branches superiorly from the terminal splenic artery or its branches or from the left gastroepiploic artery to supply the gastric cardia and fundus. In addition, a large gastric branch (posterior gastric artery) is present in 60 per cent of individuals (Fig. 13–22).

The left gastroepiploic artery is usually the largest branch originating from the distal splenic artery. In 72 per cent, it originates just proximal to the superior and inferior terminal divisions, and less frequently it arises from the inferior terminal branch. It descends along the greater curvature of the stomach in the anterior portion of the greater omentum to join the right gastroepiploic artery (arcus arteriosus ventriculi inferiori of Hyrtl) in the majority of individuals.

PANCREATIC ARTERIES (Figs. 13–9, 13–16, 13–22, and 13–24 to 13–26; Table 13–7)

The main pancreatic vessels are the dorsal pancreatic artery, arteria pancreatic magna, caudal pancreatic artery, and short pancreatic branches off the splenic artery. These form a diffusely anastomosing network, especially in

TABLE 13–7. Pancreatic Arteries: Normal and Variant Anatomy

Type	Incidence	Illustration
Pancreaticoduodenal arcade		
Two arcades	80%	
Three arcades	15%	
Four arcades	5%	
Dorsal pancreatic artery		
From splenic artery	40%	Fig. 13–24
From celiac artery	22%	Fig. 13–25
From common hepatic artery	20%	
From superior mesenteric artery or from aorta	14%	Fig. 13–26
Gives off middle colic, accessory middle colic, or jejunal branches	4%	Fig. 13–26
Transverse pancreatic artery		
From dorsal pancreatic artery	75%	Fig. 13–24
From anterior pancreaticoduodenal arcade	10%	
From superior mesenteric artery	10%	

the head of the pancreas, and communicate with branches of the pancreatico-duodenal arcades.

The dorsal pancreatic is the largest pancreatic artery. Its origin is quite variable (Table 13–7). It courses along the dorsal aspect of the pancreas and gives off the transverse pancreatic artery, which courses along the inferior aspect of the pancreas through the length of the gland to the tail, where it is joined by the arteria pancreatica magna and caudal pancreatic arteries. It provides several fine, long posterior epiploic (omental) branches. To the right, the transverse pancreatic artery branches anastomose with those of the pancreaticoduodenal arcades. A relatively constant vessel is the uncinate branch (Figs. 13–7*A* and 13–24*B*).

The dorsal pancreatic artery may also give off the middle colic or accessory middle colic artery or anastomose with these branches (proximally) from the superior mesenteric artery and function as an important collateral between the celiac and superior mesenteric arteries (Fig. 13–26). Rarely, proximal jejunal branches may originate from the dorsal pancreatic artery.

The pancreatica magna is the largest pancreatic branch to the body and usually originates from the mid to distal one third of the splenic artery and supplies the distal body and tail. Typically, it courses to the left and then divides into several right and left branches. The former anastomose with the transverse pancreatic artery, and the latter branches anastomose with the caudal pancreatic artery.

The caudal pancreatic artery is a small, short vessel and often comprises not a single vessel but multiple short vessels. It usually arises from the distal splenic artery and sometimes from the left gastroepiploic artery and supplies the tail of the pancreas. In addition, the splenic artery provides numerous small pancreatic arteries to the body and tail along its course.

SUPERIOR MESENTERIC ARTERY (SMA) (Figs. 13–27 to 13–31)

The SMA provides blood supply to the distal duodenum, small intestine, and large intestine to the splenic flexure. In addition, it provides branches to the head and body of the pancreas. In its proximal course it lies behind the pancreas (giving off its first branch, the inferior pancreaticoduodenal artery) and then passes anterior to the fourth portion of the duodenum. In this region, the left renal vein also lies behind the duodenum, between the SMA and aorta. The SMA origin is located around L_1, slightly below (range: 2 mm to 2 cm) the celiac artery.

INFERIOR PANCREATICODUODENAL ARTERY(IES) (IPDA) (Fig. 13–28; Table 13–7)

This is a single vessel in 60 per cent of individuals. It divides into anterior and posterior branches, which join the corresponding superior pancreaticoduodenal arteries to complete the pancreaticoduodenal arcades. In about 40 per cent of individuals both branches have separate origins. Occasionally, they may originate together with (or from) a jejunal branch (usually first or second), a dorsal pancreatic or hepatic artery originating from the SMA. The pancreaticoduodenal arcades show many variations. There are usually two arcades, but there may be a single, three, or four arcades in each location (anterior or posterior).

JEJUNAL AND ILEAL ARTERIES (Figs. 13–26, 13–27, 13–29, and 13–30)

Their numbers vary, but most commonly 10 to 15 vessels are present. They usually arise from the left side of the SMA as it gently curves toward the right lower quadrant. Each vessel divides into two branches coming off almost at right angles, each one communicating with similar branches from other adjacent vessels. This gives rise to a series of arcades that parallel the intestine. Further branching from each one of these arcades gives rise to successive arcades (up to three to six). The arcades closest to the intestine give off relatively straight vessels (vasa recta). These divide to supply the anterior and posterior surfaces of the intestine and do not anastomose and are oriented perpendicular to the long axis of the intestine (Fig. 13–30). Occasionally, a jejunal branch may originate from the dorsal pancreatic and rarely from the gastroduodenal artery (Figs. 13–7 and 13–26).

MIDDLE COLIC ARTERY (Figs. 13–26, 13–27, 13–30, and 13–31)

This is usually the second branch of the SMA and arises from the anterior aspect. It turns to the right and after a variable distance divides into right and left branches. The former anastomoses with the ascending branch of the right colic and the latter with the ascending branch of the left colic artery to form the marginal artery.

The middle colic or an accessory middle colic artery may originate from the dorsal pancreatic artery. In addition, the middle colic may be duplicated with both vessels arising in close proximity. Rarely it may originate from the celiac artery or replaced right hepatic (off SMA).

RIGHT COLIC ARTERY (Figs. 13–27, 13–29, and 13–31)

This vessel takes off from the mid-portion of the SMA and at the ascending colon it bifurcates into an ascending branch (anastomoses with the middle colic) and descending branch (joins the ileocolic artery). Similar to the jejunal and ileal arteries, these also form several arcades to the ascending and a portion of the transverse colon. The arcade closest to the colon provides the vasa recta.

The right colic artery may be absent or may arise together with (or from) the ileocolic artery.

ILEOCOLIC ARTERY (Figs. 13–27 and 13–29)

This vessel normally arises distal to the right colic artery. It also bifurcates into ascending and descending branches and also contributes to a series of arcades. The ascending branch joins the descending branch of the right colic. The descending branch anastomoses with the ileal arteries. Branches of the ileocolic arteries include cecal (anterior and posterior) and appendicular arteries.

VARIANT ANATOMY OF THE SMA

Aberrant hepatic and pancreatic branches may arise from the SMA and have been discussed earlier in this chapter (also see Tables 13–1 to 13–6).

ACCESSORY MIDDLE COLIC ARTERY (Fig. 13–32)

This vessel occurs in about 10 per cent of individuals and originates from the SMA above the origin of the middle colic artery. It has also been observed to originate from the celiac, splenic, or hepatic arteries. In this setting it frequently arises from the dorsal pancreatic artery. Typically it courses to the left. Its branches anastomose with the middle colic artery.

MIDDLE MESENTERIC ARTERY (Fig. 13–33)

This is an extremely rare congenital variant. It represents the persistence of an additional ventral root between the thirteenth and twenty-first segments. The middle mesenteric artery appears to be distinct from the accessory middle colic artery but may represent a variant thereof. It arises from the infrarenal aorta, above the inferior mesenteric artery. It supplies a portion of the transverse and descending colon and may anastomose with the left colic and middle colic arteries.

INFERIOR MESENTERIC ARTERY (IMA) (Figs. 13–34 to 13–37)

The IMA arises from the anterior lateral aspect of the aorta at L_3. It has a sharply inferior course paralleling the aorta. It provides blood supply to the very distal transverse colon, descending colon, sigmoid, and upper rectum. Its major branches are the left colic, sigmoid, and superior hemorrhoidal arteries.

LEFT COLIC ARTERY (Figs. 13–30 and 13–34 to 13–37)

The left colic artery is the first branch, which shortly divides into ascending and descending branches. The former joins the left branch of the middle colic, whereas the latter anastomoses with the upper sigmoid artery.

SIGMOID ARTERIES (Figs. 13–34 to 13–37)

These are two or three in number. They communicate with the left colic superiorly and with the superior hemorrhoidal artery below.

SUPERIOR HEMORRHOIDAL ARTERY (Figs. 13–35 to 13–37)

This is the end branch of the IMA which supplies the proximal rectum. It divides into two branches (to the left and right side) that are widely intercommunicating and also anastomoses with branches of the middle hemorrhoidal artery from the internal iliac artery (see Chapter 4).

ARC OF BÜHLER (Fig. 13–38)

Ventrally located communication between the celiac and superior mesenteric arteries represents the persistence of the embryonal ventral anastomosis.

ARC OF BARKOW (Fig. 13–39)

The epiploic arc lying in the omentum parallels the gastroepiploic vessels. The left epiploic artery arises from the left gastroepiploic artery near the spleen and descends in the posterior greater omentum below the transverse colon and frequently forms the left branch of the arc of Barkow. The right branch of the arc of Barkow arises from the right epiploic artery, which usually originates from the right gastroepiploic or less often the transverse pancreatic artery. The arc of Barkow provides small branches to the transverse colon.

MARGINAL ARTERY OF DRUMMOND (Figs. 13–27, 13–30, and 13–40)

It comprises a series of longitudinally anastomosing vessels lying adjacent and parallel to the colon originating from the arcades of the ileocolic, right, middle, and left colic arteries.

ARC OF RIOLAN (Figs. 13–27, 13–30, and 13–41)

This vessel lies in the mesentery and provides a direct connection between the SMA and IMA via the middle and left colic arteries at the splenic flexure. It may occasionally involve the accessory middle colic artery.

REFERENCES

1. Benton RS, Cotter WB: An unusual variation of the arterial supply of the transverse and descending colon. Anat Rec 142:215, 1962.
2. Cho KJ, Lunderquist A: The peribiliary vascular plexus: The microvascular architecture of the bile duct in the rabbit and in clinical cases. Radiology 147:357–364, 1983.
3. Diemel H, Schmitz-Draeger HG: Intraabdominelle Kollateralbahnen bei Verschlusskrankheiten der Eingeweidearterien. Zugleich ein Beitrag zur Auswertungsmethodik der Abdominellen Aortographie. Fortschr Roentgenstr 103:652–664, 1965.
4. Didio LJA, Christoforidis AJ, Chandnani PC: Posterior gastric artery and its significance as seen in angiograms. Am J Surg 139:333–337, 1980.
5. Didio LJA, Diaz-Franco C, Schemainda R, et al: Morphology of the middle rectal arteries. A study of 30 cadaveric dissections. Surg Radiol Anat 8:229–236, 1986.
6. El Eishi HI, Ayoub SF, Abd El, Khalek M: The arterial supply of the human stomach. Acta Anat 86:565–580, 1973.
7. Gmelin E, Weiss HD, Swoboda G: Seltene arterielle Variationen bei der Oberbauch und Pancreasangiographie. Fortsch Rontgenstr 129:77–82, 1978.
8. Hannoun L, LeBreton C, Bors V, et al: Radiological anatomy of the right gastroepiploic artery. Anat Clin 5:265–271, 1984.
9. Inoue K, Yamaai T, Odajima G: A rare case of anastomosis between the dorsal pancreatic and inferior mesenteric arteries. Okajimas Folia Anat Jpn 63:45–46, 1986.

10. Lawdahl RB, Keller FS: The middle mesenteric artery. Radiology 165:371–372, 1987.
11. Lippert H, Pabst R: Arterial variations in man. Classification and frequency. Munchen, JF Bergmann Verlag, 1985.
12. Michels NA: Blood supply and anatomy of the upper abdominal organs with a descriptive atlas. Philadelphia, JB Lippincott, 1955.
13. Northover JMA, Terblanche J: A new look at the arterial supply of the bile duct in man and its surgical implications. Br J Surg 66:379–384, 1979.
14. Patricio J, Bernades A, Nuno D, et al: Surgical anatomy of the arterial blood supply of the human rectum. Surg Radiol Anat 10:71–75, 1988.
15. Pierson JM: The arterial blood supply of the pancreas. Surg Gynecol Obstet 77:426–432, 1943.
16. Suzuki K, Prates JC, Didio LJA: Incidence and surgical importance of the posterior gastric artery. Ann Surg 187:134–136, 1978.
17. Suzuki T, Nakayasu A, Kawabe K, et al: Surgical significance of anatomic variations of the hepatic artery. Am J Surg 122:505–512, 1971.

Figures 13–1 through 13–41 on following pages.

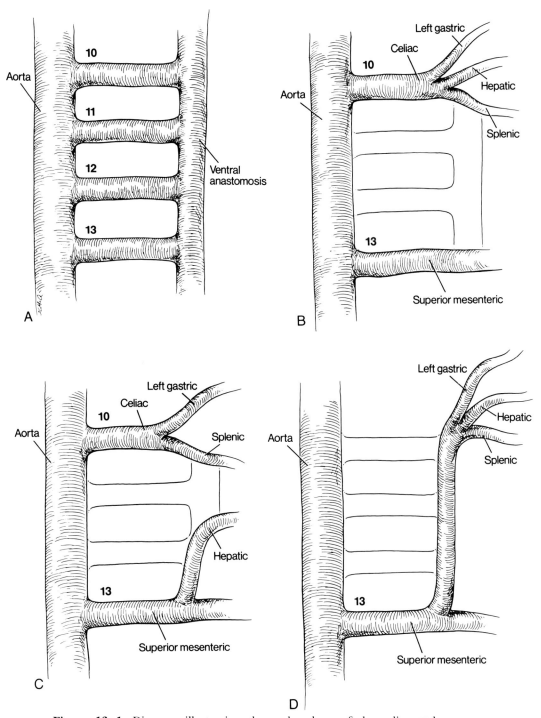

Figure 13–1. Diagram illustrating the embryology of the celiac and superior mesenteric arteries. *A*, All segmental arteries and a ventral anastomosis are present. *B*, The eleventh and twelfth segmental arteries regress, leaving the tenth to form the celiac and the thirteenth to form the superior mesenteric artery. *C*, Formation of a replaced right hepatic. *D*, Obliteration of the tenth segmental artery and persistence of the ventral anastomosis give rise to a celiacomesenteric trunk.

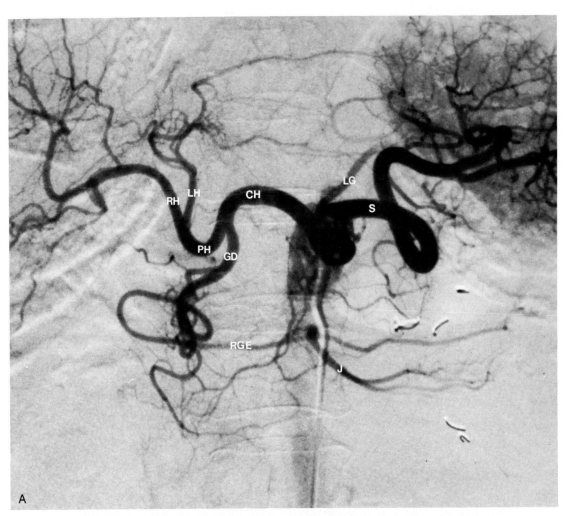

Figure 13–2. Celiac arteriogram. *A,* Subtraction film shows the classic celiac artery anatomy. Jejunal branches opacify via the pancreaticoduodenal arcades. *B,* Arteriogram from another individual shows a sharp upward course of the celiac branches. The right gastroepiploic artery has a high course, corresponding to the location of the stomach.

CH	Common hepatic
GD	Gastroduodenal
J	Jejunal
LG	Left gastric
LH	Left hepatic
PH	Proper hepatic
RGE	Right gastroepiploic
RH	Right hepatic
S	Splenic

Illustration continued on opposite page.

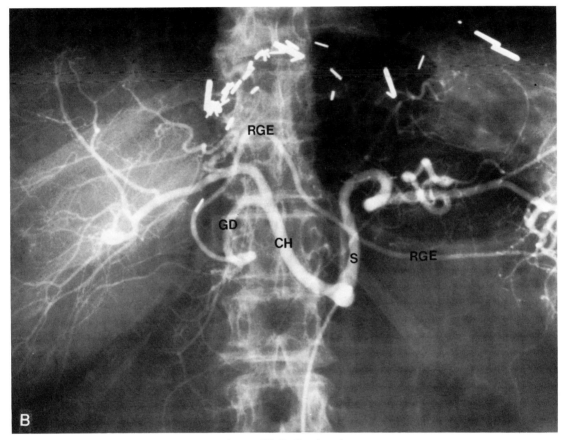

Figure 13–2. *Continued.*

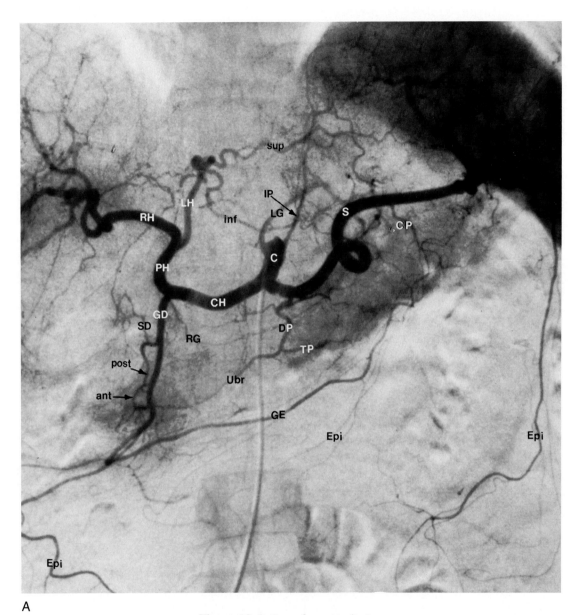

A

Figure 13–2. *Legend on opposite page.*

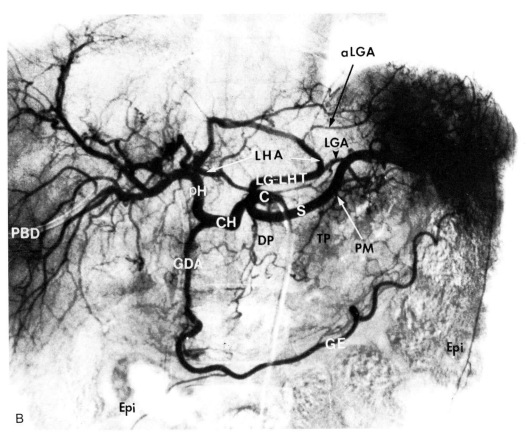

Figure 13–3. *A* and *B*, Celiac arteriograms from different persons. Subtraction film in *B* shows a common trunk of the left gastric and left hepatic arteries. (From Kadir S: Diagnostic Angiography. Philadelphia, WB Saunders Company, 1986.)

aLGA	Accessory left gastric (from left hepatic) artery
ant	Anterior superior pancreaticoduodenal
C	Celiac
CH	Common hepatic
CP	Caudal pancreatic artery
DP	Dorsal pancreatic
Epi	Epiploic
GD/GDA	Gastroduodenal
GE	Right gastroepiploic
inf	Inferior branch of left hepatic
ip	Inferior phrenic
LG/LGA	Left gastric
LG-LHT	Left gastric–left hepatic trunk
LHA	Left hepatic
PBD	Percutaneous biliary drainage catheter
pH	Proper hepatic
PM	Pancreatica magna
post	Posterior superior pancreaticoduodenal
RG	Right gastric
RH	Right hepatic
S	Splenic
SD	Supraduodenal
sup	Superior branch of left hepatic
TP	Transverse pancreatic
Ubr	Uncinate branch

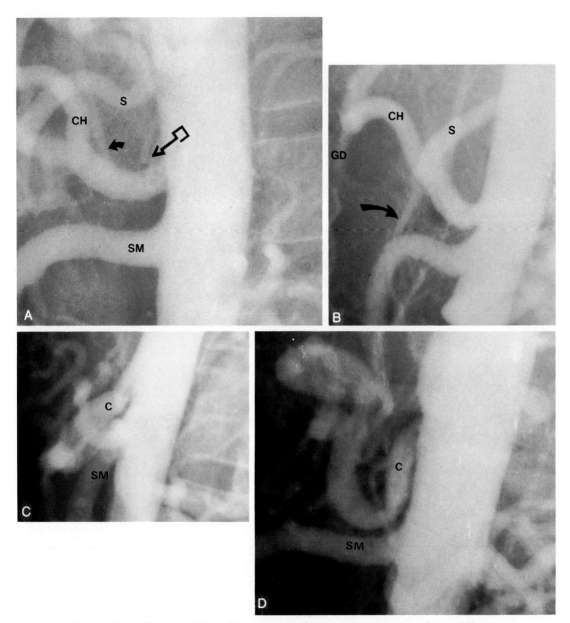

Figure 13–4. Course of the celiac artery. *A–D,* Lateral aortograms from different individuals show a horizontal, upward, and downward course. In *A,* open arrow points to inferior phrenic artery. Closed arrow points to left gastric artery. In *B,* arrow points to the accessory right hepatic artery.

C   Celiac
CH   Common hepatic
GD   Gastroduodenal
S   Splenic
SM   Superior mesenteric

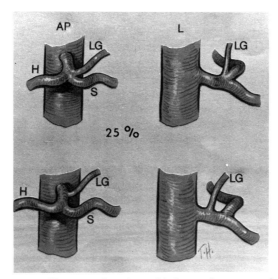

Figure 13–5. Diagram illustrates location of left gastric artery origin on the celiac artery. (From Kadir S: Diagnostic Angiography and Interventional Therapy: Abdominal-Visceral Biliary. RSP—103, RSNA, 1983. Reproduced with permission.)

AP   Anteroposterior view
H   Hepatic
L   Lateral view
LG   Left gastric
S   Splenic

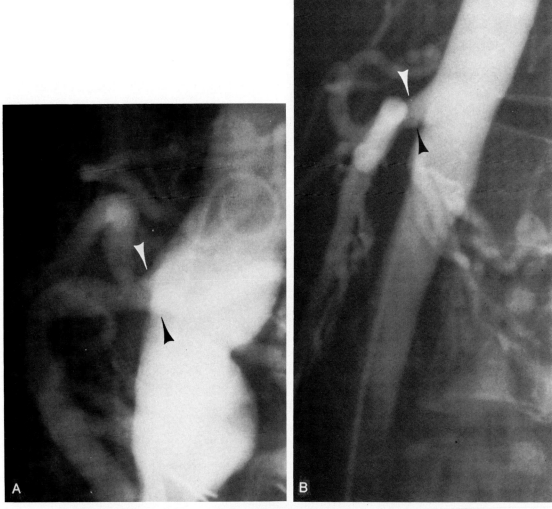

Figure 13–6. Celiacomesenteric trunk. *A* and *B*, Lateral aortograms from different individuals show a common origin of the celiac and superior mesenteric arteries (*arrowheads*). *C*, Anteroposterior aortogram from another individual shows a celiacomesenteric trunk (*arrowheads*). Right hepatic artery arises from the superior mesenteric artery. *D*, Anteroposterior arteriogram of the common trunk (*arrowheads*).

c	Celiac
CH	Common hepatic
GD	Gastroduodenal
LH	Left hepatic
R	Renal
RGE	Right gastroepiploic
RH	Right hepatic
S	Splenic
SM	Superior mesenteric

Illustration continued on opposite page.

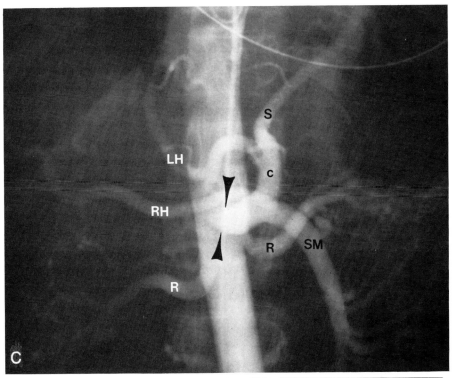

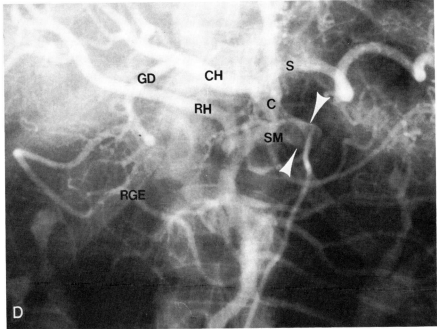

Figure 13–6. *Continued.*

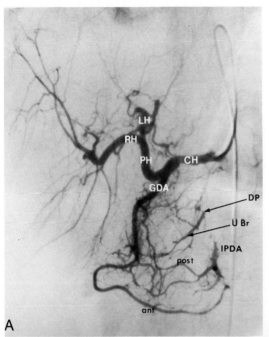

Figure 13–7. Common hepatic artery. *A*, Subtraction film from a common hepatic arteriogram. (From Kadir S: Diagnostic Angiography. Philadelphia, WB Saunders Company, 1986.) *B*, Arteriogram from another person. There is flash opacification of the splenic artery. The common hepatic artery ends in a trifurcation. The right gastric artery also arises from this trifurcation. Arrow points to cystic artery that arises from a right hepatic branch. *C*, Celiac arteriogram from another person. The right gastric is a branch of the left hepatic artery. The middle hepatic arises from the left hepatic artery. Arrow points to the cystic artery. *D*, Celiac arteriogram from another person shows independent origins of the middle (*black arrow*) and left hepatic (*white arrowhead*) from the proper hepatic artery. *E*, Celiac arteriogram showing the anterior and posterior right hepatic branches. Jejunal branch is seen arising from the gastroduodenal artery.

Illustration continued on opposite page.

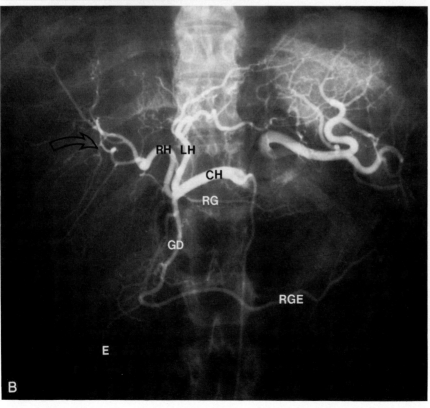

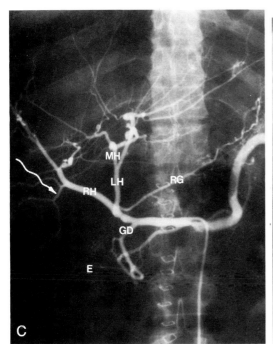

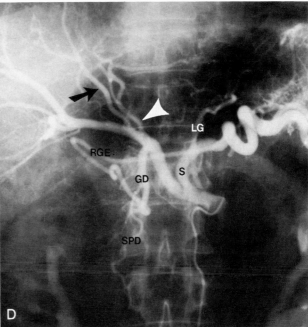

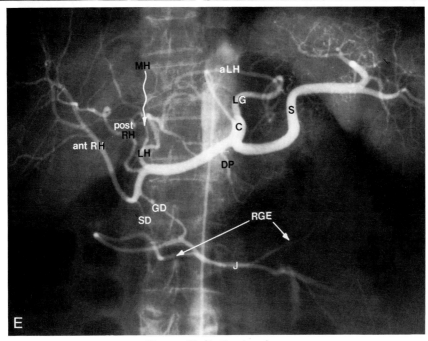

Figure 13–7. *Continued.*

aLH	Accessory left hepatic		MH	Middle hepatic
ant	Anterior pancreaticoduodenal arcade		PH	Proper hepatic
ant RH	Anterior branch of right hepatic		post	Posterior pancreaticoduodenal arcade
C	Celiac		post RH	Posterior branch of right hepatic
CH	Common hepatic		RG	Right gastric
DP	Dorsal pancreatic		RGE	Right gastroepiploic
E	Epiploic		RH	Right hepatic
GD/GDA	Gastroduodenal		S	Splenic
IPDA	Inferior pancreaticoduodenal		SD	Supraduodenal
J	Jejunal		SPD	Superior pancreaticoduodenal
LG	Left gastric		U Br	Uncinate branch
LH	Left hepatic			

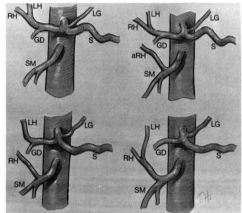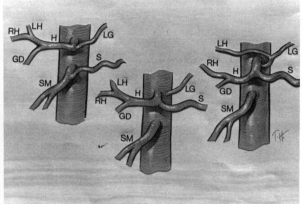

Figure 13–8. Diagram illustrating the variation of the hepatic artery origin. (From Kadir S: Diagnostic Angiography and Interventional Therapy: Abdominal-Visceral Biliary. RSP—103, RSNA, 1983. Reproduced with permission.)

aRH	Accessory right hepatic
GD	Gastroduodenal
LG	Left gastric
LH	Left hepatic
RH	Right hepatic
S	Splenic
SM	Superior mesenteric

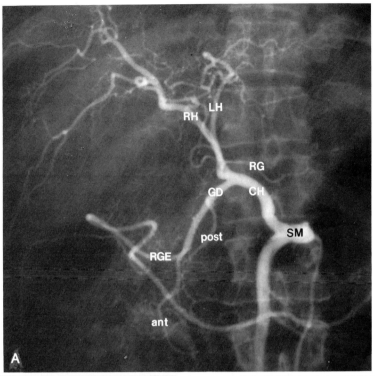

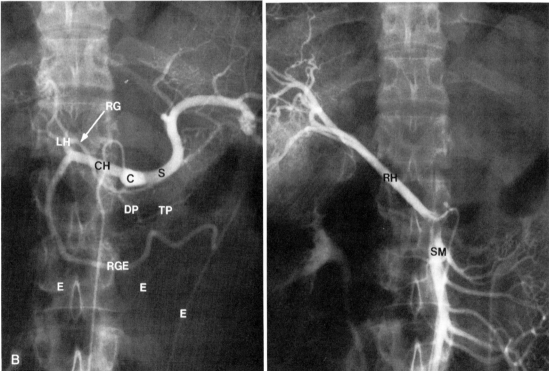

Figure 13–9. Hepatic artery originating from the superior mesenteric artery. *A*, Common hepatic artery arising from the superior mesenteric artery. *B*, Celiac arteriogram (*left*). The common hepatic artery terminates in the left hepatic and gastroduodenal arteries. Superior mesenteric arteriogram (*right*). The right hepatic artery arises close to the origin of the superior mesenteric. The right gastric artery arises from the left hepatic artery.

Illustration continued on following page.

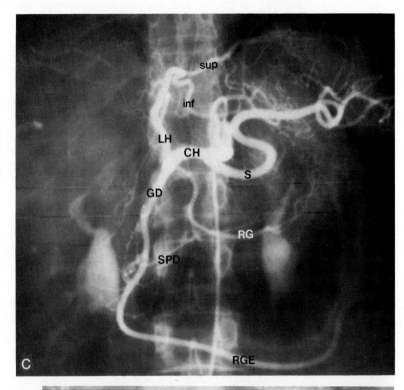

Figure 13–9. *Continued. C,* Celiac and superior mesenteric arteriograms. The right hepatic arises at a distance from the superior mesenteric orifice. The right gastric artery arises from the common hepatic artery.

ant	Anterior superior pancreatico-duodenal
C	Celiac
CH	Common hepatic
DP	Dorsal pancreatic
E	Epiploic
GD	Gastroduodenal
inf	Inferior segmental branch of left hepatic
LH	Left hepatic
post	Posterior superior pancreatico-duodenal
RG	Right gastric
RGE	Right gastroepiploic
RH	Right hepatic
S	Splenic
SM	Superior mesenteric
SPD	Superior pancreatico-duodenal
sup	Superior segmental branch of left hepatic
TP	Transverse pancreatic

Illustration continued on opposite page.

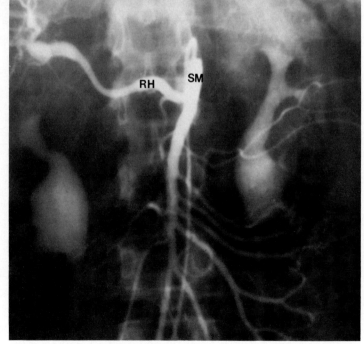

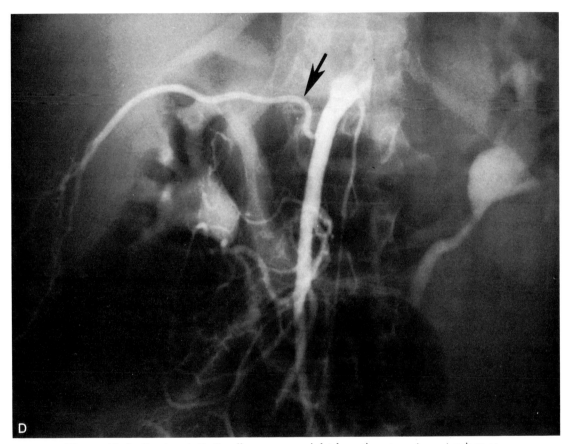

Figure 13–9. *Continued. D,* Small, accessory right hepatic artery *(arrow)* arises at some distance from the superior mesenteric artery origin.

GD	Gastroduodenal
IPDA	Inferior pancreaticoduodenal
RGE	Right gastroepiploic
SM	Superior mesenteric
S	Splenic

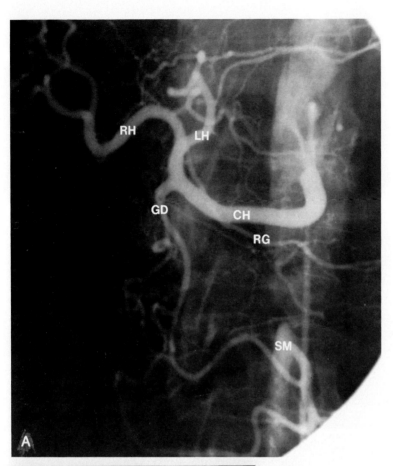

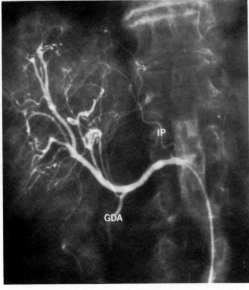

Figure 13–10. Common hepatic artery arising from the aorta. *A,* There is reflux of contrast into the aorta. The superior mesenteric artery is opacified via the pancreaticoduodenal arcades. *B,* Hepatic arteriogram from another patient. The inferior phrenic artery arises from this vessel. (*B* reproduced from Kadir S: Diagnostic Angiography. Philadelphia, WB Saunders Company, 1986.)

CH	Common hepatic
GD/GDA	Gastroduodenal
IP	Inferior phrenic
LH	Left hepatic
RG	Right gastric
RH	Right hepatic
SM	Superior mesenteric

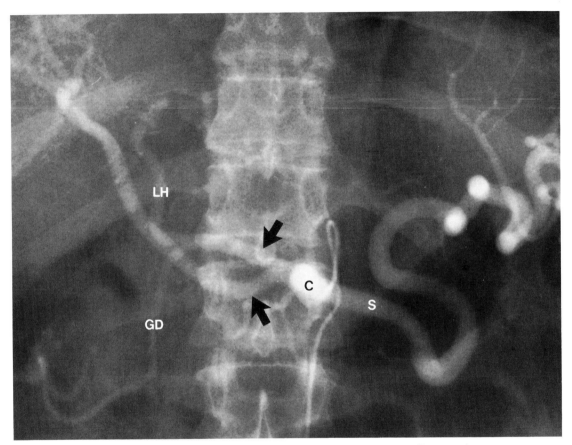

Figure 13–11. Early division of the common hepatic artery. Celiac arteriogram. The common hepatic artery divides into a right and left hepatic artery (*arrows*) shortly after its origin from the celiac artery.

C	Celiac
GD	Gastroduodenal
LH	Left hepatic
S	Splenic

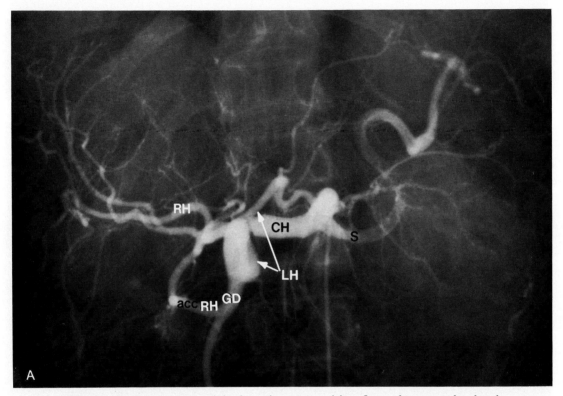

Figure 13–12. Accessory right hepatic artery arising from the gastroduodenal artery. *A*, Anteroposterior and *B*, right anterior oblique common hepatic arteriograms.

accRH	Accessory right hepatic
C	Celiac
CH	Common hepatic
GD	Gastroduodenal
LH	Left hepatic
RH	Right hepatic
S	Splenic

Illustration continued on opposite page.

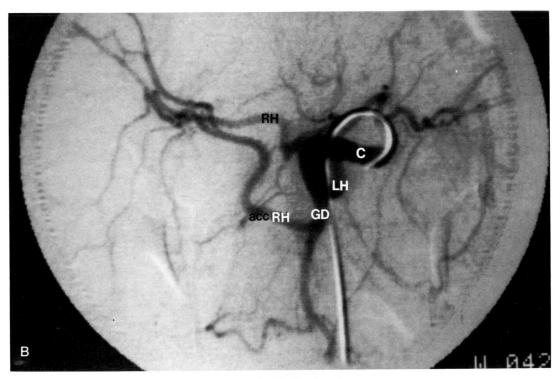

Figure 13–12. *Continued.*

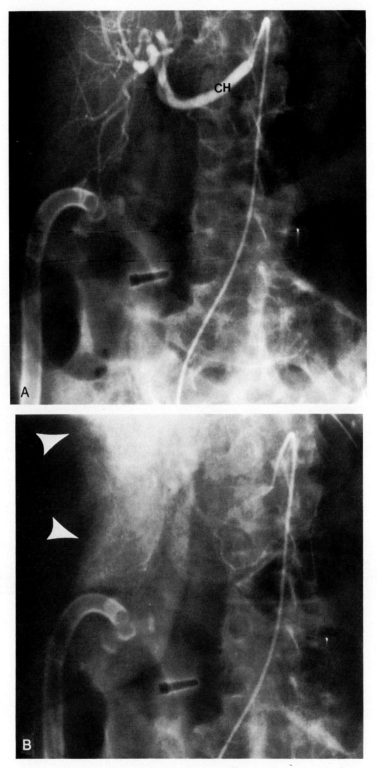

Figure 13–13. Accessory right hepatic artery off superior mesenteric artery. *A*, Arterial phase and *B*, parenchymal phase of a common hepatic arteriogram. The lateral portion of the right lobe of the liver is not opacified. Arrowheads *(B)* point to lateral margin of parenchymal opacification.

Illustration continued on opposite page.

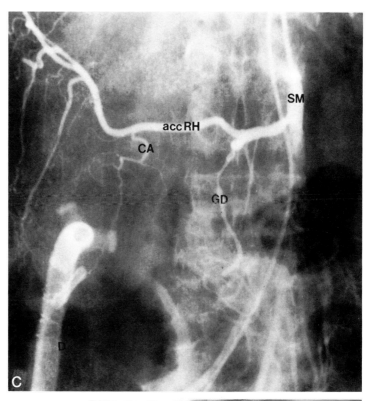

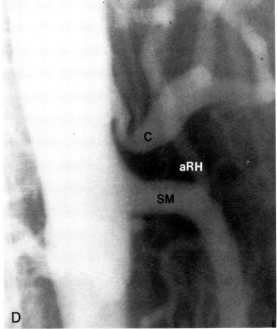

Figure 13–13. *Continued C,* Arteriogram of the accessory right hepatic artery shows branches to the segment unopacified on the arteriogram shown in *B*. The gastroduodenal artery arises from this accessory vessel. *D,* Lateral aortogram from another patient shows the accessory right hepatic artery arising from the superior mesenteric artery.

accRH/aRH	Accessory right hepatic
C	Celiac
CA	Cystic
CH	Common hepatic
GD	Gastroduodenal
SM	Superior mesenteric

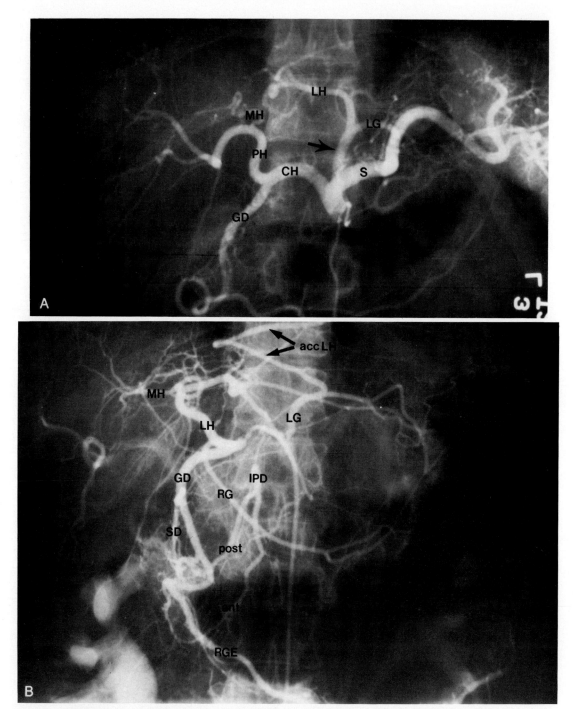

Figure 13–14. Left hepatic–left gastric artery trunk. *A,* Celiac arteriogram shows a common trunk of the left gastric and left hepatic arteries (*arrow*). *B,* Common hepatic arteriogram. There is retrograde opacification of the left gastric artery via the right gastric artery. The left gastric gives off an accessory left hepatic artery.

accLH	Accessory left hepatic	MH	Middle hepatic
ant	Anterior pancreaticoduodenal arcade	PH	Proper hepatic
CH	Common hepatic	post	Posterior pancreaticoduodenal arcade
GD	Gastroduodenal	RG	Right gastric
IPD	Inferior pancreaticoduodenal	RGE	Right gastroepiploic
LG	Left gastric	S	Splenic
LH	Left hepatic	SD	Supraduodenal

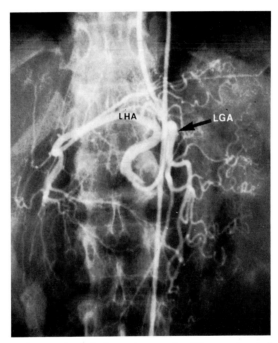

Figure 13–15. Left gastric–left hepatic trunk. The entire left hepatic artery originates from this vessel. (From Kadir S: Diagnostic Angiography. Philadelphia, WB Saunders Company, 1986.)

LGA   Left gastric
LHA   Left hepatic

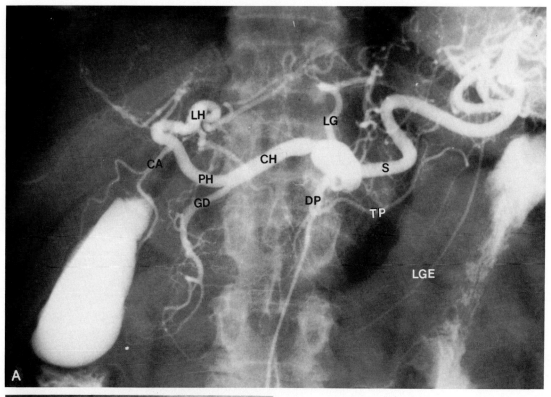

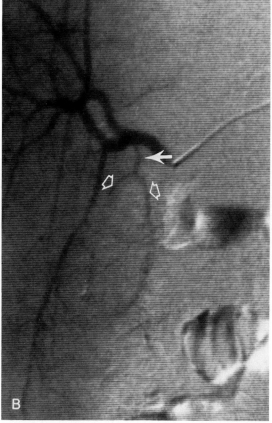

Figure 13–16. Cystic artery. *A*, Gallbladder opacified by intraductal contrast injection. Celiac arteriogram demonstrates a large cystic artery. *B*, Intra-arterial digital subtraction angiogram shows the cystic artery (*solid arrow*), anterior and posterior branches (*open arrows*).

CA	Cystic artery
CH	Common hepatic
DP	Dorsal pancreatic
GD	Gastroduodenal
LG	Left gastric
LGE	Left gastroepiploic
LH	Left hepatic
PH	Proper hepatic
S	Splenic
TP	Transverse pancreatic

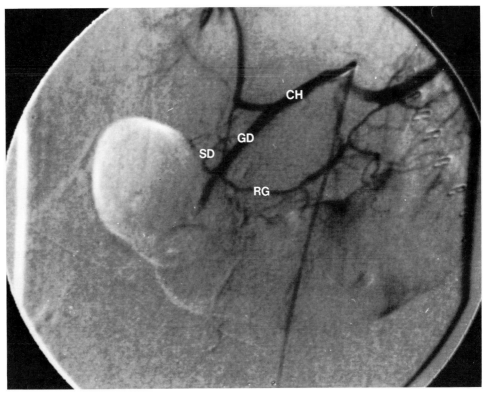

Figure 13–17. Right gastric artery arising from the gastroduodenal artery.

CH   Common hepatic
GD   Gastroduodenal
RG   Right gastric
SD   Supraduodenal

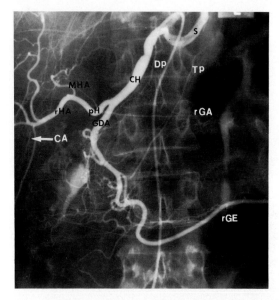

Figure 13–18. Gastroduodenal artery and pancreatic branches. Common hepatic arteriogram shows the gastroduodenal and pancreatic branches. (From Kadir S: Diagnostic Angiography. Philadelphia, WB Saunders Company, 1986.)

CA	Cystic artery
CH	Common hepatic
DP	Dorsal pancreatic
GDA	Gastroduodenal
MIIA	Middle hepatic artery
rGA	Right gastric artery
rGE	Right gastroepiploic
rHA	Right hepatic artery
pH	Proper hepatic
S	Splenic
TP	Transverse pancreatic

Figure 13–19. Gastroduodenal artery and pancreatic branches. Common hepatic arteriogram shows the gastroduodenal and pancreatic branches. (From Kadir S: Diagnostic Angiography. Philadelphia, WB Saunders Company, 1986.)

ant	Anterior pancreaticoduodenal arcade
CH	Common hepatic
Epi	Epiploic
GDA	Gastroduodenal
IPDA	Inferior pancreaticoduodenal
J	Jejunal
LHA	Left hepatic
post	Posterior pancreaticoduodenal arcade
rGA	Right gastric
rGE	Right gastroepiploic
rHA	Right hepatic
SD	Supraduodenal

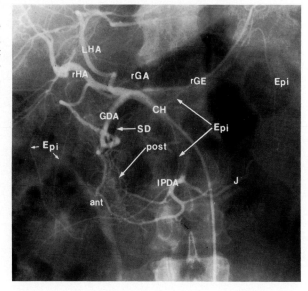

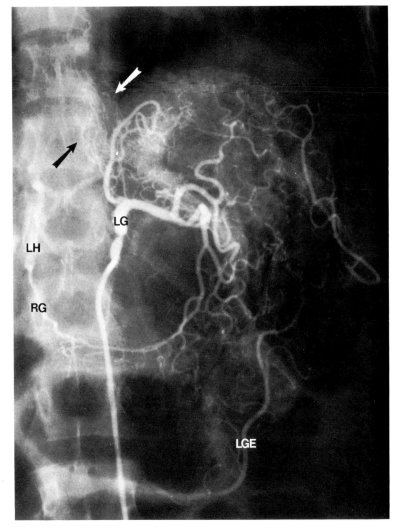

Figure 13–20. Left gastric arteriogram. Arrows point to esophageal branches.

LG   Left gastric
LGE   Left gastroepiploic
LH   Left hepatic
RG   Right gastric

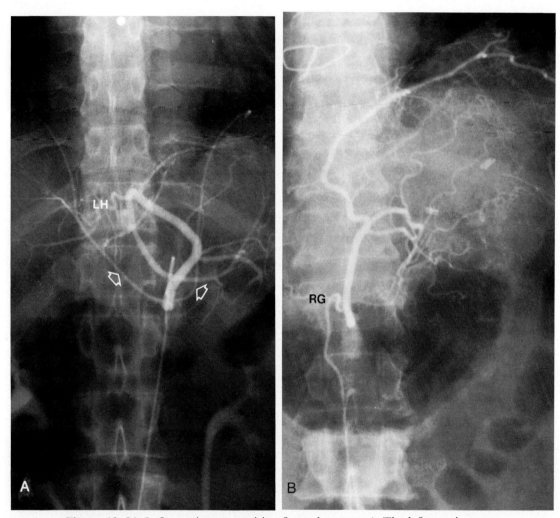

Figure 13–21. Left gastric artery arising from the aorta. *A,* The left gastric artery gives off a left hepatic (LH) branch. Arrows point to inferior phrenic arteries. *B,* There is retrograde opacification of the right gastric artery (RG).

Illustration continued on opposite page.

Figure 13–21. *Continued C,* Lateral aortogram from another individual showing the left gastric artery originating from the aorta *(arrow).*

C   Celiac
S   Superior mesenteric

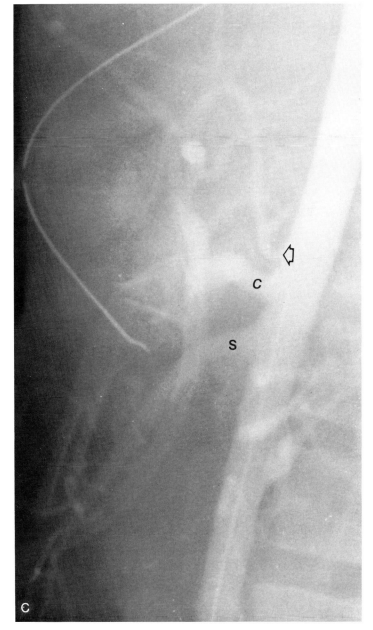

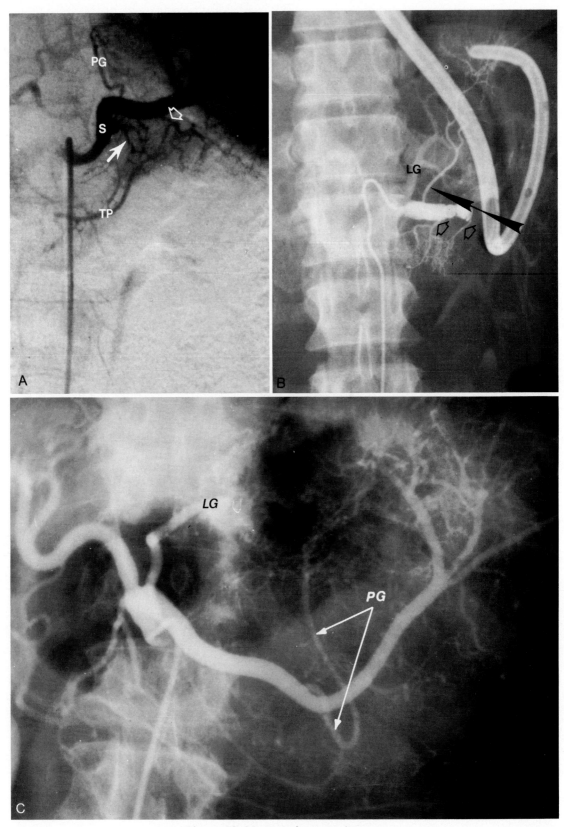

Figure 13–22. *Legend on opposite page.*

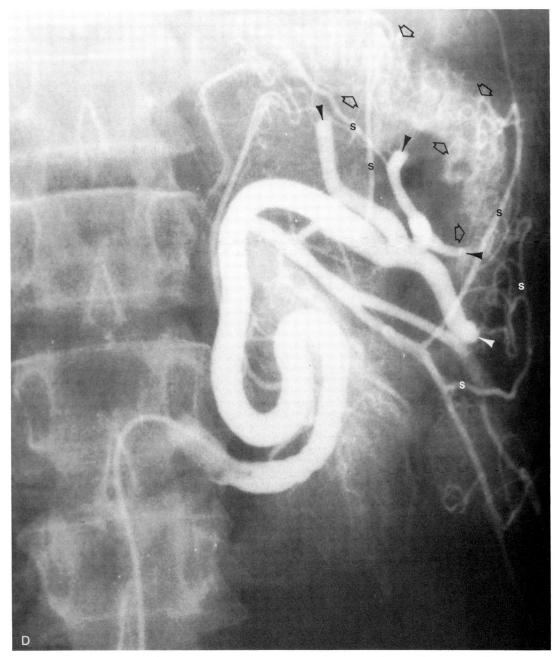

Figure 13–22. Splenic artery branches. *A*, Closed arrow points to the pancreatica magna. Open arrow points to the caudal pancreatic artery. *B*, Splenic arteriogram after embolization in another individual demonstrates the posterior gastric artery *(arrow)*. Open arrows point to pancreatic arteries. *C*, Celiac arteriogram in an individual with a gastric leiomyosarcoma shows a large posterior gastric artery. *D*, Splenic arteriogram after splenic artery embolization *(arrowheads)* in another individual shows the short gastric arteries. Open arrows outline the gastric wall.

LG	Left gastric
PG	Posterior gastric
S	Splenic
TP	Transverse pancreatic

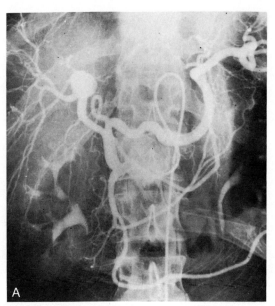

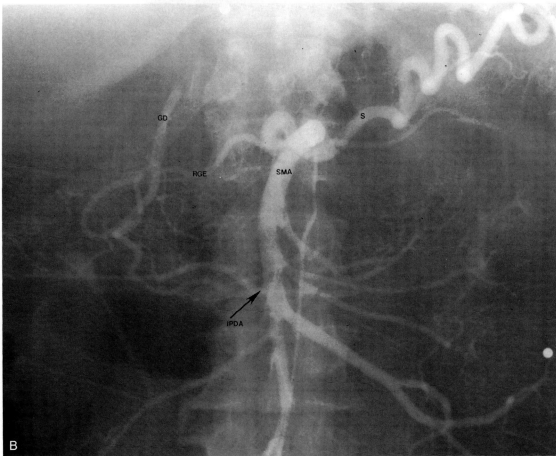

Figure 13–23. Variant origin of the splenic artery. *A,* Splenic artery arising from the proper hepatic artery. There is a mycotic aneurysm of the right hepatic artery. *B,* Splenic artery arising from the superior mesenteric artery. (From Kadir S: Diagnostic Angiography. Philadelphia, WB Saunders Company, 1986.)

S   Splenic artery
SMA Superior mesenteric artery

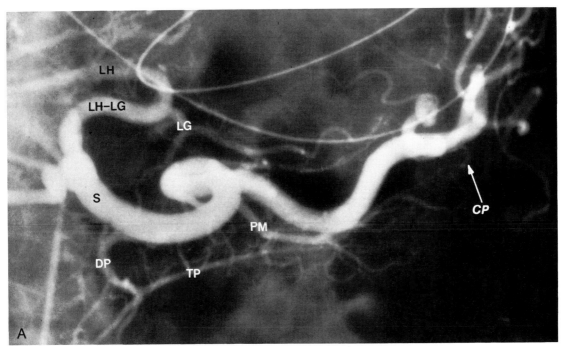

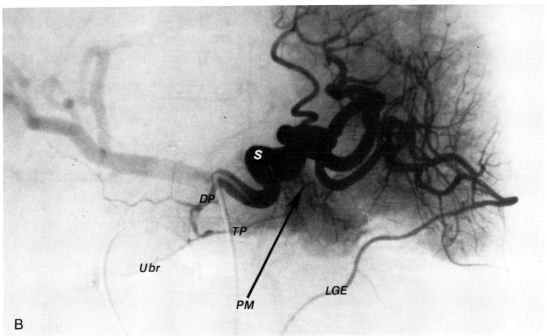

Figure 13–24. Pancreatic arteries. Splenic arteriograms show the pancreatic branches.

CP	Caudal pancreatic	LH-LG	Left hepatic–left gastric trunk
DP	Dorsal pancreatic	PM	Pancreatica magna
LG	Left gastric	S	Splenic
LGE	Left gastroepiploic	TP	Transverse pancreatic
LH	Left hepatic	Ubr	Uncinate branch

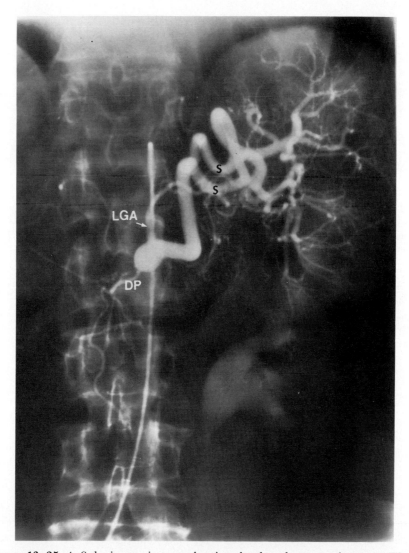

Figure 13–25. *A,* Splenic arteriogram showing the dorsal pancreatic artery. There is an early division of the splenic artery. *B,* Celiac arteriogram showing the splenic artery branches. *Arrow* points to the pancreatica magna artery.

CH	Common hepatic
CP	Caudal pancreatic
DP	Dorsal pancreatic
LGA	Left gastric
LH	Left hepatic
S	Splenic

Illustration continued on opposite page.

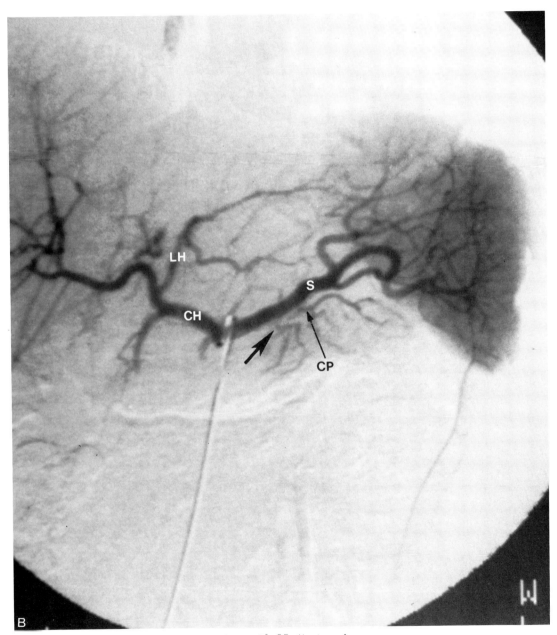

Figure 13–25. *Continued.*

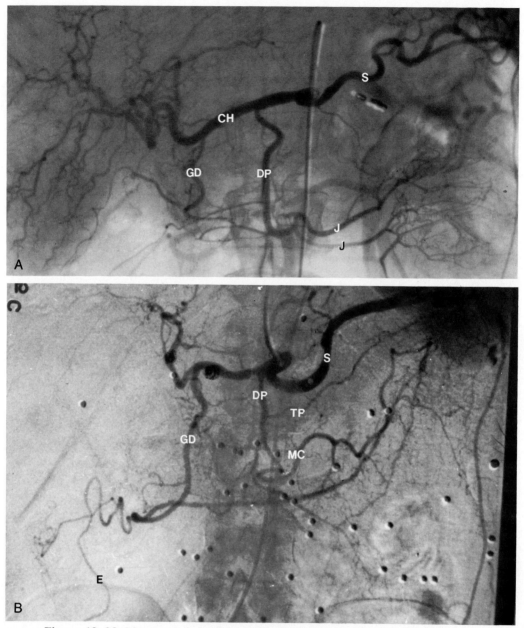

Figure 13–26. Mesenteric branches arising from the dorsal pancreatic artery. *A,* Celiac arteriogram shows a large dorsal pancreatic artery giving off jejunal branches. *B,* Celiac arteriogram shows the dorsal pancreatic artery giving off the middle colic artery (MC).

CH	Common hepatic
DP	Dorsal pancreatic
E	Epiploic
GD	Gastroduodenal
J	Jejunal branches
MC	Middle colic
S	Splenic
TP	Transverse pancreatic

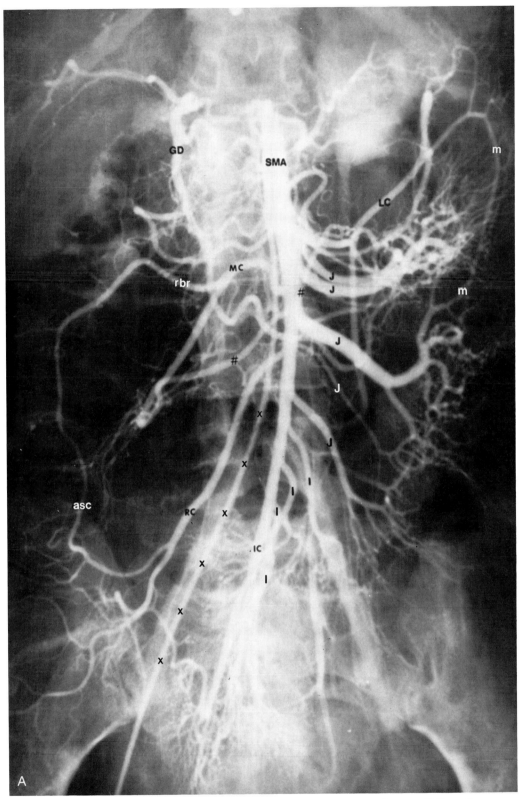

Figure 13–27. *A–C*, Superior mesenteric artery. In *B*, there is a large middle colic artery opacifying the inferior mesenteric artery via an arc of Riolan (*arrowheads*). In addition, the marginal artery is demonstrated.

Illustration continued on following page.

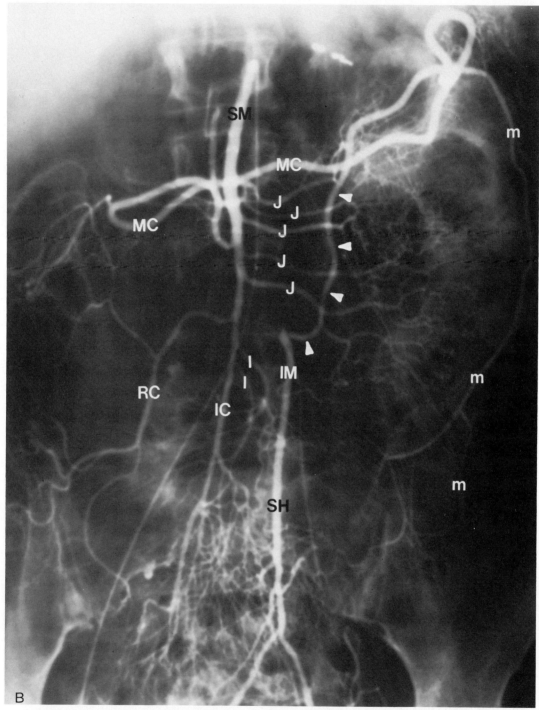

Figure 13–27. *Continued.*

asc	Ascending branch	MC	Middle colic
GD	Gastroduodenal	rbr	Right branch
I	Ileal	RC	Right colic
IC	Ileocolic	SH	Superior hemorrhoidal
IM	Inferior mesenteric	SM/SMA	Superior mesenteric
J	Jejunal	XXX	Catheter
LC	Left colic	##	Left branch of middle colic
m	Marginal		

Illustration continued on opposite page.

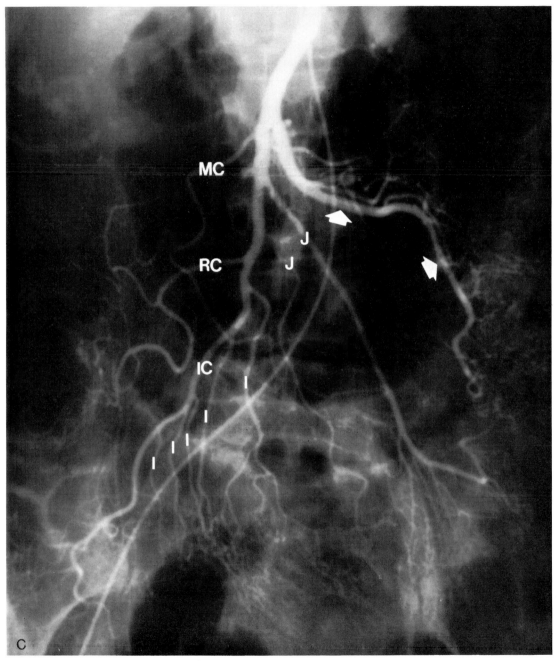

Figure 13–27. *Continued. C,* The proximal jejunal arteries arise from a separate trunk off the superior mesenteric artery (*arrows*).

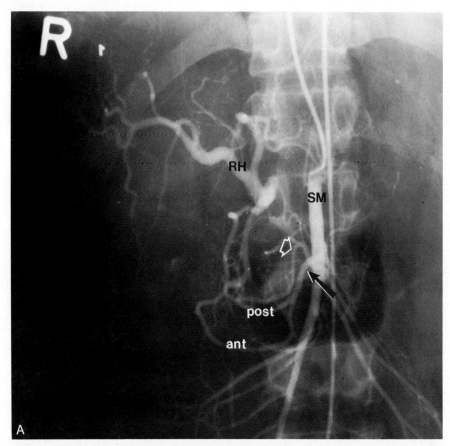

Figure 13–28. *A* and *B*, Inferior pancreaticoduodenal artery. Superior mesenteric arteriogram demonstrates the inferior pancreaticoduodenal artery (*arrow*) and the anterior and posterior pancreaticoduodenal arcades. In *A*, open arrow points to middle colic artery. In *B* there are multiple anterior and posterior pancreaticoduodenal arcades.

ant	Anterior pancreaticoduodenal arcade
GD	Gastroduodenal artery
IPD	Inferior pancreaticoduodenal artery
RGE	Right gastroepiploic artery
post	Posterior pancreaticoduodenal arcade
RH	Right hepatic artery
SM	Superior mesenteric

Illustration continued on opposite page.

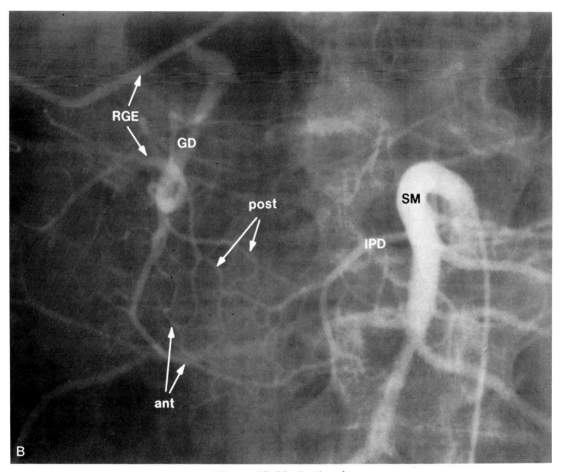

Figure 13–28. *Continued.*

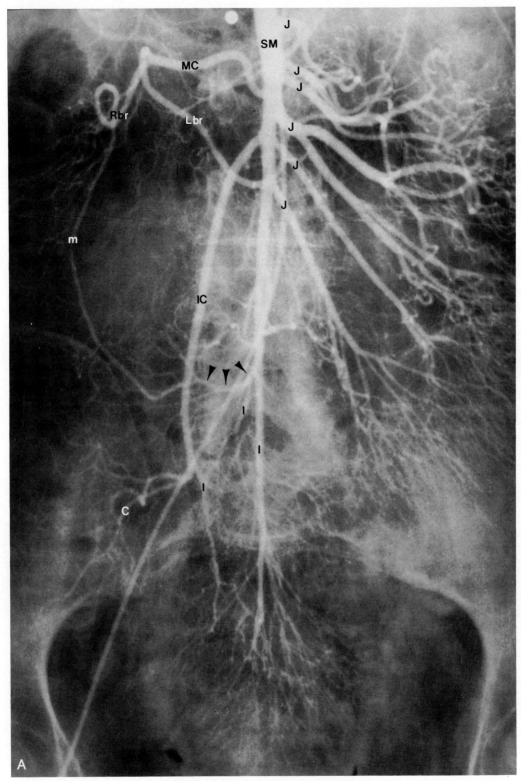

Figure 13–29. *Legend on opposite page.*

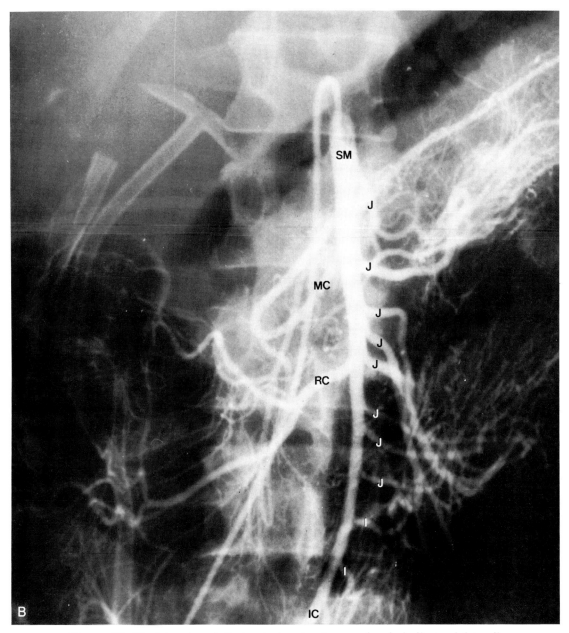

Figure 13–29. Jejunal and ileal arteries. In *A*, arrowheads indicate right colic artery. NOTE: In *A*, the ileocolic artery arises proximal to the origin of the right colic artery.

C	Cecal
I	Ileal
IC	Ileocolic
J	Jejunal
Lbr	Left branch of middle colic
m	Marginal
MC	Middle colic
Rbr	Right branch of middle colic
RC	Right colic
SM	Superior mesenteric

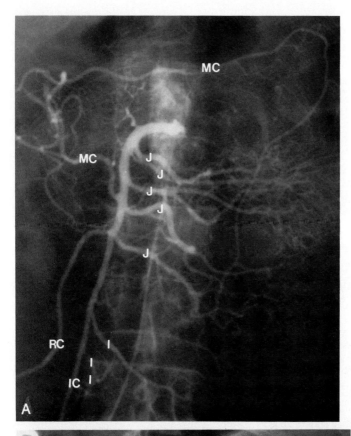

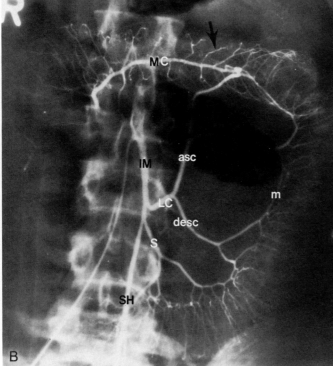

Figure 13–30. Middle colic artery. *A*, Superior mesenteric arteriogram. *B*, Inferior mesenteric arteriogram showing the middle colic artery. Arrow points to the vasa recta of the transverse colon.

asc	Ascending branch of left colic
desc	Descending branch of left colic
I	Ileal
IC	Ileocolic
IM	Inferior mesenteric
J	Jejunal
LC	Left colic
m	Marginal
MC	Middle colic
RC	Right colic
S	Sigmoid
SH	Superior hemorrhoidal

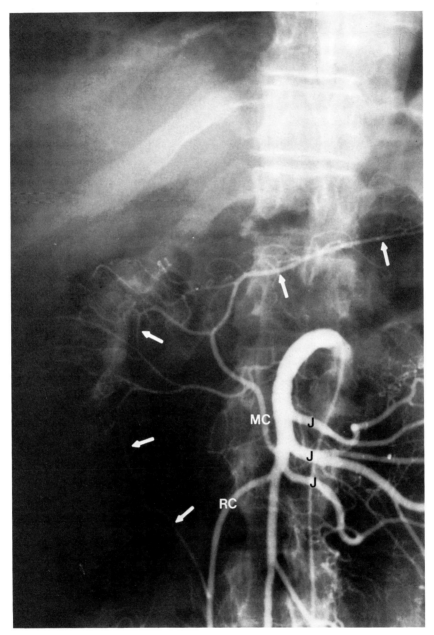

Figure 13–31. Superior mesenteric arteriogram demonstrating right colic arteries and the marginal artery (*arrows*).

J	Jejunal arteries
MC	Middle colic
RC	Right colic

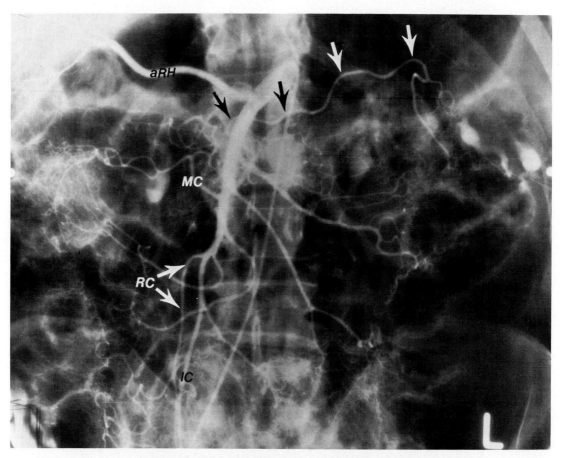

Figure 13–32. Accessory middle colic artery (*arrows*).

aRH   Accessory right hepatic off the superior mesenteric
IC   Ileocolic
MC   Middle colic
RC   Right colic

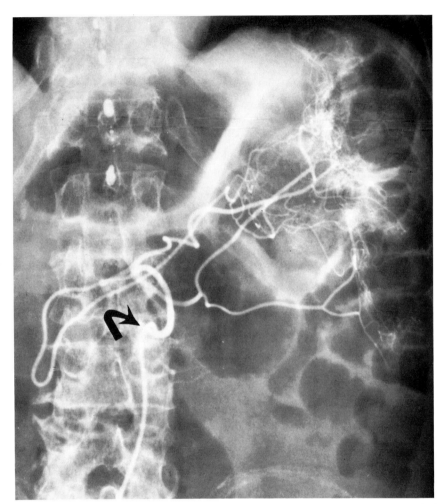

Figure 13–33. Middle mesenteric artery. Selective arteriogram of the middle mesenteric artery. Curved arrow points to its origin from the aorta. Its branches supply the distal transverse and proximal descending colon. (Courtesy of Dr. Frederick Keller. Reproduced from Radiology 165:371–372, 1987, with permission.)

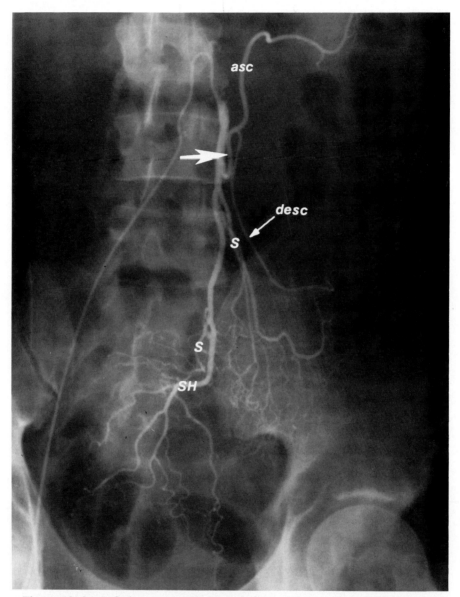

Figure 13–34. Inferior mesenteric artery. Arrow points to the left colic artery.

asc	Ascending branch of left colic
desc	Descending branch of left colic
S	Sigmoid
SH	Superior hemorrhoidal

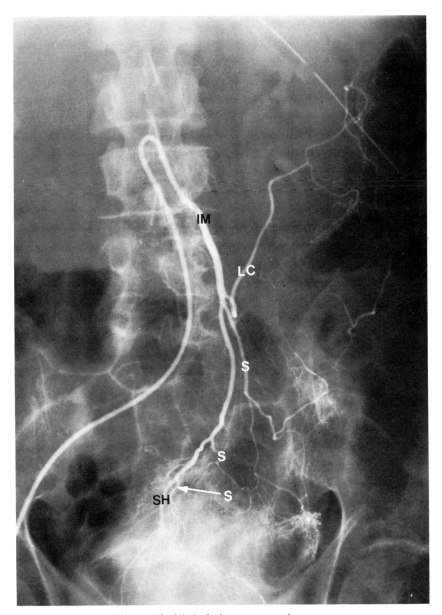

Figure 13–35. Inferior mesenteric artery.

IM Inferior mesenteric
LC Left colic
S   Sigmoid
SH Superior hemorrhoidal

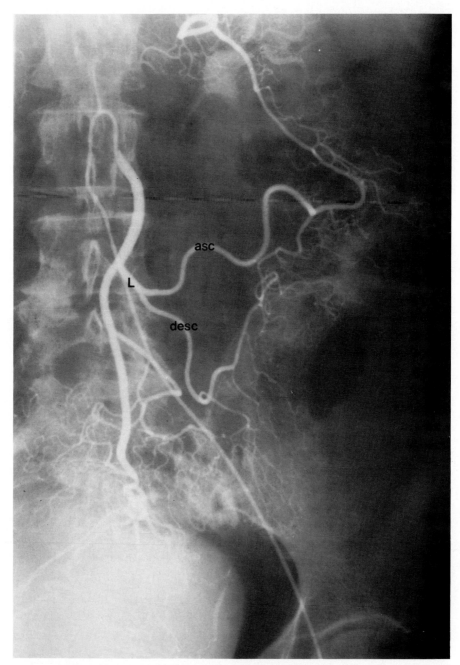

Figure 13–36. Inferior mesenteric artery. The ascending branch joins the marginal artery of the mid–descending colon; i.e., there is no arc of Riolan.

asc   Ascending branch of left colic
desc   Descending branch of left colic
L   Left colic

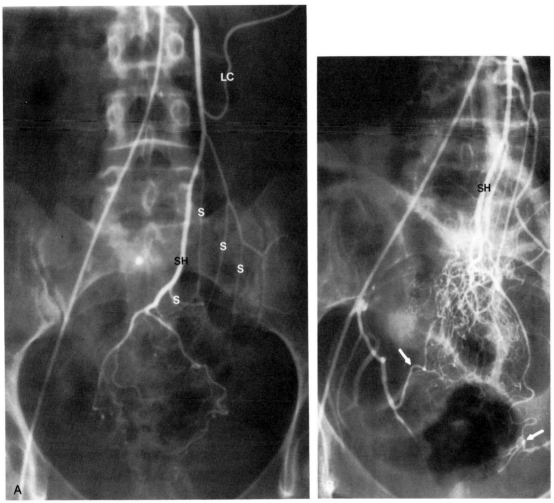

Figure 13–37. *A*, Sigmoid and superior hemorrhoidal arteries seen on an inferior mesenteric arteriogram. *B*, Inferior mesenteric arteriogram demonstrates direct communication between the superior and middle hemorrhoidal arteries (*arrows*).

LC   Left colic
S   Sigmoid
SH   Superior hemorrhoidal

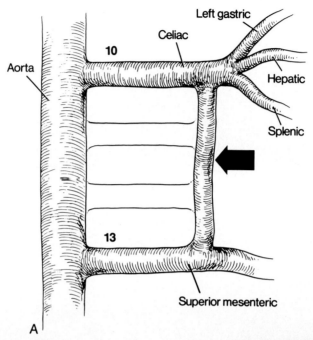

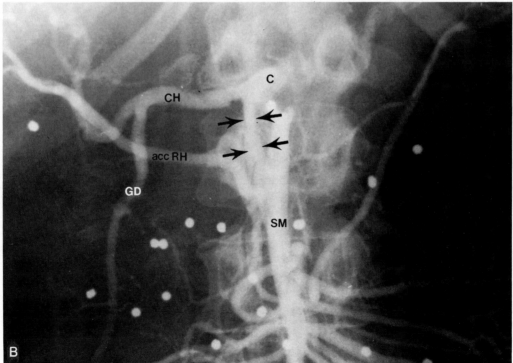

Figure 13–38. *Legend on opposite page.*

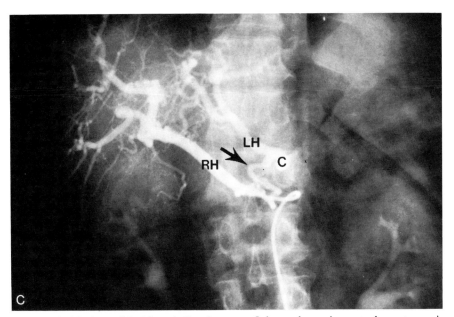

Figure 13–38. Arc of Bühler. *A*, Persistence of the embryonic ventral anastomosis (*arrow*) leads to the formation of the arc of Bühler. *B*, Superior mesenteric arteriogram opacifies the celiac artery via a large communicating vessel—the arc of Bühler (*arrows*). *C*, Arteriogram of the right hepatic artery arising from the superior mesenteric artery opacifies a large arc of Bühler (*arrow*).

accRH	Accessory right hepatic
C	Celiac
CH	Common hepatic
GD	Gastroduodenal
LH	Left hepatic
RH	Right hepatic
SM	Superior mesenteric

Illustration continued on following page.

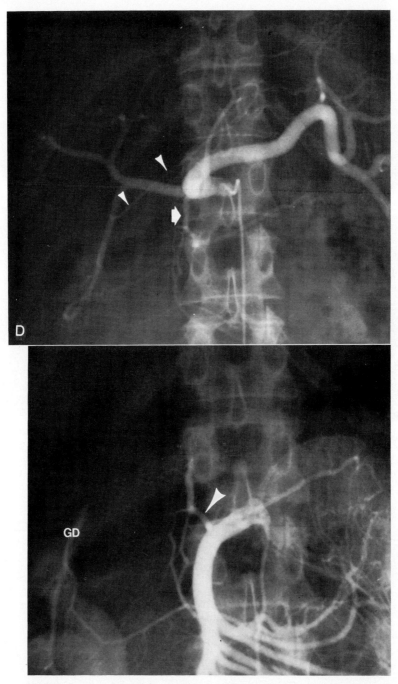

Figure 13–38. *Continued D,* Celiac and superior mesenteric arteriograms show a large anastomosing vessel (*large arrowhead*). Short arrow points to the dorsal pancreatic artery. The small arrowheads point to the right gastric artery.

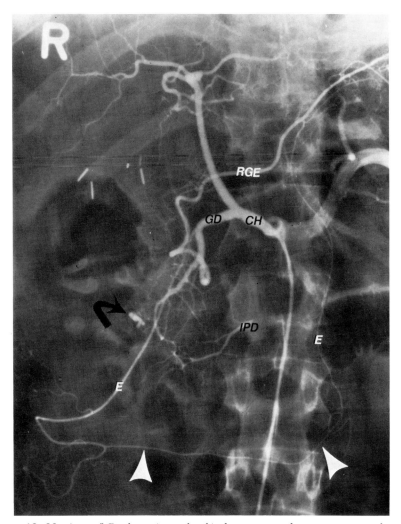

Figure 13–39. Arc of Barkow (*arrowheads*) demonstrated on a common hepatic arteriogram in a patient with postendoscopic sphincterotomy bleeding (*arrow*).

CH	Common hepatic
E	Epiploic
GD	Gastroduodenal
IPD	Inferior pancreaticoduodenal
RGE	Right gastroepiploic

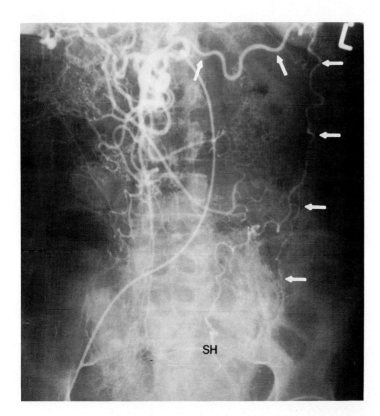

Figure 13–40. Marginal artery of Drummond (*arrows*) demonstrated on a superior mesenteric arteriogram. SH = Superior hemorrhoidal artery.

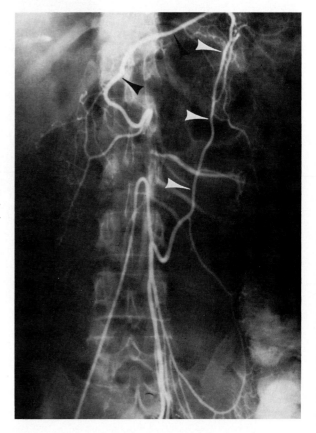

Figure 13–41. Arc of Riolan (*arrowheads*) demonstrated on an inferior mesenteric arteriogram.

Chapter Fourteen

THE PORTAL VENOUS SYSTEM AND HEPATIC VEINS

CAROLINE LUNDELL, M.D.
SAADOON KADIR, M.D.

EMBRYOLOGY

The paired vitelline veins (or omphalomesenteric veins) are the earliest precursors to the formation of the portal venous system and hepatic veins. The vitelline veins course craniocaudad along each side of the primitive duodenum and liver, forming a venous plexus around the duodenum, and then drain into the hepatic sinusoids, which subsequently enter the sinus venosus. In later development, the venous plexus around the duodenum becomes a single large vessel, the portal vein. The right and left branches of the portal vein originate from the right and left vitelline veins, respectively. The distal portion of the right vitelline vein becomes the superior mesenteric vein, which drains the primitive intestine. The left distal vitelline vein forms the splenic vein. The right and left hepatic veins are derived from the proximal right and left vitelline veins. In addition, the proximal right vitelline vein enlarges to form the right hepatocardiac channel, which becomes the suprahepatic portion of the inferior vena cava in the adult.

Initially, the umbilical veins lie along each side of the liver and develop connections with the hepatic sinusoids. As the placental circulation increases, the ductus venosus develops from the hepatic sinusoids and functions to shunt blood through the liver from the left umbilical vein to the right hepatocardiac channel. The proximal portion of the left umbilical vein and the right umbilical veins disappears, and only the left umbilical vein remains and serves to carry blood from the placenta to the liver. In the adult, the obliterated left umbilical vein and the ductus venosus form the ligamentum teres and ligamentum venosum, respectively.

PORTAL VENOUS SYSTEM (Figs. 14–1 to 14–4)

The portal venous system draws blood from the mesenteric, splenic, gastroduodenal, pancreatic, and cystic veins. It provides approximately 75 to 80 per cent of the hepatic inflow, and the hepatic veins provide the entire venous outflow of the liver into the systemic circulation. The portal venous system is demonstrated on the venous phase of the celiac (especially splenic) or superior mesenteric arteriograms (indirect portography). Direct opacification of the portal system is obtained through transhepatic or transjugular portography, splenoportography, and umbilical vein catheterization. The hepatic veins are best studied by direct contrast injection.

PORTAL VEIN

The portal vein is formed by the confluence of the superior mesenteric and splenic veins at approximately the L_1–L_2 level anterior to the inferior vena cava and behind the isthmus of the pancreas. The extrahepatic portal vein is approximately 8 cm long (range 8 to 10 cm) and measures 8 to 10 mm in diameter. The main portal vein lies between the common bile duct on the right and the hepatic artery on the left and is posterior to both in the hepatoduodenal ligament. Rarely, it may be ventral to a hepatic artery; originating from the superior mesenteric artery; it may be duplicated or absent congenitally. In the latter case, mesenteric venous return is via the inferior vena cava and the splenic vein joins the left renal vein. It divides into right and left branches at the porta hepatis. These branches accompany the segmental hepatic artery branches into the liver. The distal portal venous radicles and hepatic arteries then drain into the hepatic sinusoids.

Numerous venous connections exist within the portal venous system (portoportal anastomoses) and others that connect the portal with the systemic circulation (portosystemic anastomoses). The right portal vein branch is 2 to3 cm in length and divides into anterior and posterior segmental branches to the right lobe. These further subdivide into superior and inferior branches. Rarely, the right anterior segmental vein arises from the left branch of the portal vein. The cystic vein(s) usually joins the right branch of the portal vein before it enters the liver parenchyma.

The left portal vein branch is 2 to 4 cm in length. It consists of a transverse portion (extending from the porta hepatis) and the more distal umbilical portion. The transverse portion supplies branches to the caudate and quadrate lobes. The umbilical portion divides into superior and inferior branches to supply the entire lateral segment and inferior portion of the medial segment. The superior portion of the medial segment is supplied by either left or right portal vein branches.

The left portal vein branch joins both the obliterated umbilical vein (ligamentum teres) and the obliterated ductus venosus (ligamentum venosum). The umbilical vein courses vertically in the falciform ligament along the ligamentum teres to the anterior abdominal wall veins at the umbilicus. It is patent only when it provides collateral shunting. It is between 8 and 20 cm (average 12 cm) in length and does not have branches.

CYSTIC VEINS

Veins draining the extrahepatic biliary system most often join the right branch of the portal vein outside of the liver or less frequently the main portal vein. Usually, a single cystic vein drains the anterior surface of the gallbladder. One or two veins drain the posterior gallbladder surface and unite at the gallbladder neck; these cystic veins frequently join inferiorly with veins draining the common hepatic and upper common bile ducts. The intrahepatic bile ducts are drained by the peribiliary venous plexus, which joins the intrahepatic portal branches.

SUPERIOR MESENTERIC VEIN (Figs. 14–1, 14–3, and 14–5)

The superior mesenteric vein (SMV) lies to the right of the superior mesenteric artery and joins the splenic vein to form the portal vein. The mesenteric veins begin distally as intramural veins, vasa recta, and mesenteric arcades and subsequently form segmental branches. The major segmental branches unite to form the SMV, accompany their respective arteries, and drain the jejunum, ileum, right and transverse colon, and pancreaticoduodenal arcades.

Segmental veins from jejunum and ileum usually join the left side of the superior mesenteric vein while the right and middle colic veins join the right side. The middle colic vein anastomoses with the left colic branch of the inferior mesenteric vein. The major nonmesenteric tributaries to the SMV include the right gastroepiploic and pancreaticoduodenal veins. The right gastroepiploic, the middle colic, and the pancreaticoduodenal veins unite to form the gastrocolic trunk, which enters the proximal SMV on the right side.

SPLENIC VEIN (Figs. 14–3 and 14–6)

The splenic vein forms at the splenic hilum from the junction of two to six segmental splenic branches. It is on the average 15 cm in length. It lies inferior and slightly posterior to the splenic artery, pancreatic body, and tail. It joins the SMV behind the pancreatic neck and slightly to the right of midline. Major tributaries include the inferior mesenteric, left gastric (coronary), short gastric and gastroepiploic veins, and veins draining the pancreatic body and tail.

INFERIOR MESENTERIC VEIN (Fig. 14–7)

The inferior mesenteric vein (IMV) lies to the right of the inferior mesenteric artery. It usually joins the splenic vein to the left of the splenic–SMV junction in about 40 per cent and at their junction in about 30 per cent of individuals. In another 30 per cent of individuals, it enters the SMV.

Occasionally the IMV is duplicated. It drains the rectosigmoid and left colon; its major tributaries include the superior hemorrhoidal, sigmoidal, and left colic veins.

GASTRIC VEINS (Figs. 14–8 to 14–10)

The left gastric (coronary) vein parallels its respective artery and courses from left to right along the lesser curvature of the stomach. It joins the superior aspect of the SMV–splenic vein junction in approximately 60 per cent, the portal vein in 25 per cent, and the splenic vein in the remainder of individuals. The gastric coronary vein drains both surfaces of the stomach and also receives lower esophageal branches at the gastroesophageal junction. The right gastric (pyloric) vein is small and parallels the right gastric artery to drain the pyloric portion of the lesser curvature. It joins the coronary or pancreatic veins, which then enter the main portal vein or a portal branch at the porta hepatis.

The short gastric veins consist of several small veins that drain into the splenic vein close to the splenic hilus or the upper, posterior part of the spleen and in only one fourth of individuals into the lower part. They drain the gastric fundus and left side of the greater curvature.

The left gastroepiploic vein joins the distal splenic vein close to the splenic hilus and receives numerous small branches from both surfaces of the gastric body and adjacent greater omentum. It lies along the greater curvature of the stomach within the greater omentum and joins the right gastroepiploic vein, which drains the inferior part of the stomach. The right gastroepiploic vein joins with the middle colic and inferior pancreaticoduodenal veins to form the gastrocolic trunk, which drains into the SMV. Rarely it joins the splenic vein or the peripheral portal vein. The epiploic veins drain into the right and left gastroepiploic veins, and may form a large epiploic arcade inferiorly, parallel to the gastroepiploic veins, known as the venous arc of Barkow. This functions as an important venous collateral in splenic vein obstruction.

PANCREATIC VEINS (Figs. 14–11 to 14–14)

The pancreaticoduodenal veins that drain the head of the pancreas parallel their respective arterial arcades. The superior and inferior pancreaticoduodenal veins anastomose with each other. The anterior superior pancreaticoduodenal vein drains into the gastrocolic trunk, which drains into the SMV. It is duplicated in about 50 per cent of individuals with a branch each joining the SMV (gastrocolic trunk) or portal vein. The anterior inferior pancreaticoduodenal vein usually drains into either the SMV or first jejunal vein. The posterior superior pancreaticoduodenal vein drains into the posterior inferior border of the portal vein about 2 cm above the junction of the portal and superior mesenteric veins. The posterior inferior pancreaticoduodenal vein is less consistent and usually drains into the first jejunal vein, often along with the anterior inferior pancreaticoduodenal vein.

The dorsal pancreatic vein drains the pancreatic head, neck, and body and usually joins the proximal splenic vein or the junction of the splenic and the portal veins. The transverse pancreatic vein is the major branch of the dorsal pancreatic vein. It courses lengthwise along the posterior inferior aspect of the pancreatic body and tail to drain primarily the body. It also communicates with the pancreaticoduodenal arcades in the pancreatic head. In addition, numerous small venous branches drain the pancreatic body and enter the splenic vein directly or occasionally the gastric coronary vein. The pancreatic tail is drained by numerous tiny veins that join the splenic vein directly and also the transverse pancreatic vein.

HEPATIC VEINS (Figs. 14–15 and 14–16)

The hepatic veins provide venous return from the liver to the systemic circulation. The central or intralobular veins originate from the coalescence of hepatic sinusoids and join to form the sublobular veins, which are tributaries to the hepatic veins. The hepatic veins lie in the fissures that divide the hepatic segments and do not follow the segmental distribution of the hepatic arteries, portal veins, or bile ducts.

Three main hepatic veins are usually present: right, left, and middle hepatic veins. All three veins may enter the inferior vena cava as a single trunk, but most commonly the right hepatic vein enters the inferior vena cava separately while the middle and left hepatic veins form a trunk.

The right hepatic vein drains the posterior segment and superior part of the anterior segment of the right hepatic lobe; it lies in the fissure dividing the anterior and posterior segments of the right lobe. The middle hepatic vein lies in the interlobar fissure dividing the right and left lobes. It drains a portion of the right lobe and the medial segment of the left lobe.

The left hepatic vein drains the entire lateral segment and the superior medial segment of the left lobe. It lies in the segmental fissure of the left lobe. The caudate lobe is usually drained separately by two or three small veins that enter the inferior vena cava approximately 2 to 3 cm below the middle and left hepatic veins. Occasionally, a separate right superior hepatic vein drains the upper portion of the liver bound by the coronary ligament.

REFERENCES

1. Couinaud C: The parabiliary venous system. Surg Radiol Anat 10:311–316, 1988.
2. Göthlin J, Lunderquist A, Tylén U: Selective phlebography of the pancreas. Acta Radiol 15:474–480, 1974.
3. Harell G: Ventral portal vein. Radiology 121:369–373, 1974.
4. Healey JE Jr: Vascular anatomy of the liver. Ann NY Acad Sci 170:8–17, 1970.
5. Heloury Y, Leborgne J, Rogez JM, Robert R, Barin JY, Hureau J: The caudate lobe of the liver. Surg Radiol Anat 10:83–91, 1988.
6. Keller FS, Niles, NR, Rösch J, et al: Retrograde pancreatic venography: Autopsy study. Radiology 135:285–293, 1980.
7. Lunderquist A, Tylén U: Phlebography of the pancreatic veins. Radiologe 15:198–202, 1975.
8. Marois D, Van Heerden JA, Carpenter HA, et al: Congenital absence of the portal vein. Mayo Clin Proc 54:55–59, 1979.
9. Marks C: Developmental basis of the portal venous system. Am J Surg 117:671–681, 1969.
10. Michels NA: Blood Supply and Anatomy of the Upper Abdominal Organs With a Descriptive Atlas. Philadelphia, J.B. Lippincott Company, 1955.
11. Miyaki T, Yamada M, Kumaki K: Aberrant course of the left gastric vein in the human. Possibility of a persistent left portal vein. Acta Anat 130:275–279, 1987.
12. Rosch J, Dotter CT: Retrograde pancreatic venography. An experimental study. Radiology 114:275–279, 1975.
13. Takayasu K, Moriyama N, Muramatsu Y, et al: Intrahepatic portal vein branches studied by percutaneous transhepatic postography. Radiology 153:31–36, 1985.

Figures 14–1 through 14–16 on following pages.

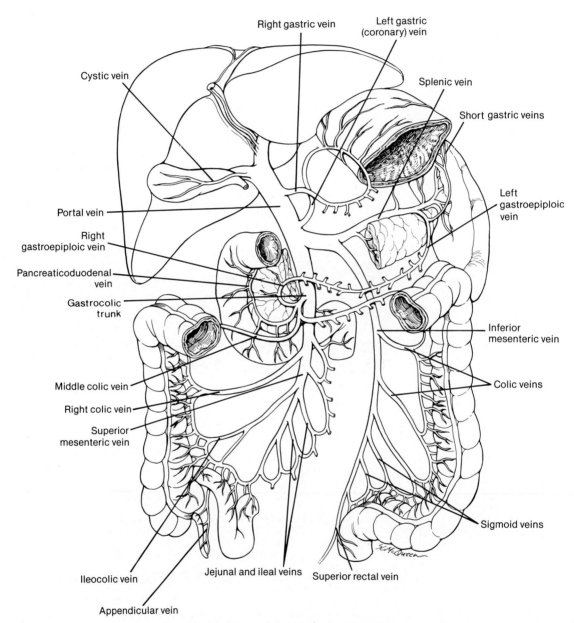

Figure 14–1. The portal venous system.

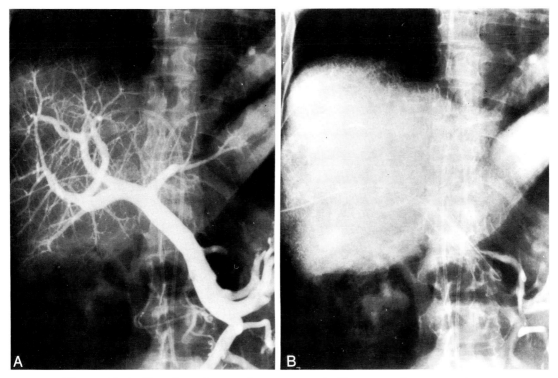

Figure 14–2. Transhepatic portal venogram. *A,* Venous and *B,* parenchymal phase. (From Kadir S: Diagnostic Angiography. Philadelphia, WB Saunders Company, 1986.)

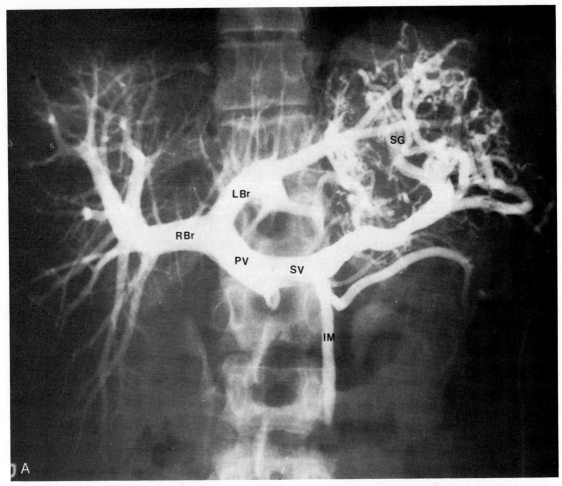

Figure 14–3. Portal system. *A*, Transhepatic splenic venogram (multiple gastric varices are demonstrated). *B*, Transhepatic superior mesenteric venogram. Solid arrow points to gastrocolic trunk. Open arrow points to the posterior superior pancreaticoduodenal vein.

I	Ileal
IC	Ileocolic
IM	Inferior mesenteric
J	Jejunal
LBr	Left branch of portal
PV	Portal
RBr	Right branch of portal
RC	Right colic
SG	Short gastric
SM	Superior mesenteric
S/SV	Splenic

Illustration continued on opposite page.

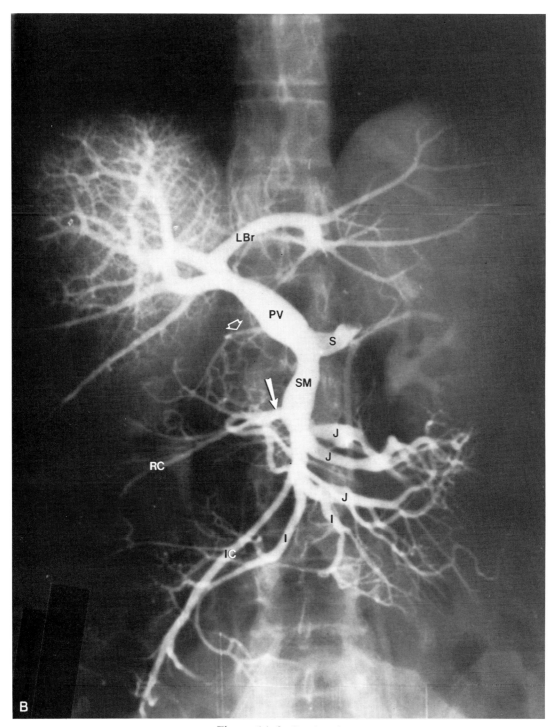

Figure 14–3. *Continued.*

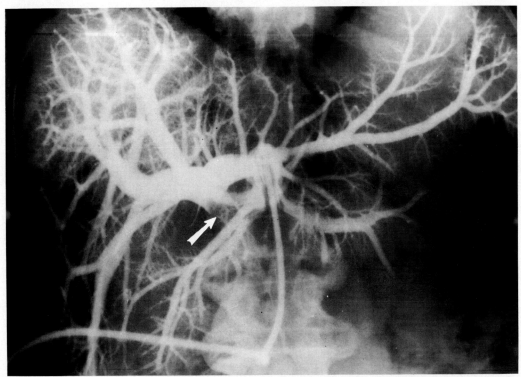

Figure 14–4. Transumbilical portogram. Arrow points to inflow of unopacified blood via the portal vein.

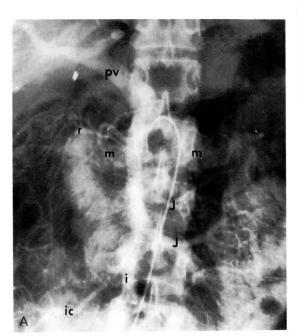
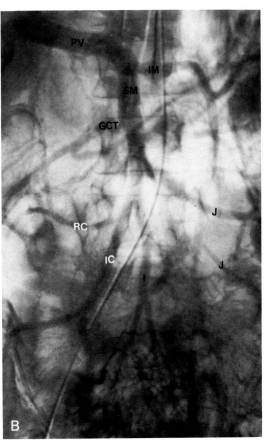

Figure 14–5. Superior mesenteric veins. *A,* Venous phase of superior mesenteric arteriogram. *B,* Venous phase of superior mesenteric arteriogram from another individual shows the inferior mesenteric vein joining the superior mesenteric vein. (From Kadir S: Diagnostic Angiography. Philadelphia, WB Saunders Company, 1986.)

GCT	Gastrocolic trunk
I, i	Ileal
IC, ic	Ileocolic
IM	Inferior mesenteric
J	Jejunal
m	Middle colic
PV, pv	Portal
RC, r	Right colic
SM	Superior mesenteric

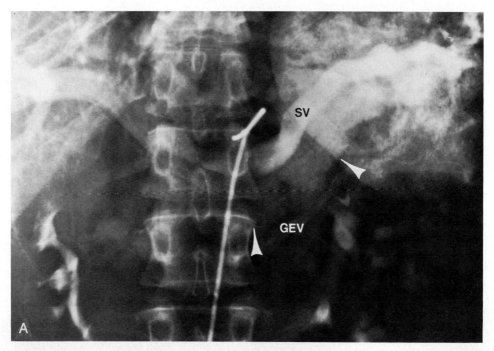

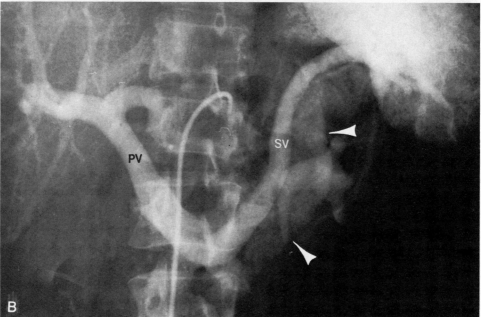

Figure 14–6. *A* and *B*, Splenic vein seen on venous phase of splenic arteriogram. In *B* the splenic vein has a vertical course. Arrowheads point to pancreatic parenchymal blush. Note how the pancreas and splenic vein remain in close proximity.

GEV   Gastroepiploic
PV   Portal
SV   Splenic

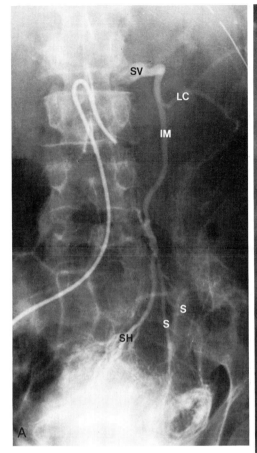

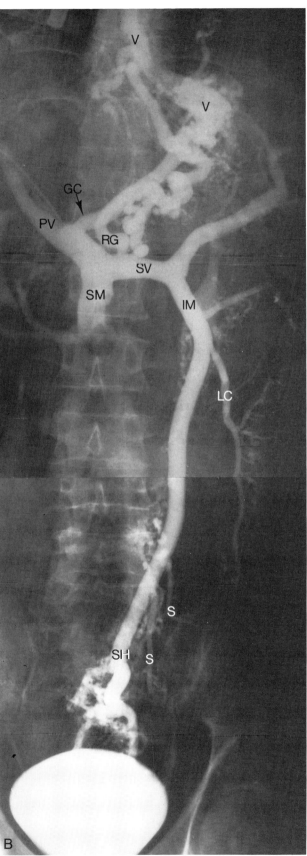

Figure 14–7. *A,* Inferior mesenteric vein seen on venous phase of an inferior mesenteric arteriogram. *B,* Transhepatic inferior mesenteric venogram.

GC   Gastric coronary
IM   Inferior mesenteric
LC   Left colic
PV   Portal
RG   Right gastric
S   Sigmoid
SH   Superior hemorrhoidal
SM   Superior mesenteric
SV   Splenic
V   Varices

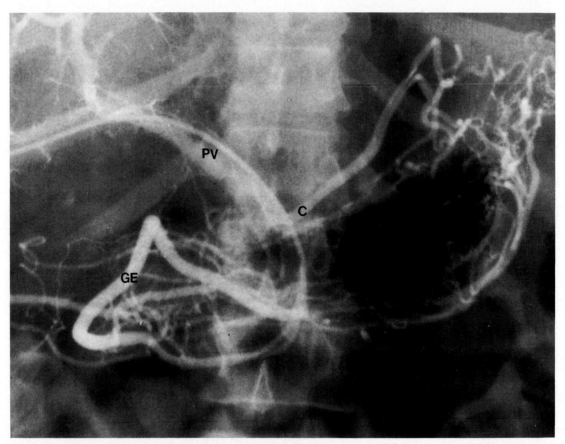

Figure 14–8. Gastric veins seen on a transhepatic gastroepiploic venogram. The coronary vein joins at the splenoportal vein junction.

C   Gastric coronary
GE   Gastroepiploic
PV   Portal

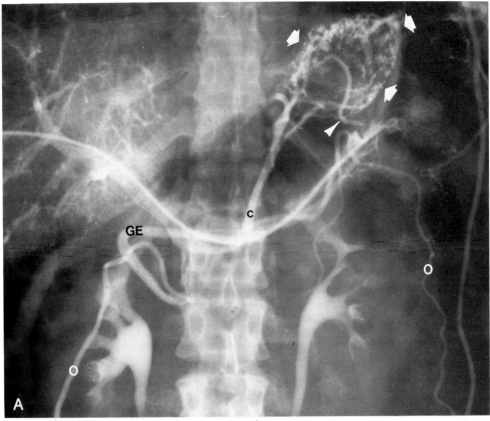

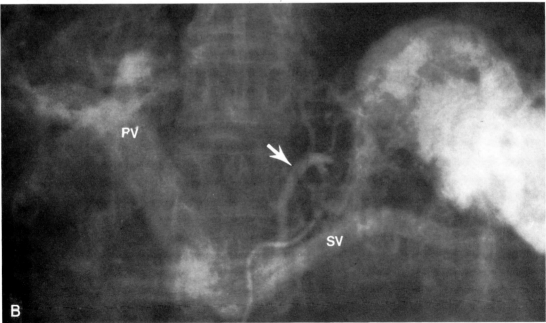

Figure 14–9. Gastric veins. *A,* Transhepatic splenic venogram opacifies the gastric fundal veins (*arrows*) via short gastric veins (*arrowhead*). *B,* Venous phase of splenic arteriogram shows the gastric coronary vein (*arrow*) in another individual.

c	Gastric coronary	PV	Portal
GE	Gastroepiploic	SV	Splenic
O	Omental (epiploic)		

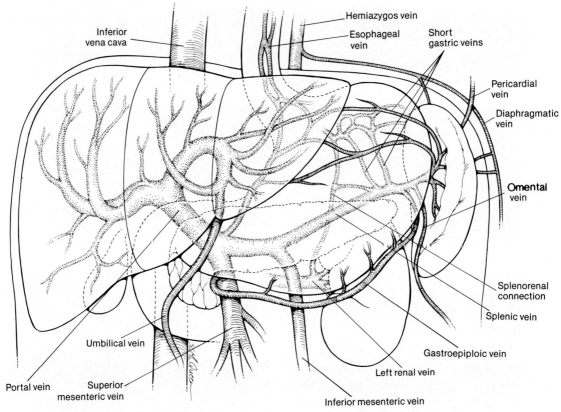

Figure 14–10. The tributaries and communications of the portal venous system.

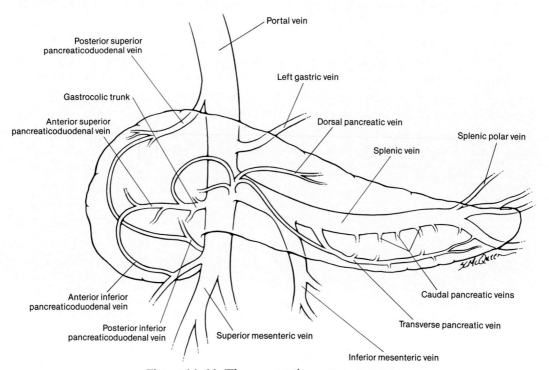

Figure 14–11. The pancreatic venous anatomy.

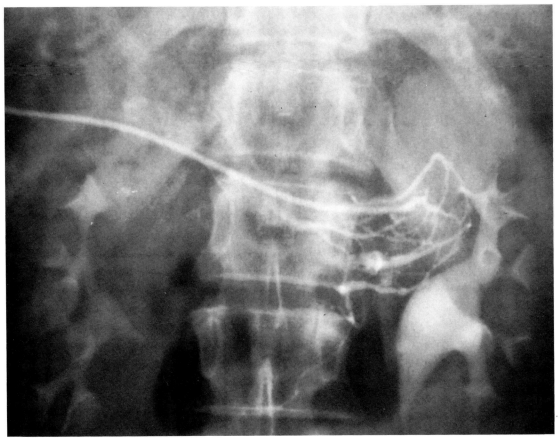

Figure 14–12. Pancreatic veins in the mid-gland seen on a transhepatic pancreatic venogram.

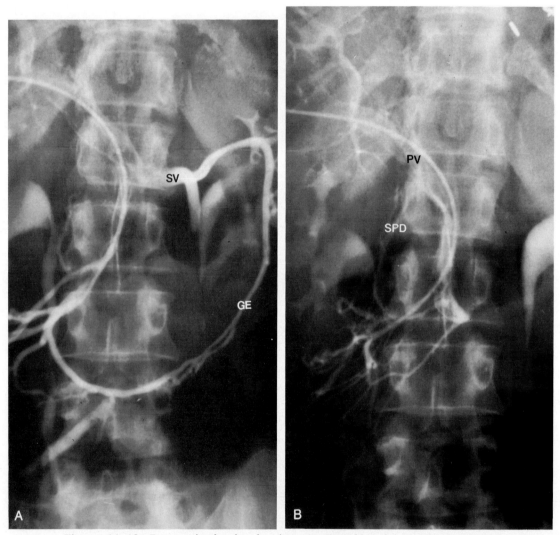

Figure 14–13. Pancreaticoduodenal veins. *A,* Transhepatic venogram of the gastrocolic trunk. The splenic vein is opacified via the gastroepiploic vein. *B,* Transhepatic–gastrocolic trunk venogram from another individual, showing the pancreaticoduodenal veins.

GE	Gastroepiploic
P	Portal
SPD	Posterior superior pancreaticoduodenal
SV	Splenic

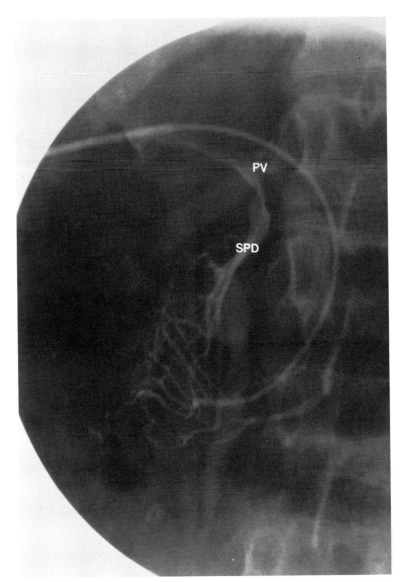

Figure 14–14. Transhepatic venogram of the posterior inferior pancreaticoduodenal vein.

PV   Portal
SPD Posterior superior pancreaticoduodenal

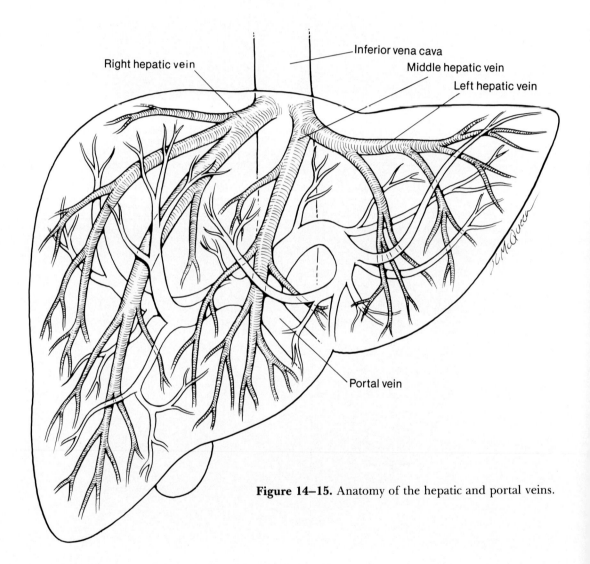

Figure 14–15. Anatomy of the hepatic and portal veins.

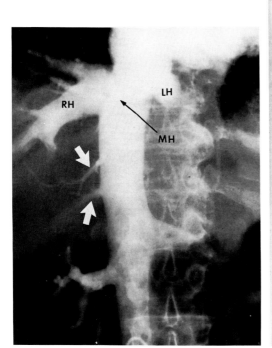

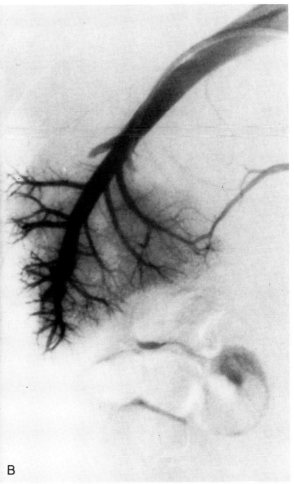

Figure 14–16. Hepatic veins. *A,* Hepatic veins seen on inferior vena cavagram. Arrows point to smaller hepatic veins joining the IVC directly. *B,* Retrograde hepatic venogram. (*A* from Kadir S: Diagnostic Angiography. Philadelphia, WB Saunders Company, 1986. *B* reproduced with permission from Miller F, et al: Hepatic venography and hemodynamics in patients with alcoholic hepatitis. Radiology 115:313–317, 1975.)

LH	Left hepatic
MH	Middle hepatic
RH	Right hepatic

Chapter Fifteen

KIDNEYS

SAADOON KADIR, M.D.

ARTERIAL ANATOMY

The Renal Arteries (Figs. 15–1 and 15–2; also see Fig. 4–1)

The renal arteries branch off the aorta immediately below the superior mesenteric artery about the L_1–L_2 intervertebral disc space in around 75 per cent of individuals. In the remainder, they may originate anywhere between the lower margins of T_{12} and L_2. They are lower in older individuals.

The renal artery orifice is located in the lateral or ventrolateral aspect of the aortic wall. The right renal artery orifice is closer to the ventral surface in more than 50 per cent, the left in around 25 per cent of individuals. Location of the orifice in the posterior lateral aortic wall is infrequent and usually involves the left renal artery.

The right renal artery passes behind the inferior vena cava, renal vein, duodenum, and pancreatic head. The left renal artery also lies behind the pancreatic body and renal and splenic veins. In around 60 per cent of individuals, the renal artery divides at the renal hilus. In approximately 15 per cent there is an early bifurcation (from the proximal or mid-portion); usually a segmental (polar) artery is present, most commonly to the upper pole.

Variant Anatomy (Figs. 15–3 to 15–12)

The overall incidence of variant arterial anatomy of the kidneys is around 40 per cent, including multiple arteries and an early division. There is a single renal artery in around 70 per cent of individuals. In the remainder, there are multiple (two to four) renal arteries, and they occur with equal frequency on both sides. Multiple arteries are unilateral in around 32 per cent and bilateral in 12 per cent of individuals. Approximately 10 per cent are accessory vessels and 20 per cent are aberrant arteries. Multiple renal arteries on the same side may occur in the following manner:

- Two equivalent-sized renal arteries in approximately 10 per cent
- An upper pole renal artery in approximately 7 per cent
- A lower pole renal artery in approximately 6 per cent
- Both upper and lower pole renal arteries in approximately 1 per cent
- Three renal arteries in approximately 3 per cent
- Four or five or more renal arteries in less than 1 per cent

Accessory renal arteries are supernumerary vessels that enter the kidney independently at the hilus. Aberrant arteries enter the kidney outside the hilus. Accessory vessels occur in approximately 10 per cent of individuals, and 98 per cent of them originate from the abdominal aorta. The remainder most frequently originate from the common iliac arteries. Aberrant arteries originate most frequently from the aorta or renal arteries. Upper pole aberrant arteries more commonly originate from the main renal artery, whereas lower pole vessels more frequently arise from the aorta.

In addition to the aorta and iliac arteries, accessory and aberrant vessels have been observed to originate from the superior and inferior mesenteric, median sacral, intercostal, lumbar, adrenal, inferior phrenic, right hepatic, or right colic arteries. Rarely, an aberrant or accessory renal artery may originate above the celiac artery or from the lower thoracic aorta. Anomalous origins of renal arteries are seen commonly in patients with ectopic or horseshoe kidneys.

Intrarenal Branches (Figs. 15–13 to 15–17; Table 15–1)

The kidney is divided into five vascular segments (Graves): apical, upper, middle, posterior, and lower. The apical and lower segments have both an anterior and a posterior surface. The upper and middle segments are anterior, whereas the posterior segment makes up the majority of the posterior surface of the kidney.

The renal artery branching pattern shows a segmental organization. At the hilus, the renal artery divides into anterior and posterior divisions. In the typical case, the anterior division supplies the apical, upper, middle, and lower segments, and the posterior division, which courses behind the renal pelvis, supplies the posterior segment and often provides branches to the apical and occasionally to the lower segment.

The segmental artery divides into lobar arteries, which further subdivide into two or three interlobar arteries (lie between the renal pyramids). The proximal interlobar arteries are extraparenchymal. At the corticomedullary

TABLE 15–1. Origin and Branching of the Segmental Renal Arteries

Segment	Origin From		Branches
Apical	Superior branch off anterior division	40%	
	Main renal artery	25%	
	Aberrant	25%	
	Posterior division	10%	
Upper	Anterior division		Apical and lateral branches
Middle	Anterior division		
Lower	Anterior division		Anterior and posterior branches
Posterior	Posterior division		Upper, middle, and terminal branches

junction, these branch dichotomously into arcuate arteries. These latter arteries are essentially endarteries and do not anastomose with one another but subdivide into interlobular arteries. The interlobular arteries subdivide, giving off the afferent glomerular arterioles. In the cortex, the interlobular arteries have a radially oriented course toward the renal surface. In the renal columns, the course of the interlobular arteries is at right angles to that of the cortical vessels, and the arcuate arteries themselves have a radially oriented course. Some interlobar arteries penetrate the renal surface as perforating arteries.

Afferent glomerular arterioles are usually branches of the interlobular arteries. However, these may occasionally arise from the interlobar (for juxta-medullary glomeruli) and arcuate arteries. Some branches of the interlobular arteries (aglomerular arterioles) do not supply glomeruli but form a capillary network that lies between the interlobular arteries. The efferent glomerular arterioles drain into the peritubular capillary network (plexus) around the convoluted tubules.

Extrarenal Branches of the Renal Arteries (Figs. 15–1, 15–7, 15–14, 15–15, and 15–18 to 15–20 and Fig. 16–4)

During its extrarenal course, the renal artery may give off several branches, which include the following:
- Inferior adrenal arteries (one or several)
- Branches to the perinephric tissues
- Capsular arteries
- Renal pelvic branches
- Proximal ureteric branch(es); this may arise from an intrarenal branch
- Gonadal arteries

The Capsular Arteries (Figs. 15–1, 15–14, 15–15, 15–18, and 15–19)

The three capsular arteries form a capsular network that anastomoses freely with perforating arteries and other retroperitoneal arteries, especially lumbar, but also with internal iliac, intercostal, and mesenteric arteries.

Superior Capsular Artery. This is most frequently a branch of the inferior adrenal artery or arises as an independent branch from the main renal artery or aorta. It provides branches to the perirenal tissues and is prominent in the presence of abundant perirenal fatty tissue.

Middle Capsular Artery. One or more vessels originate from the main renal artery at the hilus. This divides into anterior and posterior branches, which frequently form a recurrent loop around the mid-portion of the kidney (Fig. 15–15).

Inferior Capsular Artery. This is a small vessel, usually originating from the gonadal artery, from an accessory or aberrant lower pole artery, and occasionally from the main renal artery.

Vascular Supply to the Pelvis and Ureters (Figs. 15–14, 15–15, 15–18, and 15–20)

Blood supply to the renal pelvis is provided by short branches arising directly from the interlobar and arcuate arteries and occasionally the main renal artery. These branches anastomose with each other and with ureteral branches, thus forming an important intrarenal collateral pathway. The ureters are supplied by small ureteral branches from the renal artery, directly from the aorta, and from the gonadal arteries. The lower ureter receives blood supply from branches of the common and internal iliac, vesical, and uterine arteries. The inferior vesical artery provides a constant lower ureteral branch. Longitudinal anastomoses are present along the ureteral wall and provide a collateral pathway.

Perforating Vessels (Figs. 15–21 and 15–22)

These are an important collateral pathway to the kidney in the presence of a main renal artery obstruction. The perforating arteries may arise from the interlobar, arcuate, or lobar arteries and are accompanied by a vein. These arteries are recognized by their course and uniform caliber as they exit from the kidney to anastomose with retroperitoneal arteries.

VENOUS ANATOMY

Embryology (Fig. 15–23)

The lower body is drained by three pairs of longitudinally oriented cardinal veins:

1. Posterior cardinal veins develop as vessels of the mesonephric kidneys and later regress with the formation of the permanent kidneys. A segment remains as part of the iliac veins.

2. Subcardinal veins: These are located ventromedially and communicate with each other by a preaortic anastomosis (later forms part of the left renal vein) and the posterior cardinal vein via the mesonephric sinusoids. These contribute to formation of the left renal, adrenal, and gonadal veins and a segment of the inferior vena cava (IVC).

3. Supracardinal veins. They appear as the final cardinal veins and are located posterior lateral to the aorta. The left vein regresses and the right contributes to the formation of the IVC.

The sub- and supracardinal veins are connected by multiple anastomotic channels, which form a circumaortic venous ring. Venous drainage from each kidney is via two veins that join this ring.

The left IVC regresses and the right IVC is formed by contribution from the right supra- and subcardinal veins. One right renal vein atrophies, leaving a single right renal vein. Similarly, the retroaortic component of the left renal venous system atrophies, leaving behind a single preaortic renal vein.

Normal and Variant Anatomy (Figs. 15–24 to 15–31; Table 15–2)

The renal cortex is drained by superficial cortical and stellate veins that unite to form the interlobular veins. At the corticomedullary junction the interlobular veins form the arcuate veins. The medulla is drained by the ascending vasa recta, which drain into the arcuate veins and some into the interlobular veins. The veins usually accompany the same named arteries but are usually larger. The arcuate veins join to form the larger veins. These do not have a lobar organization, and three to five such veins form the main renal vein. Anastomoses between arcuate veins exist but are infrequent.

TABLE 15–2. Normal and Variant Anatomy of the Renal Veins

	Incidence
Right renal vein	
Single vein	Approx. 72%
Single vein divides before entering inferior vena cava	4%
Multiple veins	Approx. 28%
Gonadal vein joins renal vein	Approx. 8%
Adrenal branches join renal vein	Approx. 30%
Retroperitoneal connections	Approx. 3%
Valves	16%
Left renal vein	
Single preaortic vein	80%
Single retroaortic vein	3%
Single vein divides before entering inferior vena cava	1%
Circumaortic ring	17%
Single vein at hilus (75%)	
Two veins at hilus (25%)	
Gonadal vein joins renal vein	>99%
Adrenal vein joins renal vein	100%
Retroperitoneal connections (lumbar, ascending lumbar, pancreatic, splenic)	75%
Valves	15%

The right renal vein is 2 to 4 cm in length and joins the IVC about the lower one third of L_1. Multiple right renal veins are observed in 28 per cent of individuals. Infrequently, a single vein leaves the hilus and divides before entering the IVC.

The left renal vein is 4 to 11 cm in length and has a relatively horizontal course in most individuals. It frequently joins the IVC at a slightly higher level than the right renal vein. A single vein is present in around 80 per cent of individuals. Table 15–2 lists the variant anatomy and communications of the renal veins.

REFERENCES

1. Beckmann CF, Abrams HC: Renal venography: Anatomy, technique, applications. Analysis of 132 venograms, and a review of the literature. Cardiovasc Intervent Radiol 3:45–70, 1980.
2. Fine H, Keen EN: The arteries of the human kidney. J Anat 100:881–894, 1966.
3. Garti I, Meiraz D: Ectopic origin of main renal artery. Urology 15:627–629, 1980.
4. Ionescu VM, Mihail N, Ionescu C: Blutversorgung der normalen Niere des Menschen durch mehrfache Nierenschlagadern. Anat Anz 111:398–406, 1962.
5. Milynarczyk VL, Wozniak W, Kiersz A: Varianten in der Anzahl und im Verlauf der Nierenarterien. Anat Anz 118:67–81, 1966.
6. Poisel VS, Spängler HP: Uber aberrante und akzessorische Nierenarterien bei Nieren in typischer Lage. Anat Anz 124:244–259, 1969.
7. Wicke VL, Spängler HP, Dimopoulos J, Firbas W, Olbert F: Zur Dignität der Variationen der Nierenarterienabgange im Angiogramm. Anat Anz 135:140–150, 1974.

Figures 15–1 through 15–31 on following pages.

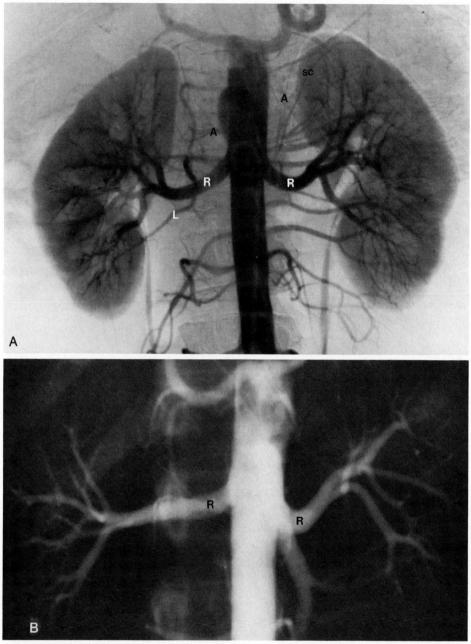

Figure 15–1. Bilateral single renal arteries. Aortograms from two different individuals.

A   Adrenal
L   Lumbar
R   Renal
sc   Superior capsular

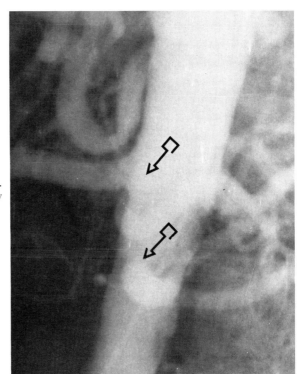

Figure 15–2. Location of renal artery orifices. Lateral abdominal aortogram shows anteriorly located origins of both renal arteries (*arrows*).

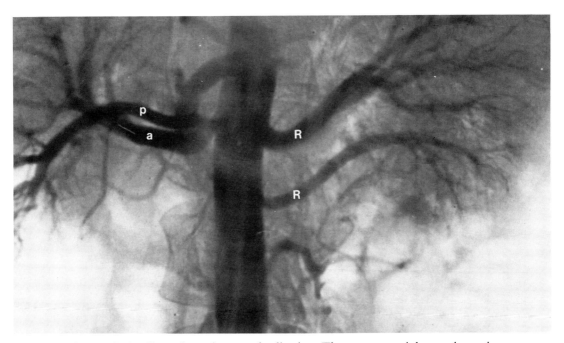

Figure 15–3. Bilateral renal artery duplication. There are two right renal arteries arising in close proximity to each other. Both vessels enter at the renal hilus. Two left renal arteries are present with an aberrant entry of the lower vessel.

a   Anterior division
p   Posterior division
R   Renal artery

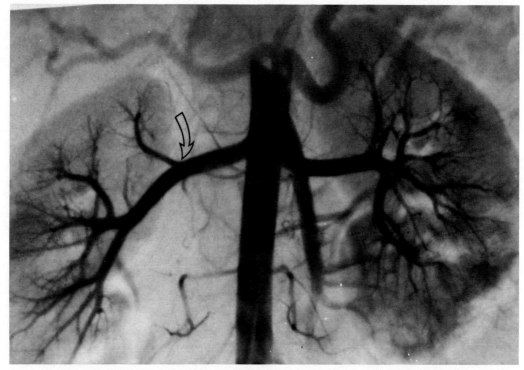

Figure 15–4. Aberrant right upper pole artery. The left renal artery divides at the hilus while the right upper pole artery is aberrant (*arrow*).

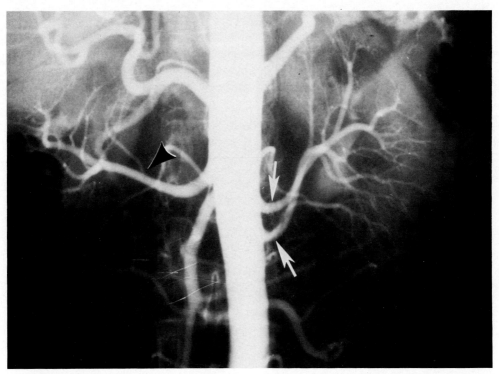

Figure 15–5. Aberrant and accessory renal arteries. Two equal-sized left renal arteries originating from aorta (*arrows*). The right upper pole artery is aberrant (*arrowhead*).

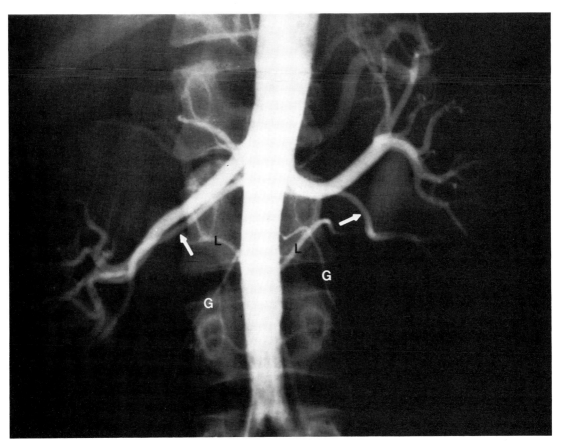

Figure 15–6. Accessory right and aberrant left renal artery (*arrows*).

G   Gonadal arteries
L   Lumbar arteries

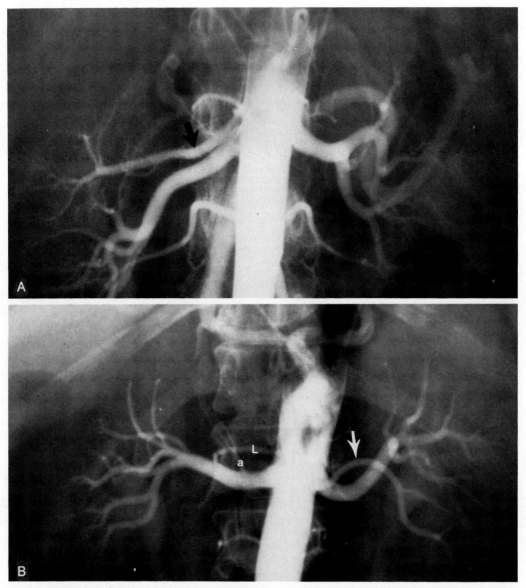

Figure 15–7. Aberrant renal artery. *A*, Large aberrant right upper pole artery arising from the aorta (*arrow*). *B*, Aberrant left renal artery (*arrow*). The proximal course is similar to that of a lumbar artery.

a   Inferior adrenal artery
L   Lumbar artery

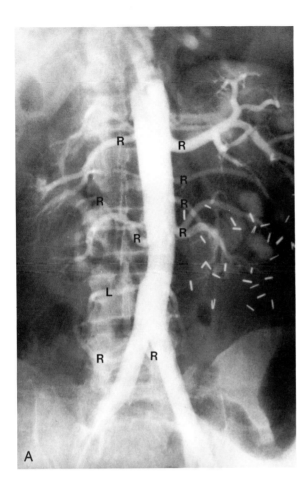

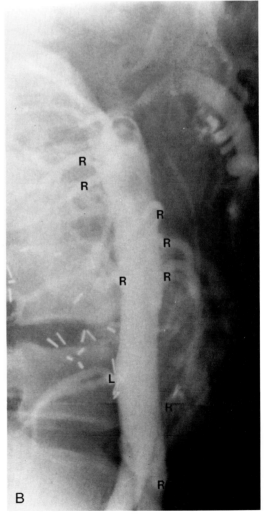

Figure 15–8. Multiple renal arteries. *A*, Anteroposterior and *B*, lateral aortogram shows multiple renal arteries in an individual with a horseshoe kidney. The lower vessels course anteriorly while the upper arteries have a normal location on the lateral aortogram. (From Kadir S: Diagnostic Angiography. Philadelphia, WB Saunders Company, 1986.)

L   Lumbar artery
R   Renal arteries

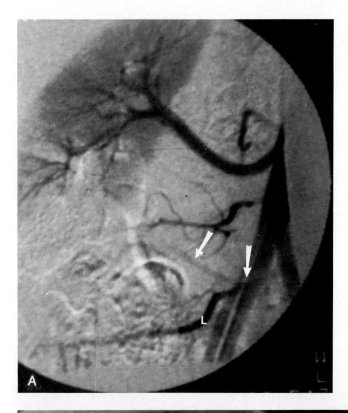

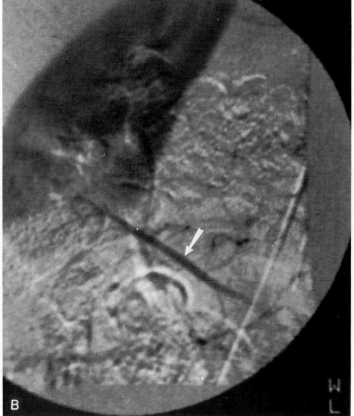

Figure 15–9. *Legend on opposite page.*

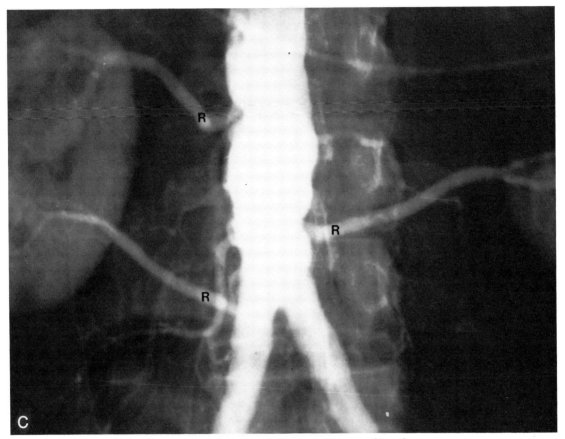

Figure 15–9. Aberrant renal artery. *A*, Early and *B*, late films from an aortogram show an aberrant right lower pole artery (*arrows*) arising from a lumbar artery. *C*, Aortogram from another individual shows a low aortic and iliac artery origin of the renal arteries.

L   Lumbar artery
R   Renal arteries

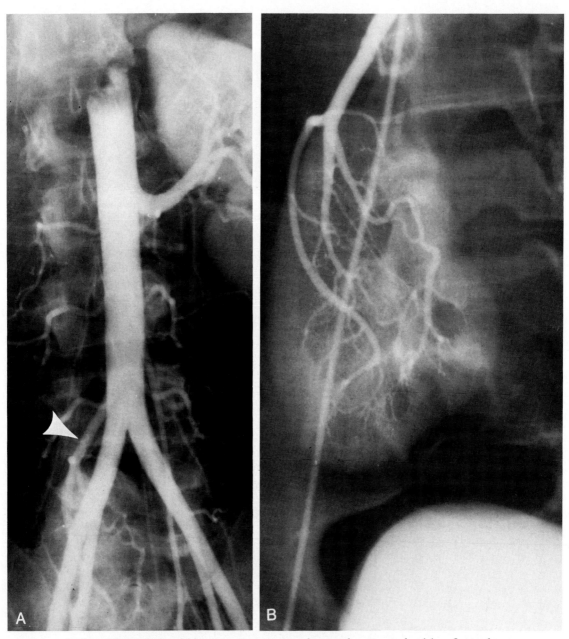

Figure 15–10. Pelvic kidney. *A,* Aortogram shows a large vessel arising from the lower aorta (*arrowhead*). The right renal artery is not present in its normal location. *B,* Early arterial and *C,* parenchymal phases of a selective arteriogram demonstrate a pelvic kidney. V = Renal veins.

Illustration continued on opposite page.

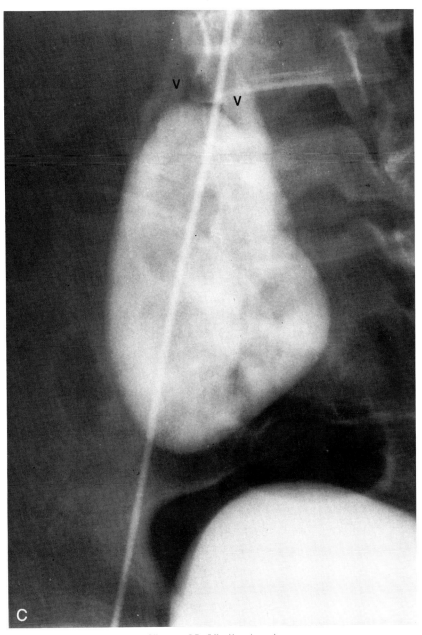

Figure 15–10. *Continued.*

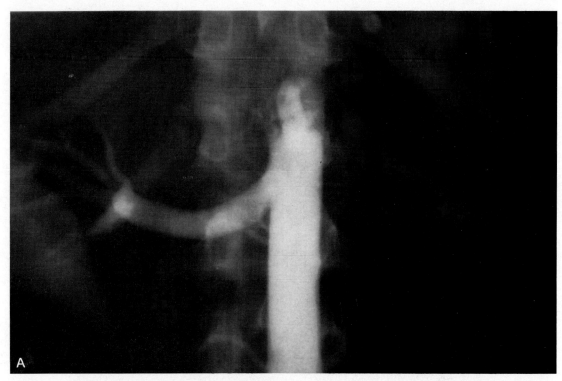

Figure 15–11. Congenitally absent left kidney. *A*, Aortogram shows a single renal artery on the right. The left aortic contour is smooth. There was no pelvic kidney. *B*, Left renal venogram shows bifurcation of the vein into an adrenal (a) and a gonadal (t) vein. This is typically seen in congenital absence of the left kidney. (From Kadir S: Diagnostic Angiography. Philadelphia, WB Saunders Company, 1986.)

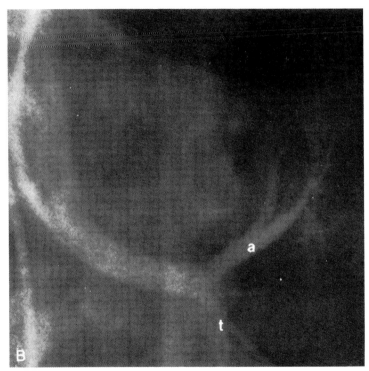

Figure 15–11. *Continued.*

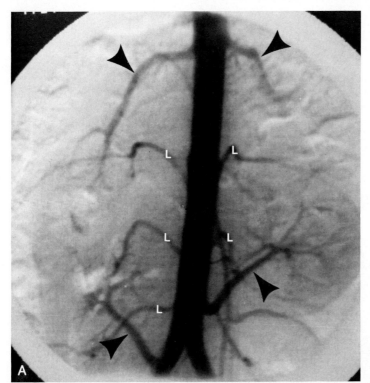

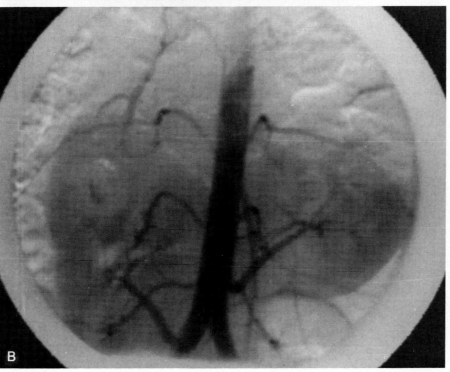

Figure 15–12. Horseshoe kidney. *A*, Early arterial and *B*, late parenchymal phase from a digital subtraction abdominal aortogram shows four large renal arteries (*arrowheads*). The lower right renal artery arises from the right common iliac and the left lower renal artery arises from the distal aorta. L = Lumbar arteries.

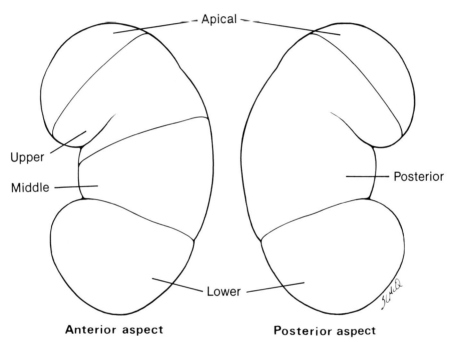

Figure 15–13. The vascular segments of the kidney.

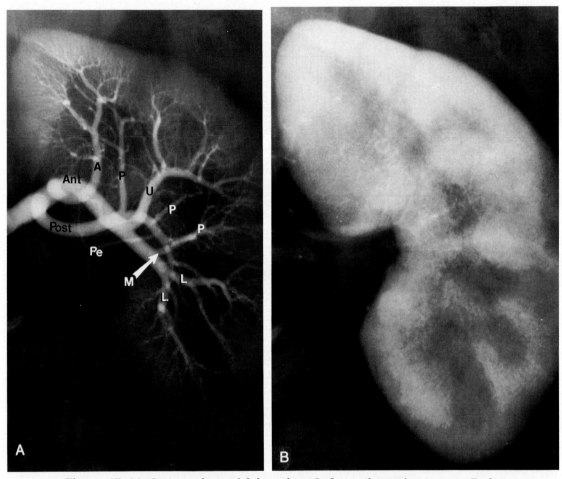

Figure 15–14. Intrarenal arterial branches. Left renal arteriogram. *A,* Early arterial. *B,* Parenchymal phase.

A	Apical segment
Ant	Anterior division
L	Lower segment branches
M	Middle segment branch
P	Posterior segment branches
Pe	Pelvic and capsular branches
Post	Posterior division
U	Upper segment branches

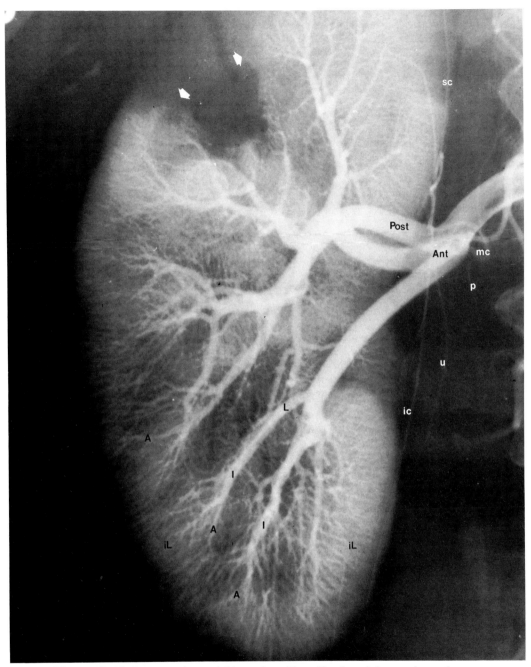

Figure 15–15. Intrarenal arterial branches. Magnification right renal arteriogram. Arrows point to an area of absent perfusion that is supplied by an accessory vessel off the aorta.

A	Arcuate	mc	Middle capsular artery
Ant	Anterior division	p	Pelvic branch
I	Interlobar	Post	Posterior
ic	Inferior capsular	sc	Superior capsular
iL	Interlobular	u	Ureteral branch
L	Lobar		

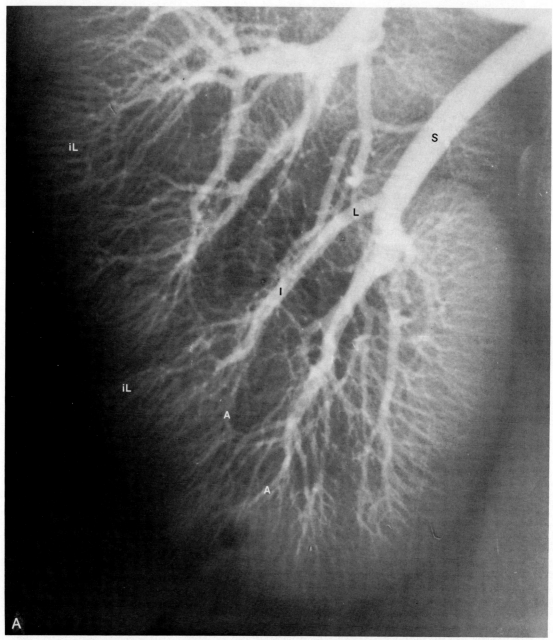

Figure 15–16. Intrarenal arterial branches. Magnification arteriogram from the same individual shown in Fig. 15–15 showing intrarenal branches. *A*, Early arterial phase. *B*, Late arterial phase.

A   Arcuate
I   Interlobar
iL Interlobular
L   Lobar
S   Segmental

Illustration continued on opposite page.

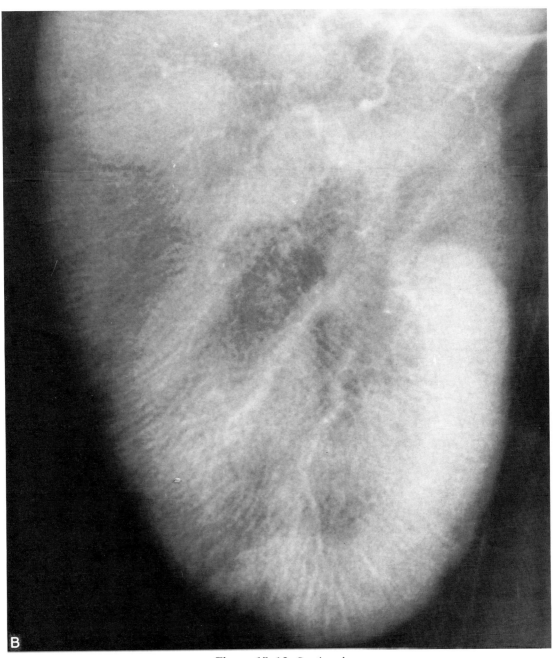

Figure 15–16. *Continued.*

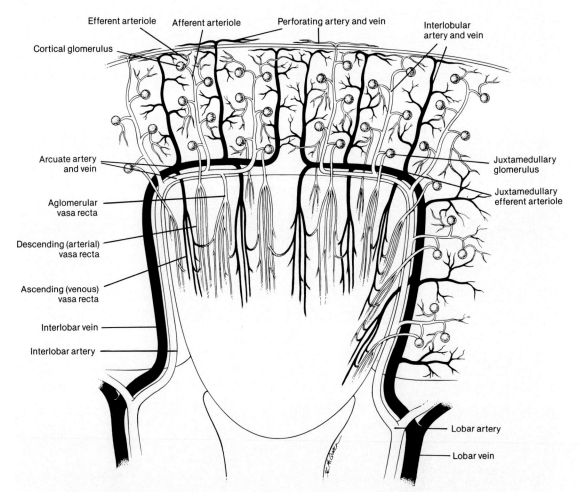

Figure 15–17. The intrarenal branching pattern. The capillary network has been omitted for clarity.

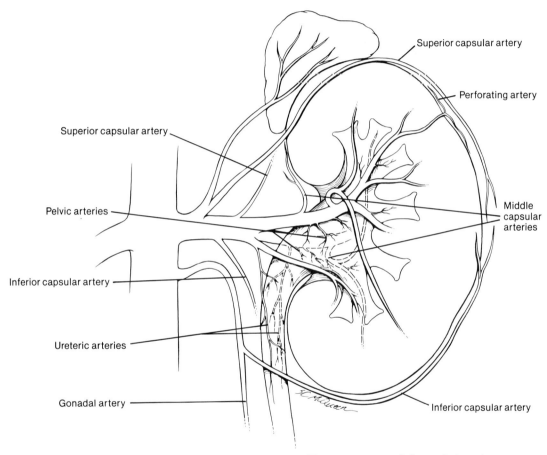

Figure 15–18. The capsular arteries. Diagram illustrates some of the variations in their origins.

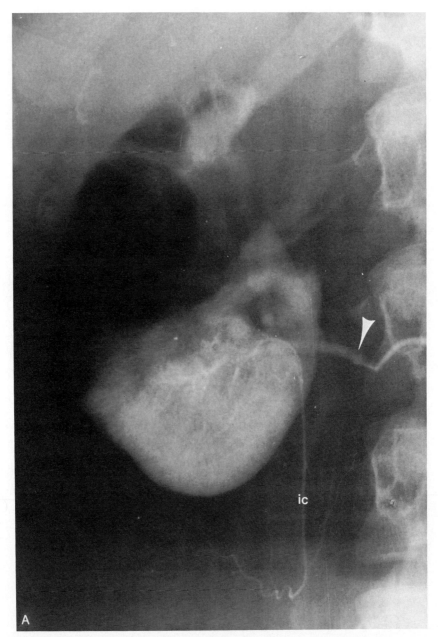

Figure 15–19. *A*, Capsular artery. Arteriogram of an aberrant lower pole artery (*arrowhead*) opacifies an inferior capsular artery (ic).

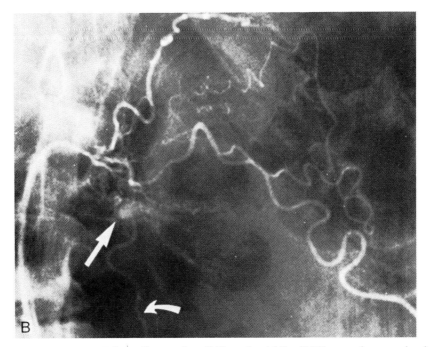

Figure 15–19. *B*, Enlarged superior (SC) and middle (MC) capsular arteries in another patient with atherosclerotic renal artery occlusion. Straight arrow points to reconstructed main renal artery. Curved arrow points to a ureteral artery. (From Kadir S: Diagnostic Angiography. Philadelphia, WB Saunders Company, 1986.)

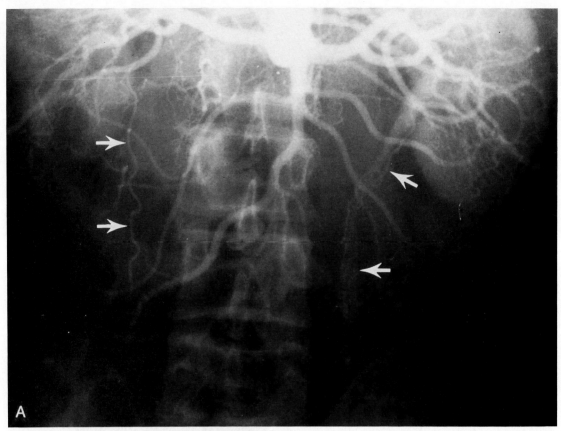

A

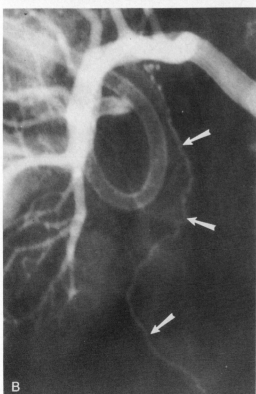

B

Figure 15–20. *Legend on opposite page.*

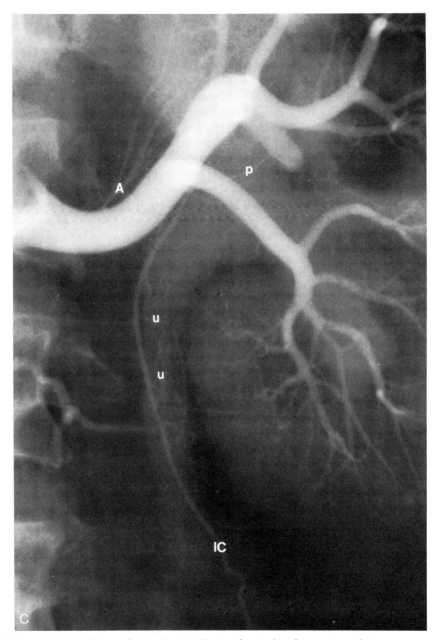

Figure 15–20. Ureteral arteries. *A,* Ureteral arteries demonstrated on a transaxillary aortogram in an individual with infrarenal aortic occlusion (*arrows*). *B,* Renal arteriogram shows an enlarged ureteral artery (*arrows*). *C,* Renal arteriogram from another individual shows ureteral arteries.

A	Inferior adrenal
IC	Inferior capsular
p	pelvic
u	ureteral

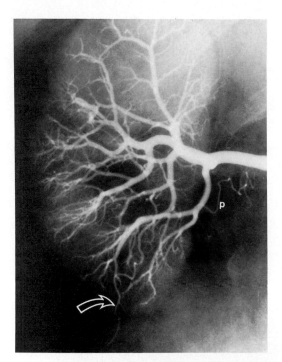

Figure 15–21. Perforating artery. Arteriogram shows a perforating artery (p) originating from a lobar artery (*arrow*). (From Kadir S: Diagnostic Angiography. Philadelphia, WB Saunders Company, 1986.)

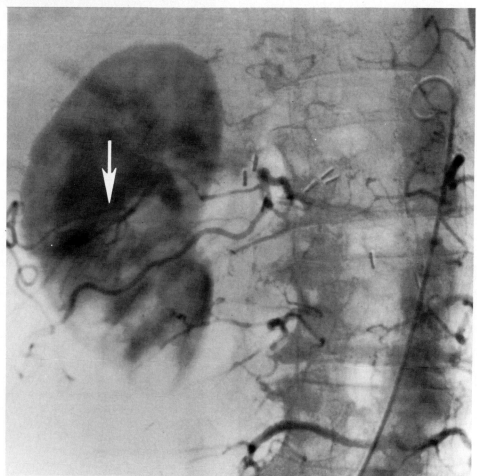

Figure 15–22. Perforating artery. Arteriogram shows a perforating artery (*arrow*) anastomosing with a lumbar artery. (From Kadir S: Diagnostic Angiography. Philadelphia, WB Saunders Company, 1986.)

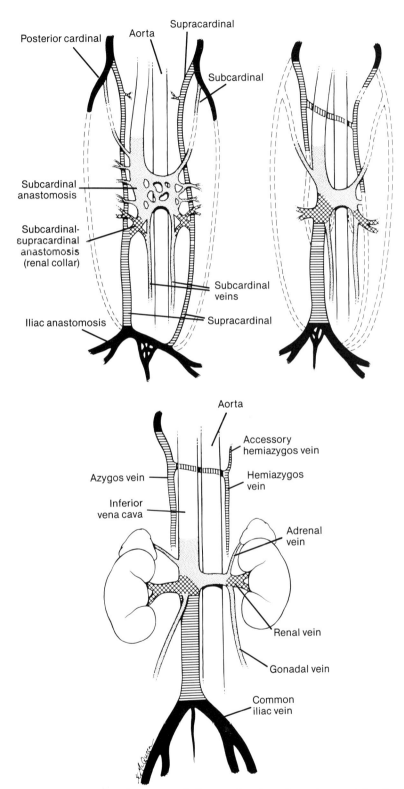

Figure 15–23. The development of the renal, adrenal, and gonadal veins and inferior vena cava.

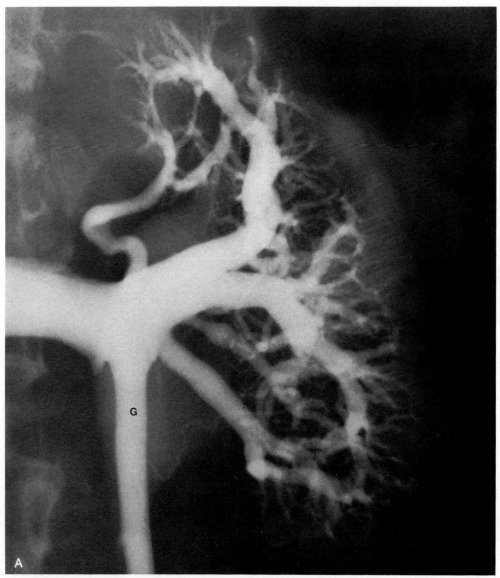

Figure 15–24. Renal veins. *A* and *B*, Retrograde renal venograms from two different individuals. In *B*, there is an upper pole renal cyst.

A   Adrenal
G   Gonadal

Illustration continued on opposite page.

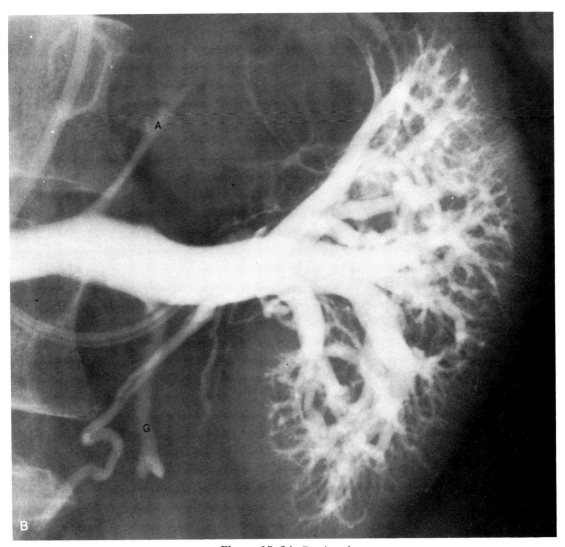

Figure 15–24. *Continued.*

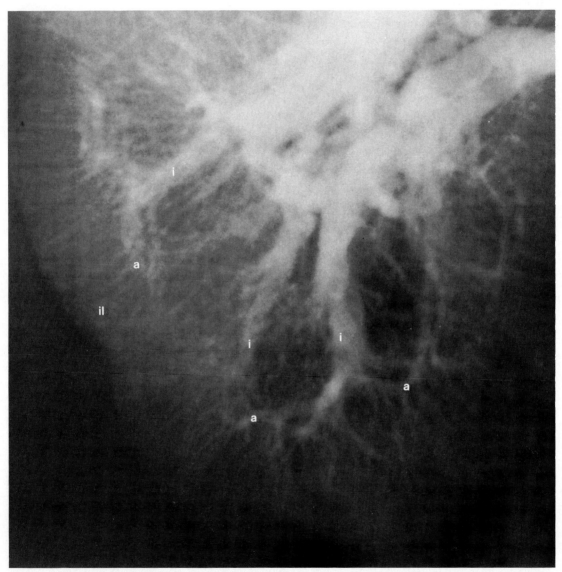

Figure 15–25. Intrarenal veins. Retrograde renal venogram shows the smaller renal vein tributaries.

a	Arcuate
i	Interlobar
il	Interlobular

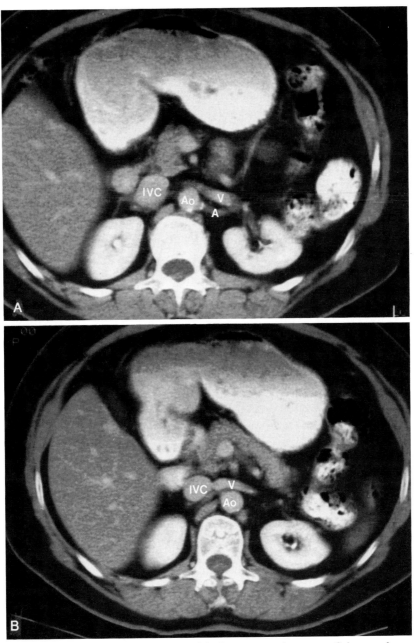

Figure 15–26. CT scans show relationship between and course of the renal artery and vein. (Courtesy of Dr. Cirrelda Cooper.)

A   Renal artery
Ao   Aorta
IVC Inferior vena cava
V   Renal vein

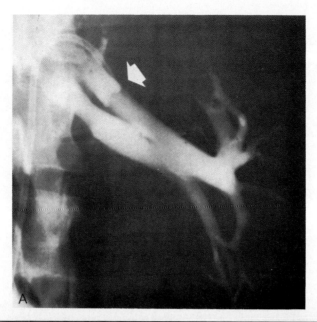

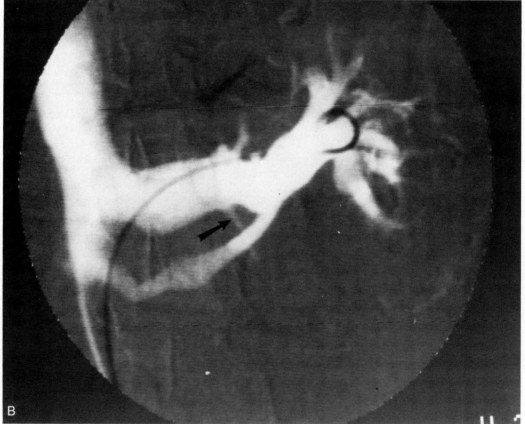

Figure 15–27. *Legend on opposite page.*

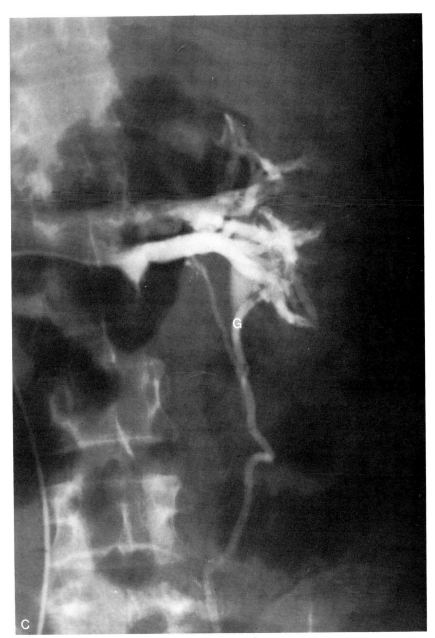

Figure 15–27. Duplicated left renal vein. *A*, Retrograde left renal venogram shows a duplicated vein with demonstration of venous valves (*arrow*). (From Kadir S, Athanasoulis CA: *In* Athanasoulis CA, et al: Interventional Radiology. Philadelphia, WB Saunders Company, 1982.) (Courtesy of Dr Carl Beckmann, Boston, MA.) *B*, Digital subtraction venogram shows a duplicated left renal vein. The gonadal vein joins the upper limb (*arrow*). *C*, Two left renal veins join before entering the inferior vena cava. G = Gonadal vein entering intrarenal branch.

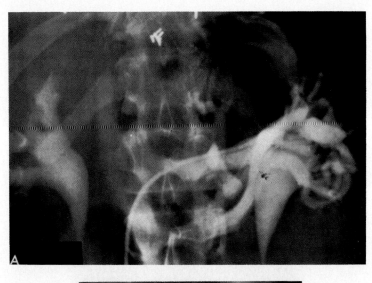

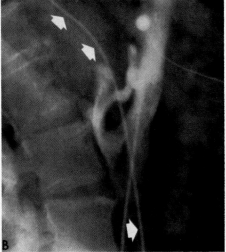

Figure 15–28. Circumaortic renal vein. *A*, Retrograde venogram opacifies two veins. The lower retroaortic vein joins the cava at a lower level. The catheter lies in the upper vein. *B*, Lateral view of a left renal venogram in another patient demonstrates the circumaortic venous ring. Arrows point to the aortic catheter. (From Kadir S, Athanasoulis CA: *In* Athanasoulis CA, et al: Interventional Radiology. Philadelphia, WB Saunders Company, 1982.)

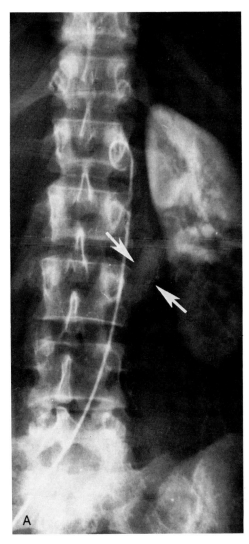

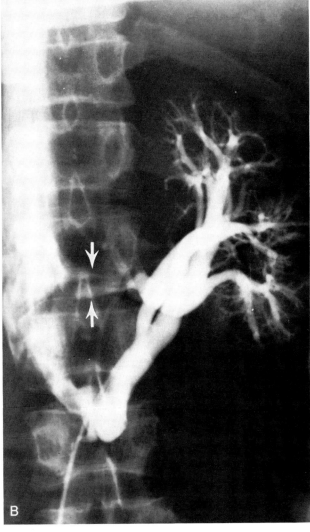

Figure 15–29. Retroaortic left renal vein. *A,* Venous phase of aortogram shows typical inferior course of the retroaortic left renal vein (*arrows*). *B,* Circumaortic left renal vein with the retroaortic component representing the major vein. The superior preaortic vein is small (*arrows*).

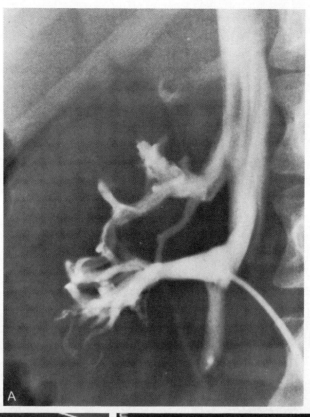

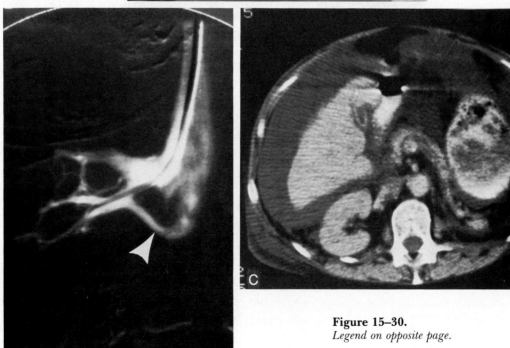

Figure 15–30.
Legend on opposite page.

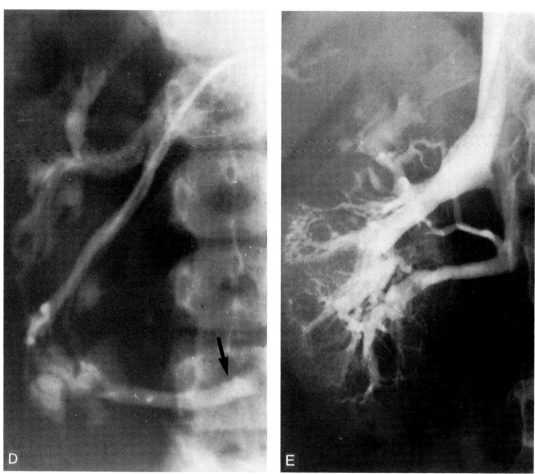

Figure 15–30. Duplicated right renal vein. *A*, Retrograde venogram via lower vein. There are multiple intrarenal connections and a large extrarenal connection. (From Kadir S, Athanasoulis CA: *In* Athanasoulis CA, et al: Interventional Radiology. Philadelphia, WB Saunders Company, 1982.) *B*, Digital subtraction venogram in another individual shows a smaller inferior channel (*arrowhead*). *C*, The computed tomogram from the patient shown in *B*. This was interpreted as showing a renal vein thrombus. *D*, Retrograde venogram in an individual with crossed renal ectopia. The lower vein (*arrow*) joins the lower inferior vena cava. The catheter enters the upper vein. *E*, Venogram from another individual. The lower vein enters the cava separately.

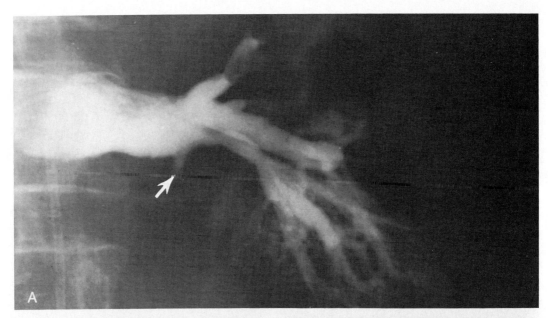

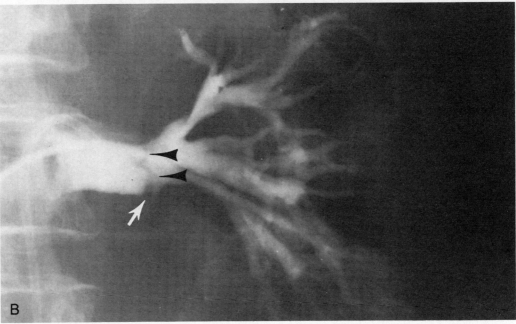

Figure 15–31. Renal vein valves. *A,* Renal vein valve leaflets are not seen during the early phase of contrast injection. Arrow points to gonadal vein. *B,* Black arrowheads point to valves. White arrow points to inflow of unopacified blood from gonadal vein.

Chapter Sixteen

ADRENALS

BENT MADSEN, M.D.

EMBRYOLOGY

The adrenal arteries develop from three mesonephric vessels near the first and second lumbar segments. By the sixth week, when the kidney has ascended to its definite position, the inferior adrenal artery becomes the renal artery but continues to furnish branches to the inferior portion of the adrenal gland. As the diaphragm develops, the superior adrenal artery or one of its branches forms the inferior phrenic artery but still supplies the superior portion of the adrenal gland.

INFERIOR ADRENAL ARTERIES (Figs. 16–1 to 16–5)

The right renal artery provides an adrenal branch in 81 per cent and the left in 60 per cent of individuals. In cases with multiple renal arteries, adrenal branches occur more frequently (right: 88 per cent; left: 62 per cent) and usually originate from the most cranial and occasionally from the second renal artery but never from a third or fourth renal artery or from a renal artery originating below the level of the second lumbar vertebra.

Only one third of the inferior adrenal arteries arise directly from the renal arteries. Two thirds are indirect; that is, they originate from either a superior capsular (Fig. 16–1), apical segmental renal branch (Fig. 16–2), or inferior phrenic artery (Fig. 16–3) arising from the main renal artery. Small direct adrenal branches may originate anywhere from the main renal artery, from its hilar divisions, or from an interlobar artery as a perforating branch to the adrenal gland (Figs. 16–4 and 16–5). Such direct inferior adrenal arteries are frequently less than 0.5 mm in diameter, whereas renal capsular arteries that provide adrenal branches measure between 1 and 2 mm in diameter.

The majority of adrenal branches, especially the larger arteries, originate from the main renal artery within 30 mm of its origin from the aorta, often very close to the orifice or from the renoaortic junction.

MIDDLE ADRENAL ARTERIES (Figs. 16–6 to 16–8)

Autopsy studies show that the right adrenal gland receives middle adrenal arteries from the aorta in 55 per cent and the left in 74 per cent, while a middle adrenal artery from the celiac or superior mesenteric artery occurs less frequently (Table 16–1). A very infrequent origin of the middle adrenal artery is from the right first lumbar or from the testicular artery.

Apart from small middle adrenal arteries originating from the aorta, larger arteries are found, which, in addition to the adrenal gland, also supply the superior renal capsule (Fig. 16–6) and sometimes a small segment of the kidney (Fig. 16–7). Such arteries measure approximately 1 mm in diameter and have been demonstrated at autopsy in 31 per cent of cases on the right and in 56 per cent on the left. Middle adrenal arteries originating directly from the aorta usually are too small for selective catheterization, unless they are enlarged owing to a tumor in the adrenal gland.

Middle adrenal arteries usually originate from the lateral aspect of the aorta at the level of the lower half of T_{12} to L_1. They occur usually less than 15 mm and never more than 30 mm above the cranial border of the renal artery. Occasionally, middle adrenal arteries may originate from the aorta below the origin of the renal arteries.

SUPERIOR ADRENAL AND INFERIOR PHRENIC ARTERIES (Figs. 16–9 to 16–14)

The inferior phrenic arteries always give off the superior adrenal arteries, which may originate from the proximal part and/or from the posterior branch. The largest adrenal branches arise from the proximal part, whereas those originating from the posterior branch of the inferior phrenic artery are minute, sometimes even too small to be identified on the arteriograms. Frequently, the superior adrenal arteries supply only a small area located in the cranial portion of the gland, but sometimes a larger portion or even the entire adrenal gland. In the latter case, a superior renal capsular branch is also present (Fig. 16–9).

The origins of the inferior phrenic arteries are shown in Table 16–2. In approximately one third of the cases they arise as a common trunk from the

TABLE 16–1. Location of the Origins of Middle Adrenal Arteries in Autopsy Studies

	Aorta	Celiac	Superior Mesenteric
Right	55%	1.2%	1.4%
Left	74%	5.4%	2.8%
No. of bodies studied	427	411	211

TABLE 16–2. Location of the Origins of Inferior Phrenic Arteries in Autopsy Studies

	Aorta	Celiac	Left Gastric	Renal
Common trunk	18.6%	13.4%		
Independent right and left	13.4%	18.3%		
Right	16.2%	7.6%		
Left	11.7%	18.9%		
Total right	48.2%	39.3%	3.1%	7.6%
Total left	43.7%	50.6%	4.1%	0.9%
No. of bodies studied	975	943	635	848

aorta or from the celiac artery (Fig. 16–10). If the right and left inferior phrenic arteries have independent origins, they may both arise from either the aorta or celiac artery, or one from the aorta and the other from the celiac artery. The diameter of the common trunk averages 2.5 mm (range 1.4 to 3.2 mm), whereas the inferior phrenic artery with an independent origin has an average diameter of 2.2 mm (range 1.2 to 2.8).

The origin of inferior phrenic arteries from the aorta is usually at the level of T_{12} or the upper half of L_1 (range: T_9 to L_2). Usually they originate from the ipsilateral wall of the aorta, sometimes from the anterior wall, or even from the contralateral side.

Inferior phrenic arteries originating from the celiac artery may arise from the proximal celiac artery close to the aorta or less frequently with independent origins of the left and right inferior phrenic arteries from the common hepatic and/or the splenic artery (Fig. 16–11). The left gastric artery originating from the aorta may also give off the inferior phrenic artery in 80 to 88 per cent of the cases and sometimes a small left middle adrenal branch (Fig. 16–12).

Origin of the right inferior phrenic artery from the right renal artery occurs in 8 per cent and rarely from the superior mesenteric artery (Fig. 16–8). Frequently it supplies the entire right adrenal gland and provides an apical segmental renal artery (Fig. 16–3). The left inferior phrenic artery may arise as a branch of the left renal artery in approximately 1 per cent of the cases. Very rarely, a right inferior phrenic artery may originate from the left renal artery (Fig. 16–13). In some cases, two inferior phrenic arteries are present on the same side, and they may both participate in adrenal supply.

The inferior phrenic arteries are easily recognized on angiograms from their characteristic cranial course alongside the spine, followed by division into anterior and posterior branches to the diaphragm. The left inferior phrenic artery is frequently seen to deliver small esophageal and gastric branches and may communicate with the internal mammary artery (Fig. 16–14). The right inferior phrenic artery represents an important collateral pathway to the liver if the hepatic artery is occluded.

COMBINATIONS OF ARTERIES SUPPLYING THE ADRENAL GLAND

In an autopsy study Busch (1954) established seven types of adrenal supply from one to three sources, i.e., aorta and renal and inferior phrenic arteries (Table 16–3). At angiography it is difficult to catheterize more than two sources

TABLE 16–3. Combinations of Adrenal Supply in 93 Cases Studied by Busch in 1954

Combination	Type	Side	Frequency in per cent
Renal, aorta and inferior phrenic	I	Right	33.3
		Left	33.3
Aorta and inferior phrenic	II	Right	16.1
		Left	36.6
Renal and inferior phrenic	III	Right	43.0
		Left	24.7
Renal and aorta	IV	Right	1.1
		Left	2.2
Renal	V	Right	3.2
		Left	0
Aorta	VI	Right	0
		Left	2.2
Inferior phrenic	VII	Right	3.2
		Left	1.1

owing to the small size of middle adrenal arteries, if these do not provide renal capsular branches. On the right side selective examination therefore usually corresponds to type III, and on the left side to type II. Other combinations of adrenal supply, not mentioned by Busch, include origin of middle adrenal arteries from the celiac or superior mesenteric artery.

ADRENAL VEINS

The anatomy of the adrenal veins is very constant. A single adrenal vein is present on each side in most individuals. It is formed by intraglandular branches that communicate with each other. It also collects blood from adrenal capsular, renal capsular, and retroperitoneal veins and the inferior phrenic vein on the left side.

RIGHT ADRENAL VEIN (Fig. 16–15)

The right adrenal vein is a short (1 to 5 mm) trunk that is between 1.5 and 2 mm in diameter. The venous hilum is located at the anterior surface of the gland, above its midpoint. The vein takes a short craniad-medial directed course and joins the inferior vena cava on the posterolateral aspect. The location of the orifice is, on the average, 45 mm above the right renal vein (range 20 to 60 mm), at the level of the twelfth rib (between 1 cm above and 1.5 cm below the rib).

Anatomic variations include the following:

1. An accessory hepatic vein joins the adrenal vein to form a common trunk. This is observed in approximately 10 per cent of individuals.

2. An accessory adrenal vein from the inferomedial pole of the gland. This was observed by Clark (1959). It joins the renal vein or, less frequently, the inferior vena cava.

LEFT ADRENAL VEIN (Figs. 16–16 to 16–18)

The left adrenal vein exits the adrenal gland from the anterior surface, near the inferomedial pole. It courses to the renal vein in a caudad and slightly medial direction. The length averages 18 mm (range 4 to 41 mm), and the diameter is between 2 and 4 mm. The orifice is located in the cranial wall of the renal vein, on average 35 mm from the inferior vena cava (range 20 to 50 mm). The adrenal vein is joined by the inferior phrenic vein 15 to 20 mm from the gland, and the length of the common trunk may vary from 1 to 31 mm. The inferior phrenic vein may run separately to the renal vein and, in rare instances, the adrenal vein may be joined by another small retroperitoneal vein.

Variations are rare and include the following:

1. An additional adrenal vein, joining the renal vein.
2. An accessory vein communicating with the renal capsular veins.
3. The inferior phrenic, adrenal, and testicular veins form a common trunk, which opens into the inferior vena cava. The renal vein joins the inferior vena cava more caudally than usual (Field and Saxton, 1974).

Two additional variations that I have observed are the following:

4. A normal adrenal gland with two adrenal veins. One drained directly into the inferior vena cava 1 cm proximal to a normally positioned renal vein. The other joined the renal vein in the usual place and received a renal capsular vein to form a short common stem. Selective injection of the contrast medium in either adrenal vein resulted in filling of the other adrenal vein as well as the inferior phrenic vein through anastomoses. The inferior phrenic vein drained unexpectedly to the caudal aspect of the renal vein (Fig. 16–17).
5. In another patient with a Cushing adenoma, three adrenal veins were present. The largest entered the inferior vena cava approximately 5 cm proximal to the renal vein. It was also joined by the inferior phrenic vein as well as a retroperitoneal vein, which connected it to the inferior vena cava midway between the adrenal and renal veins. Contrast injection into the second adrenal vein, which entered the renal vein, demonstrated the presence of yet another slender third adrenal or adrenal capsular vein, which entered the renal vein a few millimeters further medially (Fig. 16–18).

Knowledge of these variations in normal anatomy is important, as they may influence not only the catheterization of adrenal veins but also results from blood-sampling for hormonal assay.

REFERENCES

1. Anson BJ, Cauldwell EW: The pararenal vascular system. A study of 425 anatomical specimens. Q Bull Northw Univ Med School 21:320, 1947.
2. Anson BJ, Cauldwell EW, Pick JW, Beaton LE: The blood supply of the kidney, suprarenal gland, and associated structures. Surg Gynecol Obstet 84:919, 1947.
3. Arey LB: Developmental Anatomy. 7th ed. Philadelphia, WB Saunders Company, 1965, p 519.
4. Busch W: Die arterielle Gefässversorgung der Neben nieren (Zugleich ein Beitrag zur Anatomie der Nierenarterien). Z Mikrosk Anat Forsch 61:159, 1955.
5. Clark K: The blood vessels of the adrenal gland. J R Coll Surg Edinb 4:257, 1959.
6. Gagnon R: The arterial supply of the human adrenal gland. Rev Canad Biol 16:421, 1957.
7. Gagnon R: Middle suprarenal arteries in man: A statistical study of two hundred human adrenal glands. Rev Canad Biol 23:461, 1964.

8. Gérard G: Contribution a l'étude morphologique des artères des capsules surrénales de l'homme. J Anat (Paris) 49:269, 1913.

9. Kahn PC: Selective angiography of the inferior phrenic arteries. Radiology 88:1, 1967.

10. Madsen B: Selective adrenal angiography. A study of adrenal and related arteries in normal and pathological conditions. Vols 1 & 2 FADL's Forlag, Kobenhavn Århus. Odense, 1980.

11. Merklin RJ, Michels NA: The variant renal and suprarenal blood supply with data on inferior phrenic, ureteral and gonadal arteries. A statistical analysis based on 185 dissections and review of the literature. J Int Coll Surg 29:41, 1958.

12. Merklin RJ: Arterial supply of the supra-renal gland. Anat Rec 144:359, 1962.

13. Pick JW, Anson BJ: The inferior phrenic artery: Origin and suprarenal branches. Anat Rec 78:413, 1940.

14. Field S, Saxton H: Venous anomalies complicating left adrenal catheterization. Br J Radiol 47:219, 1974.

15. Joffre F, Carcy JB, Putois J, Suc JM, Conte J: La phlebographie surrenalienne. Ann Radiol 14:709, 1971.

16. Johnstone FRC: The suprarenal veins. Am J Surg 94:615, 1957.

17. McLachlan MSF, Roberts EE: Demonstration of the normal adrenal gland by venography and gas insufflation. Br J Radiol 44:664, 1971.

18. Merklin RJ, Eger SA: The adrenal venous system in man. J Int Coll Surg 35:572, 1961.

19. Mikaelsson CG: Venous communications of the adrenal glands. Acta Radiol 10:369, 1970

Figures 16–1 through 16–18 on following pages.

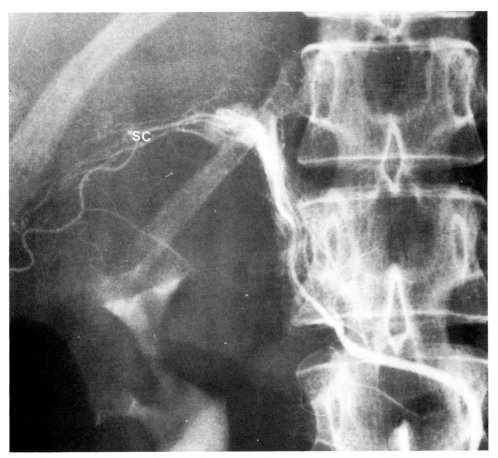

Figure 16–1. Right inferior adrenal/superior capsular artery, arising from the proximal right renal artery close to its origin from the aorta. There is a dense adrenal stain. SC = Superior capsular branches.

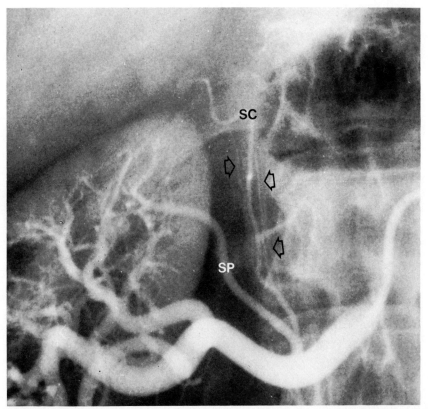

Figure 16–2. Aberrant superior polar renal artery providing inferior adrenal (*open arrows*) and superior capsular branches.

SC   Superior capsular branches
SP   Aberrant superior polar renal artery

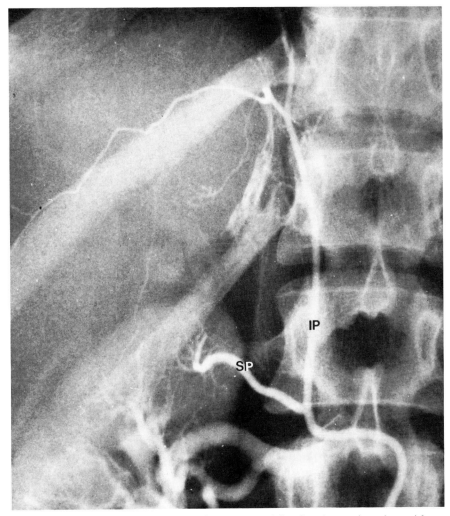

Figure 16–3. Right inferior phrenic artery, originating in conjunction with an aberrant superior polar renal artery, both of which provide adrenal branches.

IP   Inferior phrenic
SP   Superior polar renal

Figure 16–4. Subtraction right renal arteriogram shows multiple inferior adrenal arteries. Arrowheads point to branches arising from the distal main renal and the proximal segmental renal arteries. (From Kadir S: Diagnostic Angiography. Philadelphia, WB Saunders Co., 1986.)

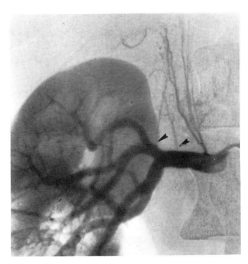

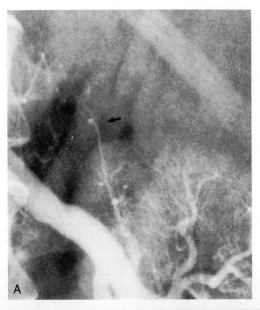

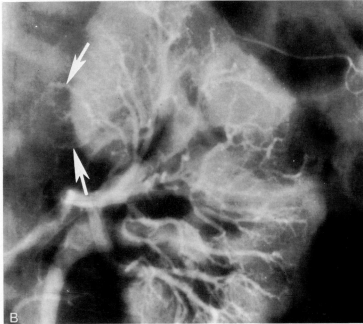

Figure 16–5. Perforating adrenal branch (*A*) from an interlobar renal artery (*arrow*). *B*, Two branches (*arrows*) from an interlobar artery in a patient with an adrenal tumor.

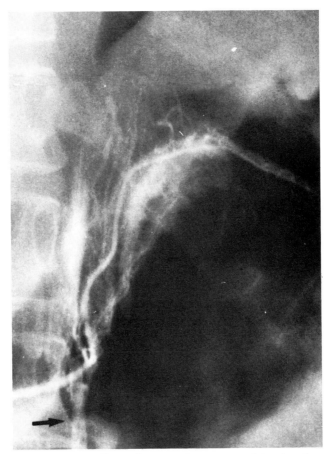

Figure 16–6. Middle adrenal/superior capsular artery, originating from the lateral aspect of the aorta. There is opacification of the adrenal vein (*arrow*).

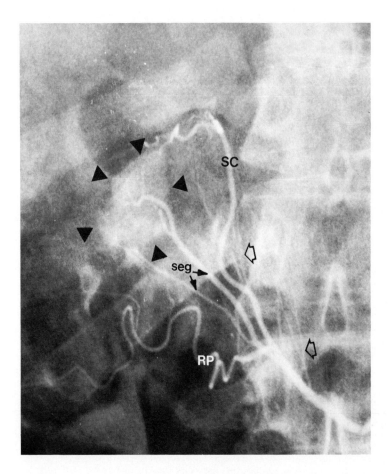

Figure 16–7. Common trunk of a middle adrenal/renal capsular/apical segmental artery. Accumulation of contrast material in a small segment of the right kidney parenchyma (*arrowheads*). Open arrows point to adrenal branches.

RP Retroperitoneal branch
SC Superior capsular branch
seg Apical segmental renal
       artery branches

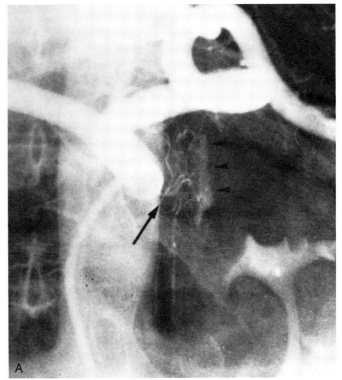

Figure 16–8. *A*, Left middle adrenal artery (*arrow*), originating from the celiac trunk, verified through accumulation of contrast material in the adrenal gland (*arrowheads*). *B*, Inferior phrenic artery (*large arrow*) originating from the superior mesenteric artery. The adrenal gland (*open arrow*) is opacified via superior adrenal arteries (*arrowheads*).

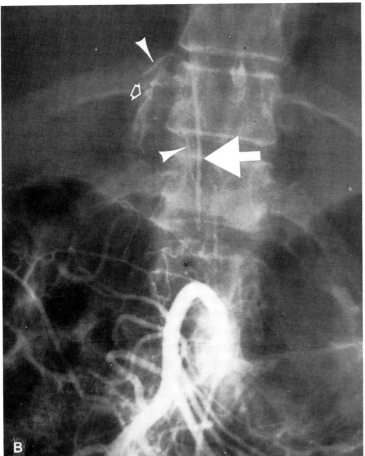

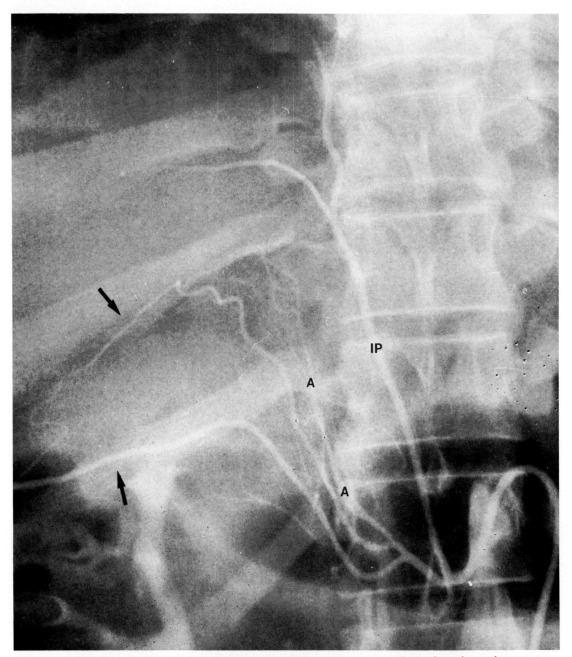

Figure 16–9. Right inferior phrenic artery, furnishing a complete adrenal supply as well as superior capsular arteries (*arrows*).

A   Adrenal branches
IP   Inferior phrenic artery

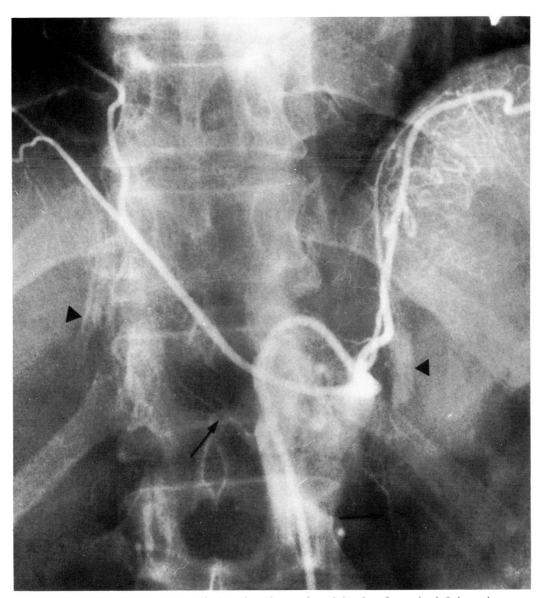

Figure 16–10. Common inferior phrenic trunk, originating from the left lateral aspect of the aorta. Adrenal supply is verified through accumulation of contrast material in both adrenal glands (*arrowheads*) as well as retrograde filling through peripheral anastomoses of the middle adrenal artery bilaterally (*arrows*).

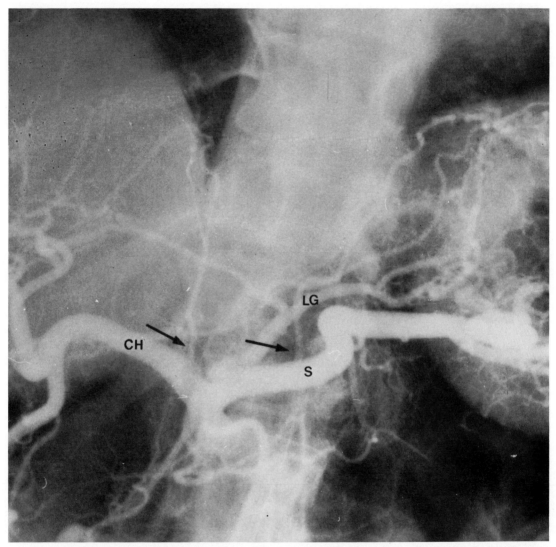

Figure 16–11. Inferior phrenic arteries (*arrows*) with independent origins from common hepatic and splenic artery.

CH Common hepatic
LG Left gastric
S Splenic

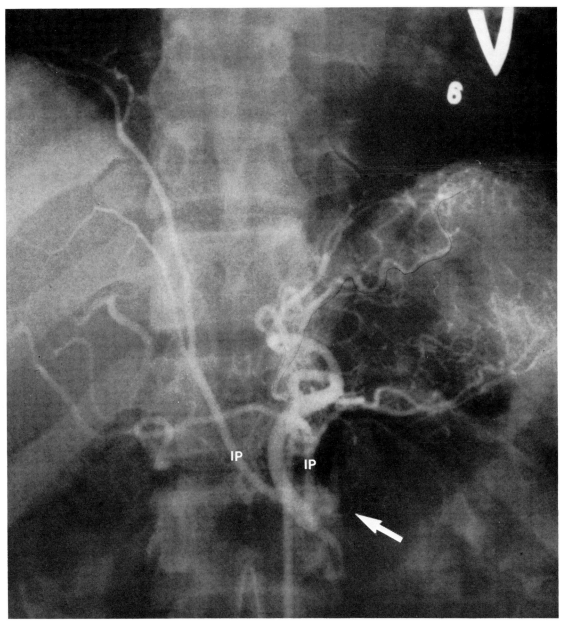

Figure 16–12. Left gastric artery branching directly from the aorta and furnishing a left middle adrenal artery (*arrow*) as well as right and left inferior phrenic arteries (IP).

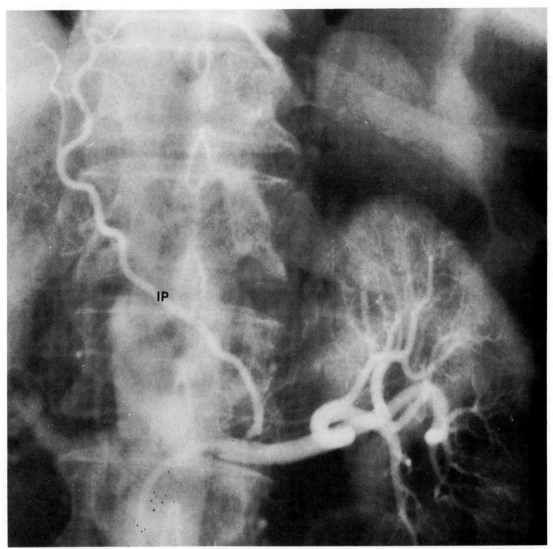

Figure 16–13. Right inferior phrenic artery originating from the left renal artery. Supply to the left adrenal gland from the main trunk (seen on later films) to the right adrenal gland from the posterior branch of the right inferior phrenic artery (IP).

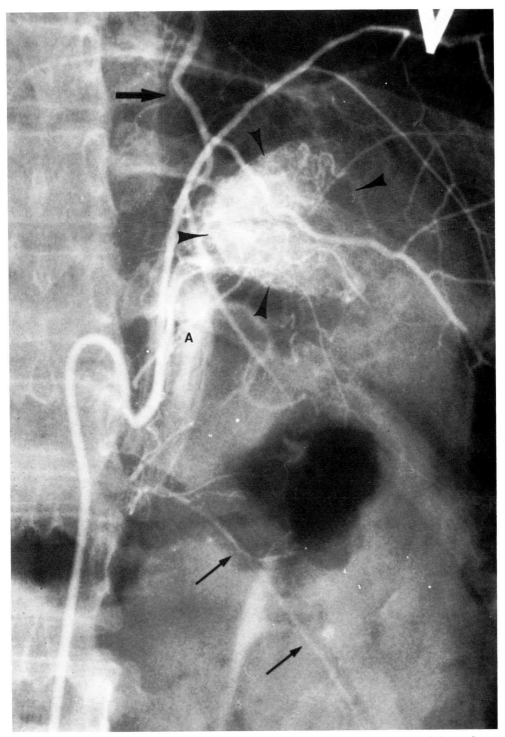

Figure 16–14. Left inferior phrenic arteriogram demonstrates accumulation of contrast material in adrenal gland (A) and gastric mucosa (*arrowheads*) and filling of internal mammary artery (*large arrow*) and subcostal artery (*long arrows*) through anastomoses.

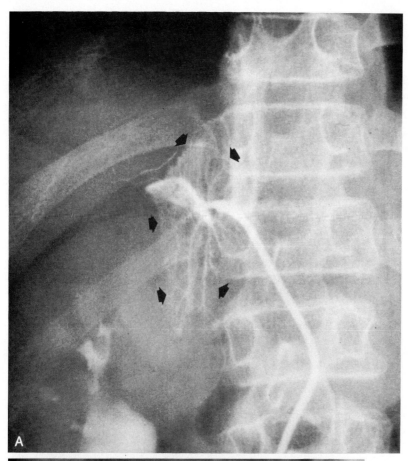

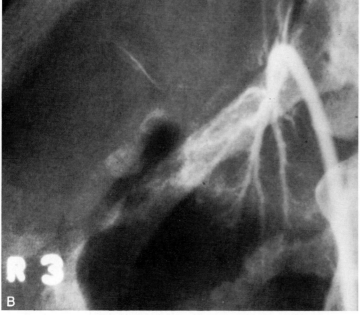

Figure 16–15. *A*, Right adrenal venogram shows the typical location of the adrenal vein orifice in the inferior vena cava at the cranial border of the twelfth right rib. Arrows outline the adrenal gland. *B*, Right adrenal venogram from another individual. (*B* From Kadir S: Diagnostic Angiography. Philadelphia, WB Saunders Company, 1986.)

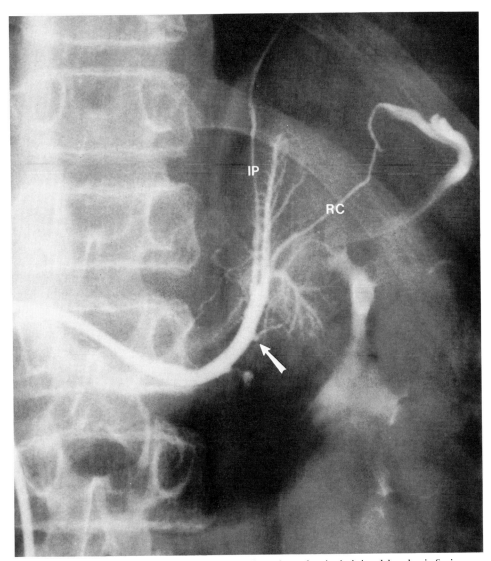

Figure 16–16. Left adrenal venogram. The adrenal vein is joined by the inferior phrenic as well as a small renal capsular vein. Typical location of the orifice in the cranial wall of the renal vein, just lateral to the spine. A small accessory adrenal vein joins the inferior phrenic–adrenal trunk (*arrow*).

IP   Inferior phrenic
RC   Renal capsular

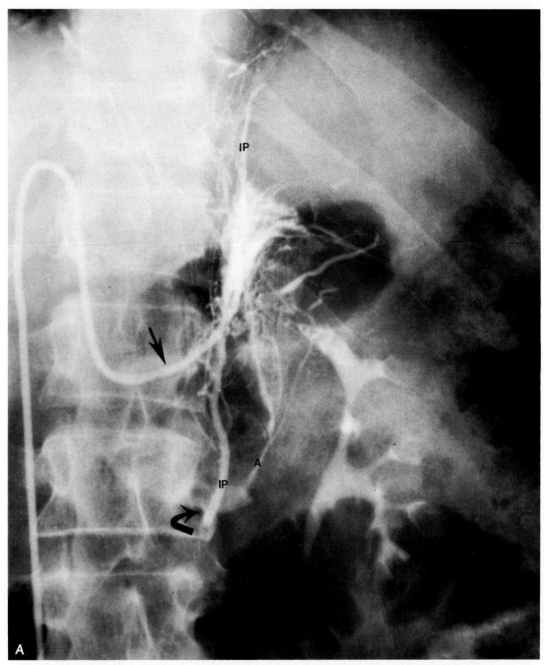

Figure 16–17. Two left adrenal veins. *A,* Contrast injection into the upper adrenal vein, which enters the inferior vena cava directly (*straight arrow*). There is opacification of the inferior phrenic vein, atypically joining the caudal aspect of the renal vein (*curved arrow*), and of a caudal adrenal vein, joining the renal vein. *B,* Contrast injection into the normally located lower adrenal vein shows that it is joined by renal capsular branches. The upper adrenal (*arrow*) and inferior phrenic veins are also opacified.

A   Adrenal vein
IP   Inferior phrenic vein
RC   Renal capsular branches

Illustration continued on opposite page.

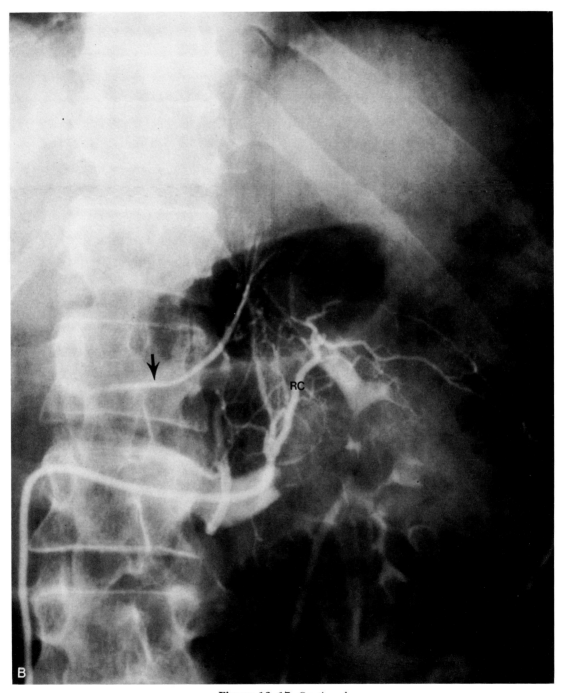

Figure 16–17. *Continued.*

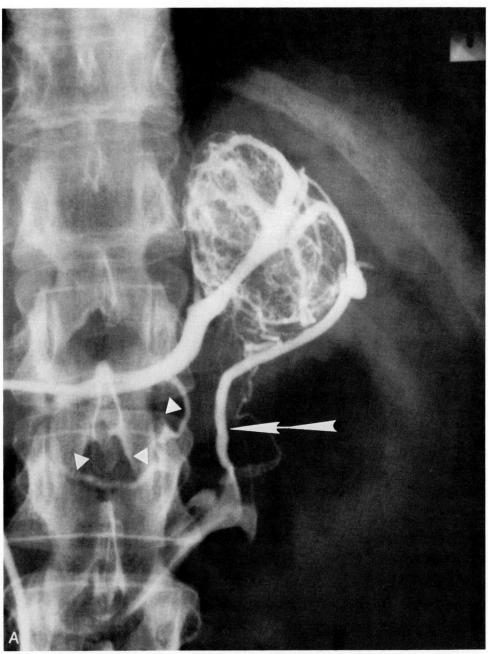

Figure 16–18. Three left adrenal veins. *A,* Contrast injection into the upper adrenal vein, which drains directly into the inferior vena cava. A lower adrenal vein (*arrow*) which joins the renal vein and a small retroperitoneal vein (*arrowheads*) which join the inferior vena cava are also seen. *B,* Contrast injection into the lower adrenal vein demonstrates a renal capsular branch (*curved arrow*) and a third adrenal or adrenal capsular vein (*short thick arrows*), joining the renal vein (*thin arrow*) medial to the one injected. In addition, another branch is seen that connects the adrenal with the renal vein further laterally.

Illustration continued on opposite page.

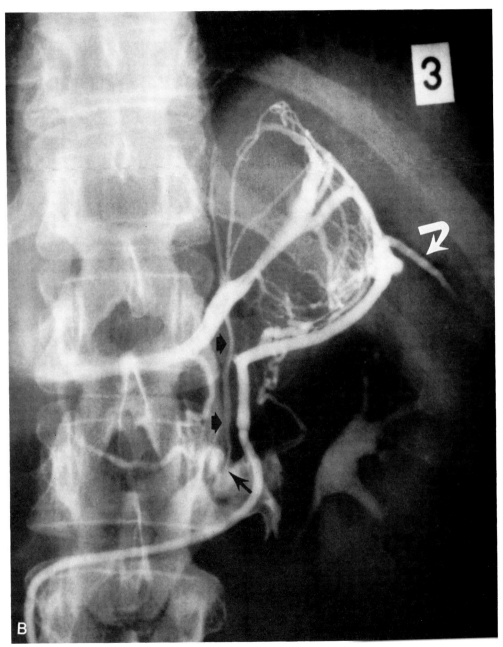

Figure 16--18. *Continued.*

Section V

ARTERIAL AND
VENOUS ANATOMY
OF THE HEAD

Chapter Seventeen

NEUROVASCULAR ANATOMY

MICHAEL F. BROTHERS, M.D.
WILLIAM PROTZER, M.D.

ARTERIAL ANATOMY

Carotid Artery (Figs. 17–1 to 17–8, Tables 17–1 to 17–6)

The common carotid artery enters the neck from below in a neurovascular bundle contained within fascia with the vagus nerve and internal jugular vein. The common carotid bifurcates (Fig. 17–1) at a level that varies widely but usually occurs at vertebrae C_3–C_4 to C_5–C_6. Typically there are no branches of the common carotid, but occasionally the superior thyroid or ascending pharyngeal arteries may originate from the bifurcation region.

Beyond the bifurcation, the external carotid artery (ECA) usually lies anterior and medial to the internal carotid. The usual sequence of branching in ascending order is outlined in Table 17–1 (Figs. 17–2 and 17–3). Proximal branches course anteriorly and medially. The ECA trunk passes deep to the angle of the mandible and terminates within the parotid gland in two large divisions, the internal maxillary artery coursing anteromedially and the superficial temporal artery heading superiorly. Variations in branching are frequently seen. The superior thyroid, lingual, and facial arteries form common variant combinations in origin. The ascending pharyngeal (APh) and posterior auricular may each arise independently from the ECA or from the occipital artery (OCC). Rarely, the APh or OCC can arise directly from the internal carotid.

The internal carotid artery (ICA) ascends medial and then anterior to the internal jugular vein in the neck before entering the carotid canal of the petrous

TABLE 17–1. External Carotid Branches in Usual Order

Artery	Major Branches
Superior thyroid	Infrahyoid, superior laryngeal, sternomastoid, cricothyroid
Ascending pharyngeal	Pharyngeal, infratympanic, neuromeningeal
Facial	Submental, ascending palatine, tonsillar, angular
Lingual	Suprahyoid, linguals
Occipital	Communicating branch to vertebral artery; mastoid; meningeal
Posterior auricular	Stylomastoid, auricular, occipital
Superficial temporal	Transverse facial, zygomatico-orbital, middle temporal, frontal, parietal
Internal maxillary	
Mandibular segment	Anterior tympanic, deep auricular, middle meningeal, accessory meningeal, inferior alveolar
Pterygoid segment	Deep temporal, pterygoid, masseteric, buccal
Pterygopalatine segment	Posterior and superior alveolar, infraorbital, greater palatine, artery to foramen rotundum, vidian, pharyngeal, sphenopalatine

bone. There are normally no branches of the cervical ICA. Within the petrous bone it passes first vertically and then anteromedially. Three branches in the petrous portion are classically described but may be recognized angiographically only when they have hypertrophied to supply a hypervascular lesion (Table 17–2). The ICA exiting the carotid canal enters the cavernous sinus. Together with the distal intradural ICA, this portion is termed the "siphon" and has five segments (numbered from above downward) (Table 17–2) (Fig. 17–4A). There are several important extra- and intradural branches of the ICA in this region. They can form anastomoses with the ECA branches (Table 17–3). Branches of the meningohypophyseal trunk (MHT) and inferolateral trunk (ILT) are frequently recognized on routine angiography (Fig. 17–4B), particularly when they have been recruited to provide collateral blood supply in ECA or ICA occlusion. The origin of the ophthalmic artery (OA) marks the approximate exit of the ICA from the cavernous sinus into the subdural space. In 80 to 90 per cent of cases, this origin is intracavernous. On an AP projection, the posterior siphon lies medial while the most lateral part is anterior (where the ICA lies medial to the anterior clinoid process). Although the ECA does not participate in supply of the cerebral hemispheres in the normal state, both the ICA and the ECA normally supply the contents of the orbit (Table 17–4) (Fig. 17–5), the dura (Table 17–5), and some of the cranial nerves (Table 17–6).

TABLE 17–2. Internal Carotid Branches in Ascending Order by Segment

Segment	Branch
Cervical	None
Petrous	Caroticotympanic, periosteal, vidian

Siphon (extradural)–C_5	Meningohypophyseal trunk (MHT): basal tentorial
	        dorsal meningeal
	        inferior hypophyseal

–C_4	Inferolateral trunk (ILT): gasserian ganglion
	        foramen rotundum
	        free margin tentorial

–C_3	McConnell's capsulars (to sella)
–C_3–C_2	Ophthalmic
Siphon (intradural)–C_2	Superior hypophyseal
–C_1	Posterior communicating, anterior choroidal, bifurcation (anterior, middle cerebral)

Note: The MHT and ILT, usually not true "trunks," are composed of separate vessel origins closely situated.

TABLE 17–3. Anastomoses Between Intra- and Extracerebral Arteries

Parent Cerebral Vessel	Branch	Extracerebral Artery Anastomosing
Internal carotid	Caroticotympanic	Ascending pharyngeal
	Vidian	Internal maxillary
	Meningohypophyseal trunk	Middle, accessory meningeals; ascending pharyngeal
	Inferolateral trunk	Internal maxillary, accessory meningeal
	Ophthalmic	Facial, superficial, temporal, internal maxillary
Vertebral	Artery of first intervertebral space	Occipital
	C₃ branch	Ascending pharyngeal (musculospinal division)
	Odontoid arch branch	Ascending pharyngeal (neuromeningeal division)

TABLE 17–4. Arterial Supply to the Orbit

Parent Vessel	Branch
Internal carotid	Ophthalmic
External carotid	Infraorbital branch of internal maxillary
	Superficial temporal
	Angular branch of facial
	Lacrimal branch of middle meningeal
	Deep temporal branch of internal maxillary

TABLE 17–5. Major Arterial Supply of the Dura

Parent Vessel	Branch
Internal carotid	Meningohypophyseal trunk
	Inferolateral trunk
	Ophthalmic artery (anterior and posterior ethmoidal)
Posterior cerebral	Davidoff-Schechter (to tentorial apex)
Vertebral	Posterior meningeal
	Odontoid arch artery
External carotid	Ascending pharyngeal
	Occipital (mastoid branch)
	Middle meningeal
	Accessory meningeal

TABLE 17–6. Arterial Blood Supply of the Cranial Nerves

Nerve	Supply
I	Anterior cerebral;* anterior communicating*
II	Internal carotid;* anterior communicating;* anterior cerebral;* ophthalmic
III, IV, VI	Perforators* (from basilar and posterior cerebral); meningohypophyseal trunk
V	Basilar;* inferolateral trunk; middle meningeal (cavernous branch)
	Ascending pharyngeal; internal maxillary (foramen rotundum branch); accessory meningeal
VII	Basilar;* middle meningeal (petrosal branch); postauricular (stylomastoid branch); internal carotid (caroticotympanic); ascending pharyngeal (inferior tympanic)
IX–XI	Vertebral;* ascending pharyngeal (jugular branch)
XII	Vertebral;* ascending pharyngeal (hypoglossal branch)

Note: Vessels marked with an asterisk refer to the part of the nerve's blood supply in its subarachnoid portions.

TABLE 17–7. Some Vertebral Artery Variations

Left dominant
Right dominant
Hypoplasia, unilateral
Terminates in posterior inferior cerebellar artery
Vertebral artery duplication
Vertebral artery fenestration
Vertebrobasilar junction fenestration

Variant Anatomy of the Carotid Artery

1. Persistent carotid-vertebrobasilar fetal anastomoses (Fig. 17–6)
2. "Anomalous" ICA (Fig. 17–7)
3. Aplasia of the ICA (Fig. 17–8)
4. Anomalous origin of the OA from the middle meningeal artery, or vice versa.

Vertebral Artery (Figs. 17–9 and 17–10; Tables 17–7 and 17–8)

The vertebral artery enters the foramen transversarium usually at C_6 and ascends through to exit via the C_1 foramen, and then courses over the superior aspect of the posterior arch of C_1 to pass intradurally, medial to the capsule of the atlanto-occipital joint and then through the foramen magnum. The two vertebral arteries join to form the basilar artery anterior to the pontomedullary junction, although the exact level is variable (Fig. 17–9).

Variations in relative size of the vertebral arteries, as well as common anomalies, are described in Table 17–7 (variations in origin are discussed in Chapter 2). Branches of the vertebral arteries by region are listed in Table 17–8 (Figs. 17–9 and 17–10).

Arterial Supply of the Brain (Figs. 17–9 to 17–18; Tables 17–9 to 17–11)

The major arteries and their branches to the brain, brain stem, and cerebellum are described in Tables 17–9 and 17–10. Cerebral vessels may have branches of up to four types. These are (1) perforating (small, penetrating

TABLE 17–8. Important Branches of Vertebral Artery

Level	Branch
C_6–C_2 (variable)	Radiculomedullary branch to anterior spinal artery
C_2–C_1	Odontoid arch branch
C_1–vertebrobasilar junction	Posterior inferior cerebellar artery; posterior meningeal; anterior spinal artery (origin); perforators to brain stem

TABLE 17–9. Arterial Supply of the Cerebrum

Parent Vessel	Major Branches
Internal carotid	Posterior communicating
	Anterior choroidal
	Anterior cerebral
	Middle cerebral
	Perforators (at bifurcation)
Anterior cerebral	
A1	Anterior communicating artery
	Perforators (medial striate group)
	Heubner (recurrent artery)
A2	Pericallosal
Beyond	Frontopolar
	Orbitofrontal
	Callosomarginal
	Internal frontals (anterior, middle, posterior)
	Paracentral
	Internal parietals (superior, inferior)
Variants	"Azygos" anterior cerebral artery
	Triple pericallosal (a. medianis corporis callosi)
Middle cerebral	
M1	Perforators (lateral striate group)
	Cortical branches: orbitofrontal and/or temporopolar (variable)
M2/beyond	*Anterior division* (variable)
	Orbitofrontal, opercular, prerolandic, rolandic
	Posterior division (variable)
	Posterior parietal, angular, posterior temporal (temporopolar)
Posterior cerebral	
P1	Perforators (to brain stem); thalamoperforators
	Medial posterior choroidal; meningeal branch (Davidoff-Schechter)
P2	Thalamogeniculate; perforators (to brain stem)
Beyond	Lateral posterior choroidal
	Cortical trunks: anterior temporal
	parieto-occipital
	calcarine
	posterior temporal

deep structures), (2) cortical, (3) choroidal (ventricular), and (4) meningeal (dural). Thus, the anterior cerebral artery (ACA) has only perforating and cortical branches, whereas the ICA and posterior cerebral arteries (PCAs), for example, provide all four types of branches.

The ICA and basilar artery (BA) have important anastomoses in the suprasellar cistern, termed collectively the circle of Willis (Fig. 17–11). Each of

TABLE 17–10. Arterial Supply of the Posterior Fossa

Parent Vessel	Branch
Vertebral	Perforators (to brain stem)
	Anterior spinal artery
	Posterior inferior cerebellar artery
Basilar	Perforators
	Posterior cerebral artery
	Superior cerebellar artery
	Anterior inferior cerebellar artery

TABLE 17–11. Some Variations in Cerebellar Arteries

Duplicated superior cerebellar artery
   Unilateral
   Bilateral
Posterior cerebral artery origin from superior cerebellar artery
Absent posterior inferior cerebellar (with large AICA)
Absent anterior inferior cerebellar (with large PICA)

its components may be variable in size. There is normally a reciprocal relationship between the size of the posterior communicating and the ipsilateral P1 segment of the PCA.

Although the various cortical branches of the anterior, middle, and posterior cerebral arteries (Figs. 17–12 to 17–18) are variable in the pattern of branching proximally, their distal territories of supply are consistent. All three major cerebral arteries have been described in terms of numbered segments (Fig. 17–12). The proximal stem of the middle cerebral artery (MCA) is termed the M1 (sphenoidal) segment. The middle cerebral branches that have entered and course within the insular region are termed the M2 segments; those descending under the operculum, M3; and those terminal branches outside of the sylvian fissure, M4. Similarly, the ACA in its proximal, horizontal precommunicator portion is termed A1. The A2 segment is that portion beyond the anterior communicating artery (ACoA), usually termed the pericallosal artery. Segments 3 through 5 describe the more distal course in front of and above the corpus callosum. For the PCA segments (see Fig. 17–11), P1 connects the basilar termination with the posterior communicating artery (PComm); P2 is the portion in the perimesencephalic cistern beyond the PComm.

The posterior fossa neural structures (Table 17–10) (see Figs. 17–9 and 17–10) are supplied by the three long cerebellar arteries—superior cerebellar (SCA), anterior inferior cerebellar (AICA), and posterior inferior cerebellar (PICA)—and the numerous perforating branches arising along the course of the intracranial vertebral artery, the basilar artery, the proximal PCA, and the proximal long cerebellar arteries (see Figs. 17–9 and 17–10). There is great variability in the normal size and appearance of the long cerebellar arteries (Table 17–11). The perforating vessels, although in many cases not angiographically visible, are by comparison much more predictable and orderly in configuration anatomically.

TABLE 17–12. Dural Venous Sinuses

Superior sagittal
Inferior sagittal
Occipital
Transverse
Straight
Superior petrosal
Inferior petrosal
Sphenoparietal
Sigmoid
Cavernous

VEINS

Face and Neck (Fig. 17–19)

The extracranial facial system can be opacified on external carotid arteriography. The most important of these veins are illustrated in Figure 17–19. They drain via the external and internal jugular veins and have anastomoses with deep extra- and intracranial venous structures.

Cerebral Venous System (Figs. 17–18 to 17–20; Tables 17–12 and 17–13)

There are 10 commonly recognized, named dural sinuses (Table 17–12). Essentially all important cerebral venous drainage occurs via these sinuses (Figs. 17–19 and 17–20). The brain drains both centrifugally into the superficial system and centripetally toward the deep cerebral system.

The superficial veins are highly variable in size and location. Only three are frequently identified by name on routine angiography (Figs. 17–21 and 17–22): (1) the superficial middle cerebral veins in the sylvian fissure; (2) the superior anastomotic vein (Trolard) connecting the sylvian veins with the superior sagittal sinus over the parietal convexity; and (3) the inferior anastomotic vein (Labbé) connecting the sylvian veins with the transverse sinus over the posterior temporal region.

The deep system can be described schematically as follows (Figs. 17–23 to 17–25). The subependymal veins of the lateral ventricle drain via the ipsilateral thalamostriate vein. These join the septal vein at the foramen of Monro to form the internal cerebral veins (ICVs). The ICVs course posteriorly in the roof of the third ventricle on each side and the two then join with the basal vein of Rosenthal as well as a number of posterior fossa veins to form the vein of Galen (VOG). The VOG ascends a short distance to join the inferior sagittal sinus forming the straight sinus. The straight and superior sagittal sinuses join at the torcula to form a transverse sinus on each side, usually larger on the right. These course anterolaterally and become the sigmoid sinuses. They drain into the internal jugular veins. Usually the right jugular vein is larger (dominant).

The posterior fossa has no true deep venous system. Instead three superficial groups of veins (Figs. 17–26 to 17–28) are present (Table 17–13).

TABLE 17–13. Veins of the Posterior Fossa

Drainage To	Venous Inflow From
Vein of Galen	Precentral cerebellar vein
	Superior vermian vein
	Mesencephalic (posterior and lateral) veins
Petrosal (Superior or inferior petrosal sinuses)	Anterior pontomesencephalic vein
	Petrosal vein
Posterior (Straight, occipital and transverse sinuses)	Brachial vein
	Inferior vermian vein
	Inferior hemispheric vein

REFERENCES

1. Huber P, Krayenbuhl H: Cerebral Angiography, 2nd ed. Stuttgart, Thieme-Stratton, 1982.
2. Lasjaunias P, Berenstein A: Surgical Neuroangiography, Vol. 1: Functional Anatomy of Craniofacial Arteries. Berlin, Springer-Verlag, 1987.
3. Newton TH, Potts DG: Radiology of the Skull and Brain, Vol. 2, Book 2: Angiography. St Louis, CV Mosby, 1974.
4. Osborne AG: Introduction to Cerebral Angiography. Philadelphia, Harper & Row, 1980.

Figures 17–1 through 17–28 on following pages.

Figure 17–1. Lateral view on a common carotid arteriogram. Atherosclerotic stenosis at internal carotid origin *(arrow)* and siphon *(arrowhead)*.

CC   Common carotid
ECA   External carotid
FA   Facial
ICA   Internal carotid
IM   Internal maxillary
LA   Lingual
OCC Occipital
ST   Superficial temporal

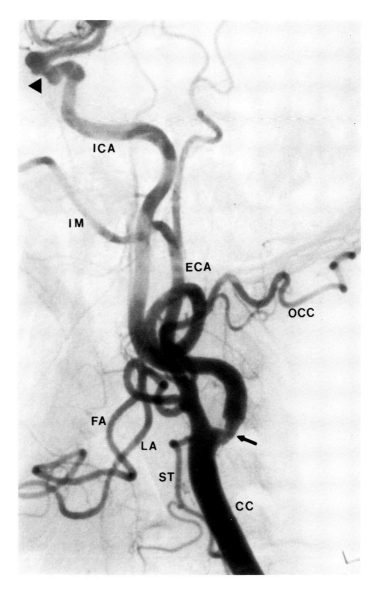

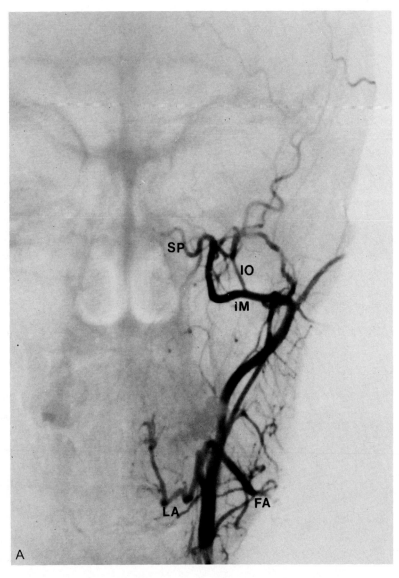

Figure 17–2. *A,* AP and *B,* lateral external carotid arteriograms showing all the branches.

AMA   Accessory
          meningeal artery
FA   Facial artery
IO   Infraorbital artery
LA   Lingual artery
MM   Middle meningeal
          artery
PAU   Posterior auricular
          artery
SP   Sphenopalatine
          artery

*Illustration continued
on following page*

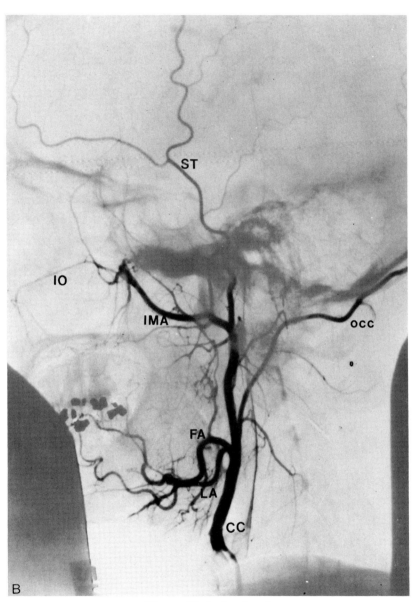

Figure 17–2. *Continued.*

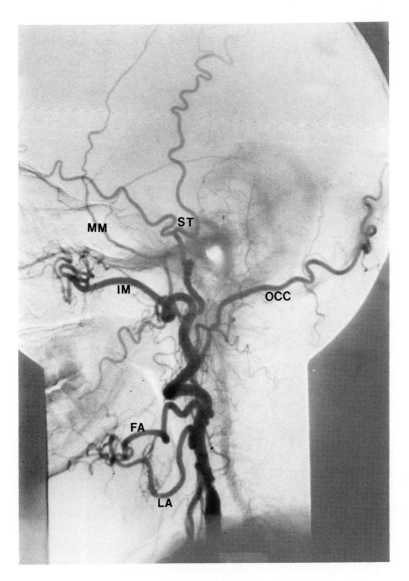

Figure 17–3. Lateral common carotid arteriogram in a patient with an internal carotid artery occlusion.

FA	Facial
IM	Internal maxillary
LA	Lingual artery
MM	Middle meningeal
OCC	Occipital
ST	Superficial temporal

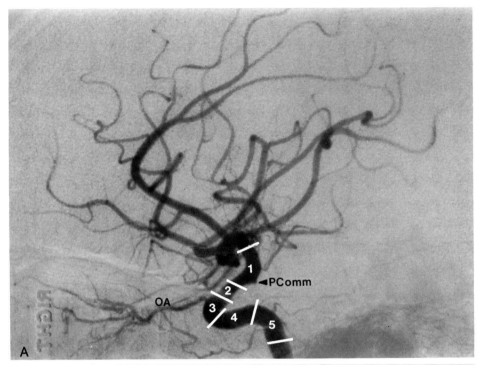

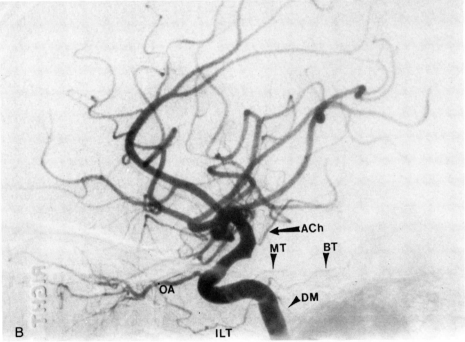

Figure 17–4. Lateral internal carotid arteriograms. *A,* Segments of siphon numbered from above downward (see text). *B,* Normal branches of the cavernous segment of the carotid artery.

ACh	Anterior choroidal	MT	Medial tentorial
BT	Basal tentorial	OA	Ophthalmic
DM	Dorsal meningeal	PComm	Posterior communicating
ILT	Inferolateral trunk		origin

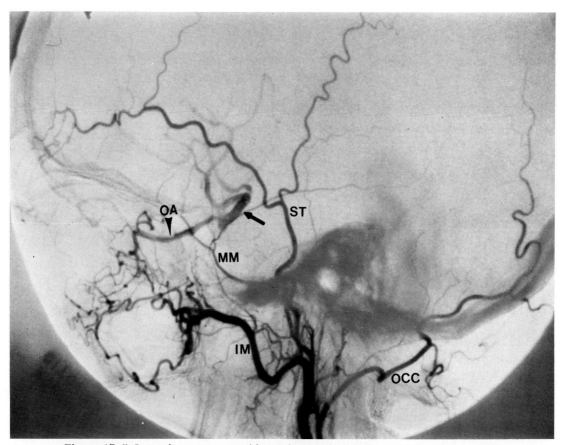

Figure 17–5. Lateral common carotid arteriogram in a patient with internal carotid occlusion. There is opacification of the supraclinoid carotid *(arrow)* via retrograde filling of the ophthalmic artery. The ophthalmic artery fills via anastomoses with several external branches around the orbit (superficial temporal and facial).

IM	Inferior maxillary
MM	Middle meningeal
OA	Ophthalmic
OCC	Occipital
ST	Superficial temporal

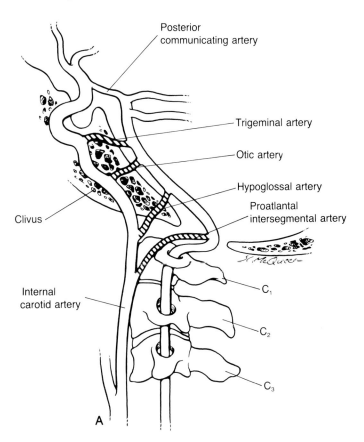

Figure 17–6. Persistent fetal carotid-vertebral anastomoses. *A*, Diagram showing the four variants. *B*, Persistent trigeminal artery *(arrow)*. This is by far the most common type seen at arteriography. On this vertebral artery injection, early filling of the carotid siphon *(arrowhead)* is seen where the trigeminal artery enters (C$_5$ portion).

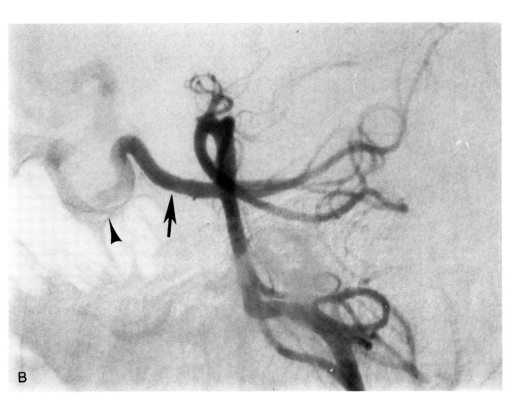

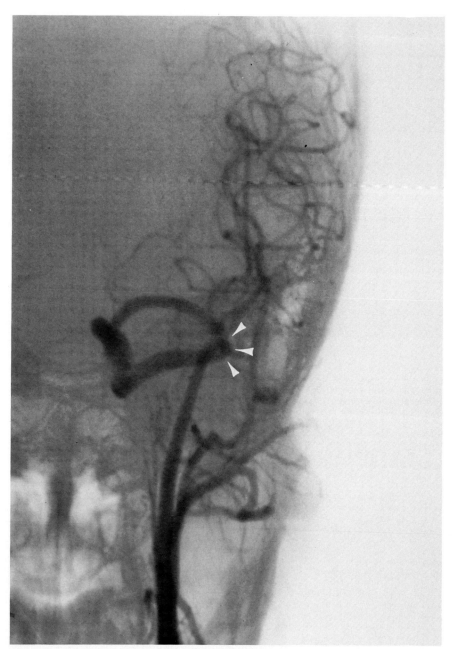

Figure 17–7. "Anomalous" course of internal carotid artery in the petrous bone. On anteroposterior view it extends further laterally than normal *(arrowheads),* often presenting in the middle ear cavity.

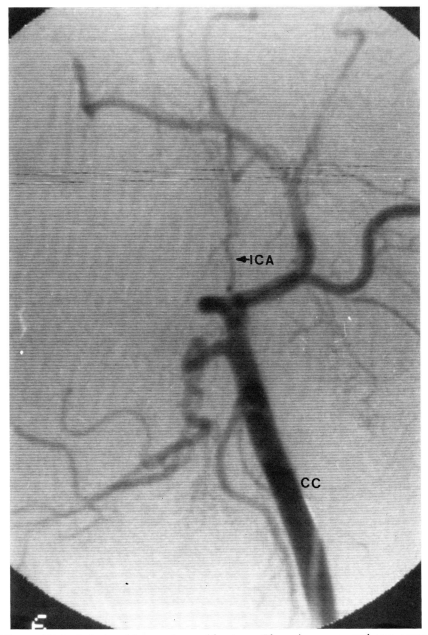

Figure 17–8. Aplasia of internal carotid artery. There is an unusual appearance of the junction of the common and external carotid arteries. In true aplasia, the carotid canal is absent.

ICA   Internal carotid (rudimentary)
CC   Common carotid

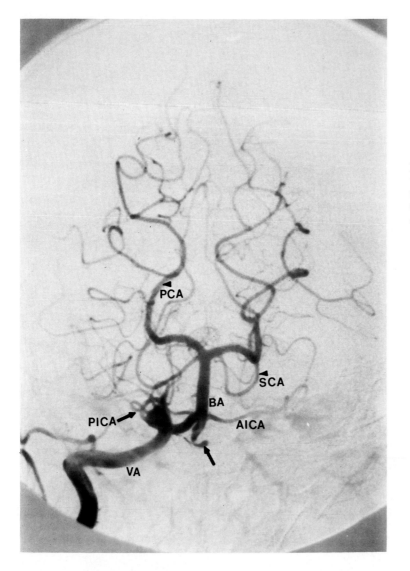

Figure 17–9. Anteroposterior view of a right vertebral arteriogram. Slight reflux down the left vertebral artery has occurred *(arrow)*.

AICA	Anterior inferior cerebellar artery
BA	Basilar artery
PCA	Posterior cerebral artery
PICA	Posterior inferior cerebellar artery
SCA	Superior cerebellar artery
VA	Vertebral artery

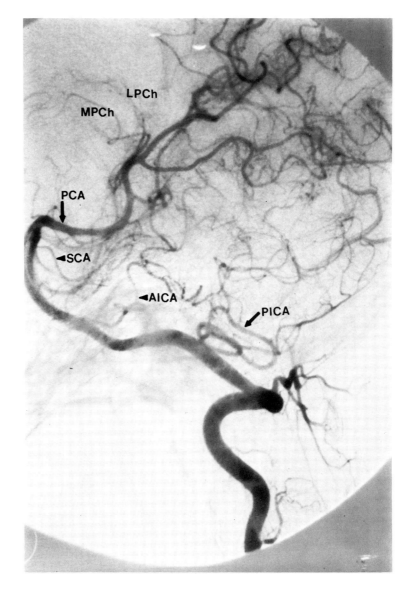

Figure 17–10. Lateral view of a left vertebral arteriogram.

AICA   Anterior inferior cerebellar artery

LPCh   Lateral posterior choroidal artery

MPCh   Medial posterior choroidal artery

PCA   Posterior cerebral artery

PICA   Posterior inferior cerebellar artery

SCA   Superior cerebellar artery

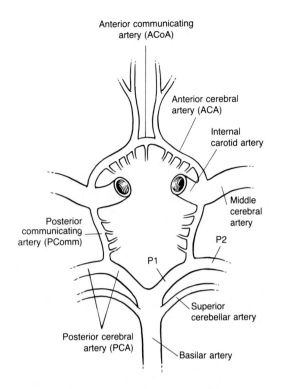

Figure 17–11. Circle of Willis and its variations. A complete intact circle occurs in less than 20 per cent of cases.

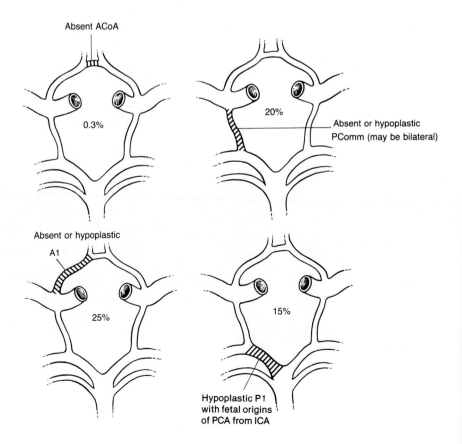

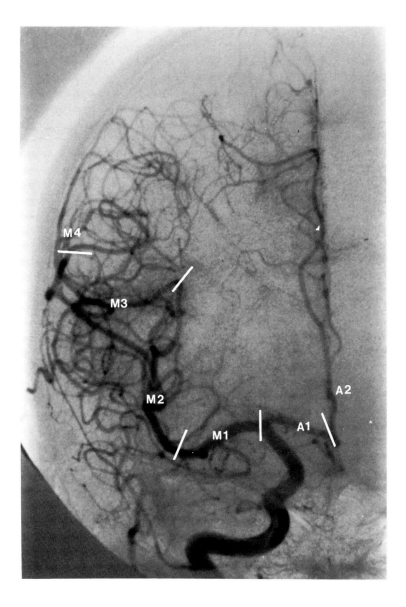

Figure 17–12. Anteroposterior view of a right common carotid arteriogram. The numbered segments of the anterior and middle cerebral arteries are identified (see text).

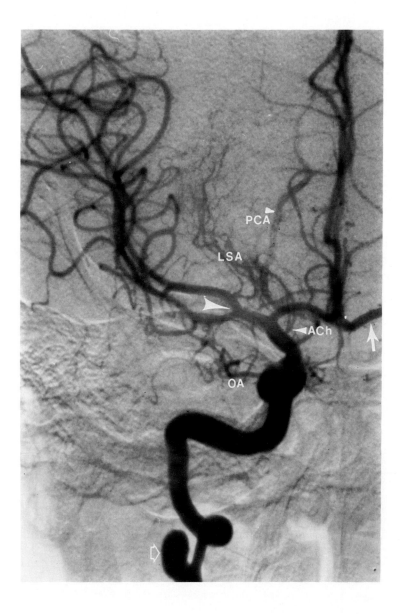

Figure 17–13. Anteroposterior view of a right common carotid arteriogram. The middle cerebral bifurcation *(arrowhead)* is seen and there is spontaneous cross-filling of the opposite anterior cerebral artery *(arrow)* through a patent anterior communicating artery; there is also faint filling of the ipsilateral posterior cerebral artery. The incidental presence of a traumatic pseudoaneurysm and stenosis of the internal carotid artery in the neck *(open arrowhead)* can also be seen.

ACh   Anterior cerebral
         artery
LSA   Lenticulostriate
         arteries
OA   Ophthalmic artery
PCA   Posterior cerebral
         artery

Figure 17–14. Lateral view of a right common carotid arteriogram. Aplasia of the ipsilateral A1 segment of the anterior cerebral artery is inferred, as only the middle and posterior cerebral arteries opacify. Note the large "fetal" type of posterior communicating artery (posterior cerebral origin) *(arrow)*. The middle cerebral artery bifurcates into an anterior *(small arrowhead)* and a posterior *(open arrow)* division. (Frequently, a trifurcation pattern is seen.) Some of the cortical branches of the middle cerebral artery are labeled as follows: 1, Orbitofrontal; 2, opercular; 3, rolandic; 4, angular; 5, posterior parietal.

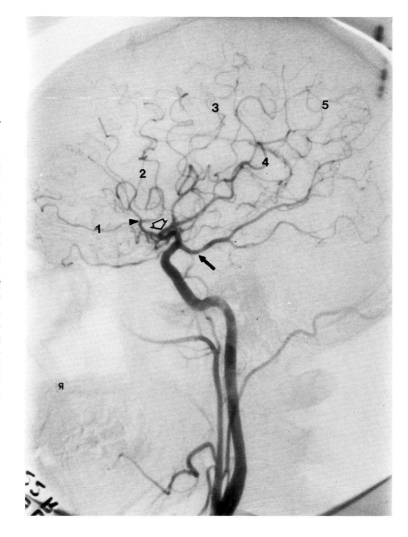

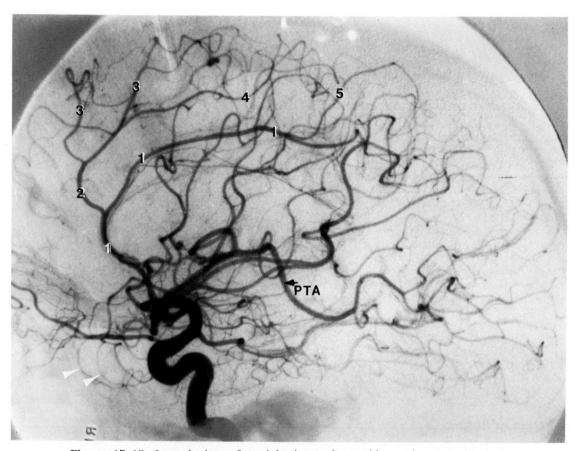

Figure 17–15. Lateral view of a right internal carotid arteriogram. Cortical branches of the anterior cerebral artery are demonstrated: 1, Pericallosal; 2, callosomarginal; 3, internal frontals; 4, paracentral; 5, internal parietals. Also well seen are the posterior temporal (PTA) and anterior temporal *(arrowheads)* branches of the middle cerebral artery.

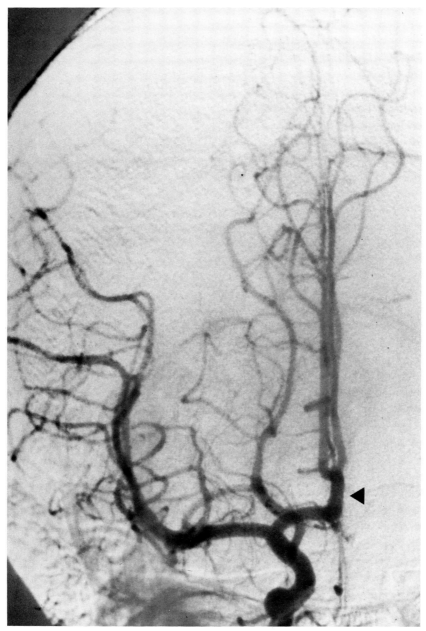

Figure 17–16. Azygos (undivided) anterior cerebral artery *(arrowhead)*. The single artery supplies both hemispheres and receives blood from both A1 segments.

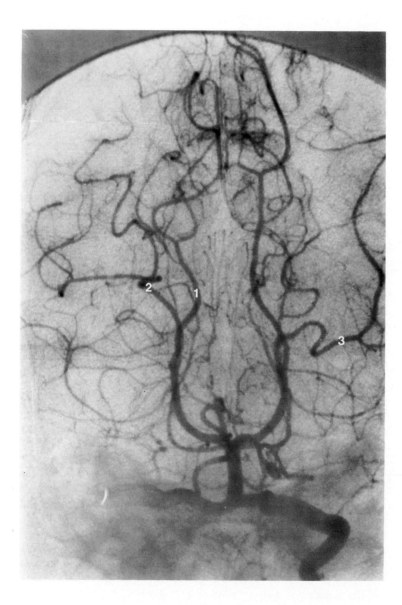

Figure 17–17. Anteroposterior Towne's view of a left vertebral arteriogram. Cortical branches of the posterior cerebral artery are seen: 1, Calcarine; 2, parieto-occipital; 3, posterior temporal.

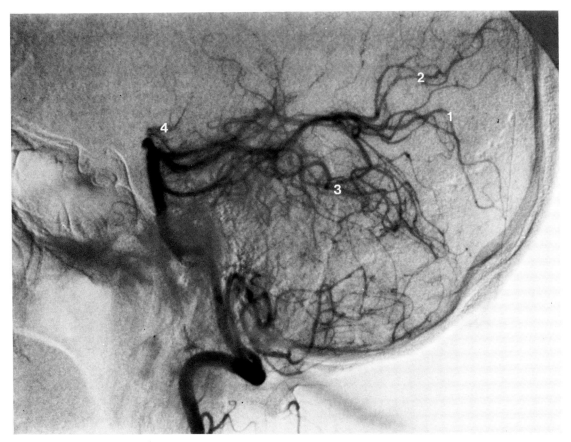

Figure 17–18. Lateral view of a left vertebral arteriogram showing the posterior cerebral artery branches: 1, Calcarine; 2, parieto-occipital; 3, posterior temporal; 4, thalamoperforators.

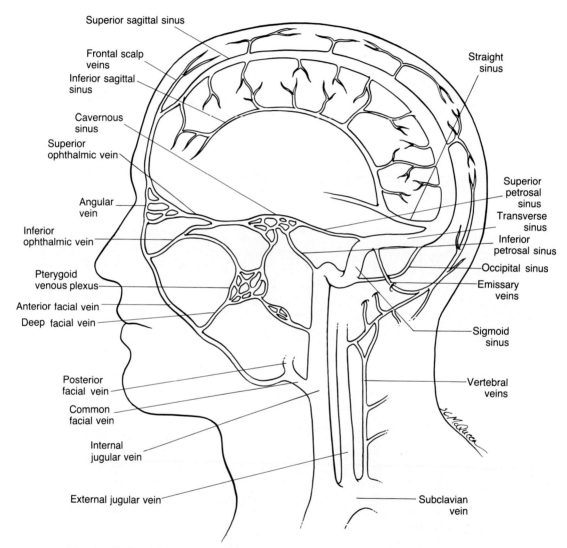

Figure 17–19. The extracranial facial venous system and its anastomoses with major dural sinuses.

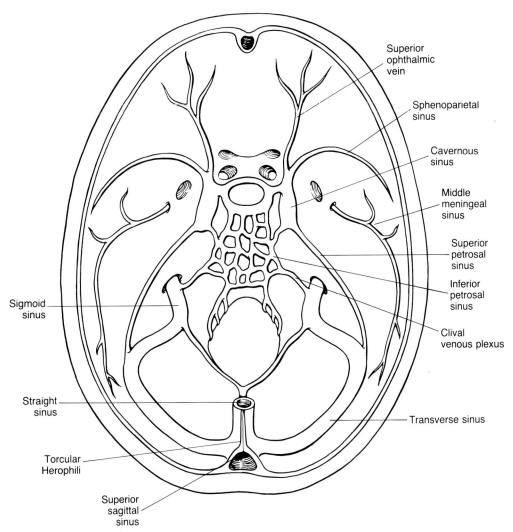

Figure 17–20. Intracranial aspect of the veins at the skull base, viewed from above, showing major dural sinuses and their anastomoses.

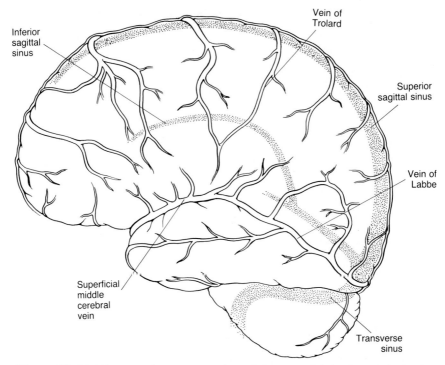

Figure 17–21. Diagramatic representation of the superficial veins of the brain.

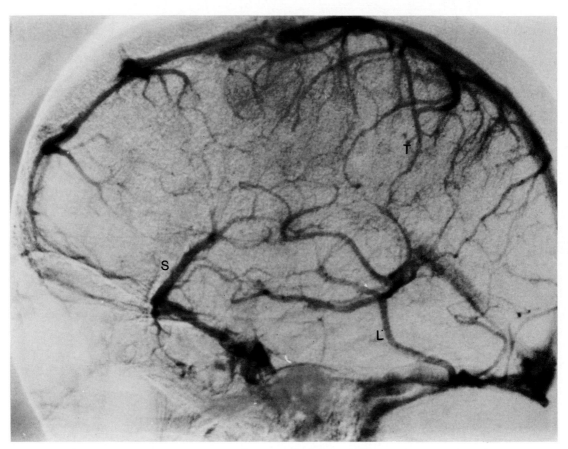

Figure 17–22. Venous phase of a lateral right carotid arteriogram: superior anastomotic vein of Trolard (T), inferior anastomotic vein of Labbé (L), and superficial sylvian veins (S).

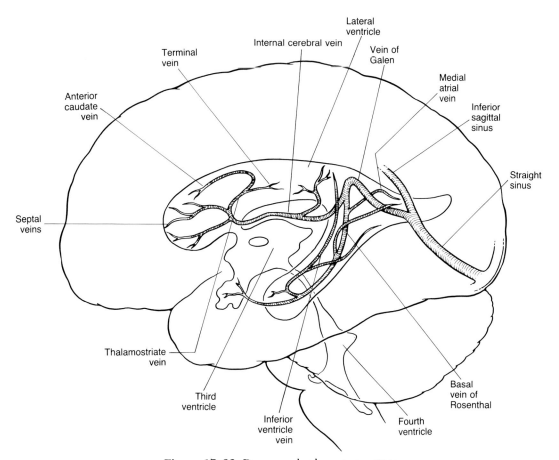

Figure 17–23. Deep cerebral venous system.

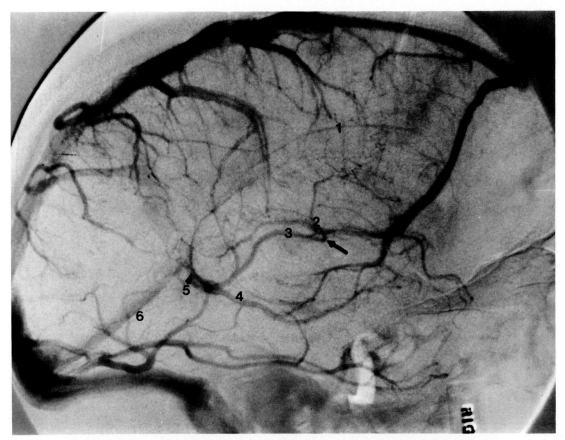

Figure 17–24. Venous phase of a lateral right carotid arteriogram: 1, Inferior sagittal sinus; 2, thalamostriate vein; 3, internal central vein; 4, basal vein of Rosenthal; 5, vein of Galen; 6, straight sinus. The "venous angle" *(arrow)* marks the position of the foramen of Monro, formed at the junction of the internal cerebral and thalamostriate veins.

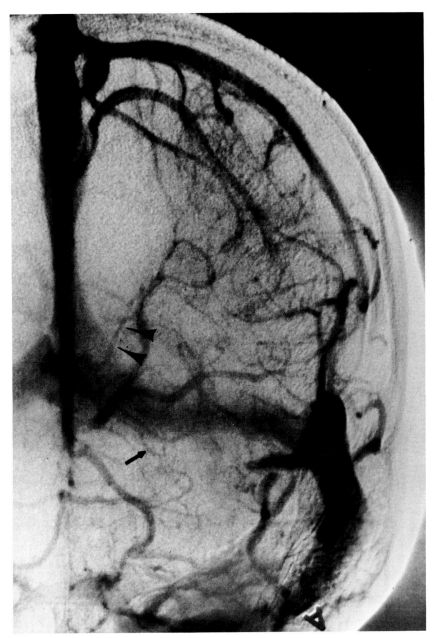

Figure 17–25. Anteroposterior view, venous phase, of a carotid arteriogram. The deep system, being mostly midline, is superimposed on itself. The basal vein of Rosenthal *(arrow)* and thalamostriate vein *(arrowheads)* are identifiable as paramedian.

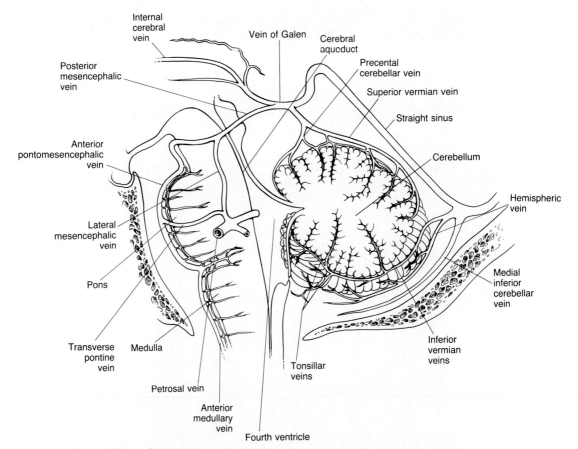

Figure 17–26. Schematic diagram of a posterior fossa venous system.

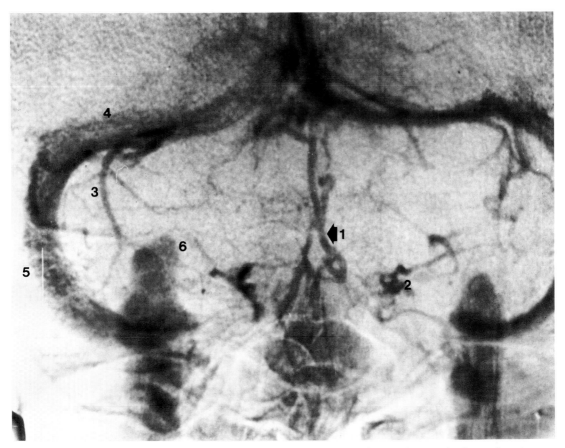

Figure 17–27. Anteroposterior Towne's view, venous phase, of a vertebral arteriogram. Precentral cerebellar vein (1), petrosal vein (2), cerebellar hemispheric veins (3), transverse sinus (4), sigmoid sinus (5), and jugular bulb (6). The right jugular bulb is unusually high-riding.

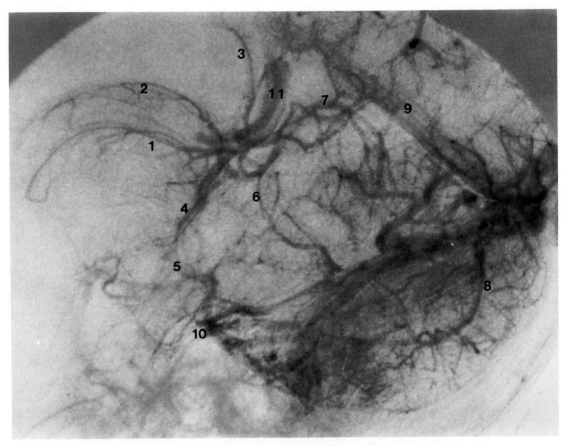

Figure 17–28. Venous phase of a lateral vertebral arteriogram. Internal cerebral vein (1), lateral choroidal plexus veins and blush (2), splenial veins (3), lateral pontomesencephalic vein (4), anterior pontomesencephalic vein (5), precentral cerebellar vein (6), superior vermian vein (7), inferior vermian vein (8), straight sinus (9), petrosal veins (10), and vein of Galen (11).

Section VI

THE LYMPHATIC SYSTEM

Chapter Eighteen

LYMPH VESSELS AND NODES

CAROLINE LUNDELL, M.D.
SAADOON KADIR, M.D.

EMBRYOLOGY

The exact origin of the lymphatic system remains in question. It is thought possibly to arise from capillary branches of the venous endothelium or from fusion of mesenchymal clefts. Probably the earliest precursors to the lymphatics are the six primary lymphatic sacs seen at the fifth to sixth week. These form the major regional lymphatics and include (1) paired jugular sacs (form lymphatics of head, neck, and upper extremities), (2) paired iliac sacs (form lymphatics of lower extremities and lower abdomen), (3) single retroperitoneal sac at the mesenteric root (forms lymphatics of the mesentery, celiac, and retroperitoneal organs), and (4) cisterna chyli (located posterior to the retroperitoneal sac). Lymphatic vessels develop from these lymphatic sacs predominantly along the major veins. Connections between the lymphatic vessels and adjacent veins may form and persist in the adult (lymphaticovenous communications). In addition, two large vessels develop anterior to the paired aorta and connect with the jugular lymph sacs and the cisterna chyli at about the seventh to eighth week. These become the right and left thoracic ducts; both may interconnect throughout their courses. The adult thoracic duct develops from the inferior part of the embryonic right duct, superior part of the left duct, and their anastomosis. Valves are present in the embryonic thoracic duct but are absent by birth. The superior portion of the cisterna chyli remains present in the adult.

Shortly after the lymphatic vessels are formed, the lymph nodes begin to develop from the lymphatic sacs, predominantly adjacent to the lymphatic sacs and along the major lymph vessels. At birth, the final lymph node components are present except for the differentiation of the germinal centers from primary to secondary lymph nodules; this occurs around birth. The lymphocytes in the lymph nodes at birth are derived from the thymus.

LYMPHATICS OF THE LOWER EXTREMITIES (Figs. 18–1 to 18–3).

The lymphatics of the lower extremities are divided into two systems: (1) a superficial prefascial group that drains the skin and subcutaneous tissue and (2) a deep subfascial group that drains the muscles and joints. Valves direct flow from the deep to superficial lymph systems; usually no interconnection is present between the superficial groups.

In the legs, two groups of superficial lymphatic vessels are present and include (1) a medial set that courses adjacent to the greater saphenous vein and (2) a lateral set that follows the lesser saphenous vein. The medial group consists of five or six vessels in the anteromedial aspect of the lower leg and 10 to 20 vessels in the thigh. The medial group also has an anterolateral component that consists of five or six vessels along the lateral leg which crosses medially at the knee to follow the greater saphenous vein, then joins the superficial inguinal lymph nodes. The lateral set consists of one to three vessels that terminate in subfascial lymph nodes in the popliteal region.

The popliteal lymph nodes predominantly drain into the deep inguinal nodes via subfascial vessels, which course along with the major vessels in the medial thigh. The popliteal nodes are small and located in the popliteal fossa; they drain the lesser saphenous vein territory, knee joint, and area adjacent to both tibial vessesls. A few popliteal nodes drain into the superficial inguinal lymph nodes.

The inguinal lymphatics are divided into superficial and deep groups. The inferior superficial inguinal lymph nodes are seen on lymphangiography and are located around the hiatus for the saphenous vein; they receive all of the superficial lower extremity lymph except for the posterior and lateral calf. One of the most constant and largest inguinal lymph nodes is the node of Rosenmüller located medial to the common femoral vein. The superior superficial group drains the gluteal region, part of the anterior abdominal wall below the umbilicus, the external genitalia, the inferior anal canal, and the uterus. The deep inguinal lymph nodes are located along the medial aspect of the femoral vein and receive drainage from the deep lymphatic vessels that course close to the femoral vessels.

LYMPHATICS OF THE PELVIS AND ABDOMEN (Figs. 18–4 and 18–5)

The lymphatics of the pelvis are divided into three groups based on their proximity to the iliac vessels and include (1) external iliac, (2) internal iliac (hypogastric), and (3) common iliac lymphatic chains. The external iliac chain is further subdivided into lateral, middle, and medial lymph nodes. The internal iliac chain is further divided into parietal and visceral groups; neither group fills on pedal lymphangiography. The parietal group consists of superior and inferior gluteal, sacral, and obturator lymph nodes. The visceral group drains the bladder, rectum, prostate, uterus, and ovaries. Efferent lymphatics of the internal iliac chain drain into the common iliac and para-aortic lymph node groups. The common iliac chain is a direct continuation of the three external iliac lymphatic groups and continues into the para-aortic region.

The lumbar lymphatics course along the anterior aspect of the lumbar vertebra surrounding both abdominal aorta and inferior vena cava and can be divided into (1) para-aortic and (2) paracaval lymph node chains. The para-aortic group directly drains the common iliac chains and represents the most consistent and largest group of lymph nodes seen on a bipedal lymphangiogram. Contrast filling of the para-aortic lymph nodes is more frequent than of the paracaval group and reaches the L_1 level in about 50 per cent, the L_2 level in 40 per cent, and the L_3 level or below in 10 per cent. Contralateral lymphatic filling at the L_4–L_5 level is seen in about 50 per cent of normal lymphangiograms and occurs more often from left to right.

Three major divisions of the para-aortic group are present, which include the (1) preaortic, (2) lateral aortic, and (3) retroaortic lymph nodes. The preaortic group is located anterior to the abdominal aorta and drains the major viscera supplied by anterior aortic branches, i.e., celiac and mesenteric lymph node groups. The celiac group is the terminal lymph node group for the stomach, duodenum, liver, gallbladder, pancreas, and spleen; it is subdivided into gastric, hepatic, and pancreaticosplenic lymph node groups. The mesenteric lymph nodes are numerous, often ranging between 100 and 150 lymph nodes that lie adjacent to their respective superior and inferior mesenteric arterial branches. This group drains the jejunum, ileum, and entire colon and rectum, including appendix. A few pararectal lymph nodes may drain via common iliac lymph nodes.

The lateral aortic group of the para-aortic lymph nodes is located lateral and posterior to the aorta and is responsible for draining the genitourinary organs. Its major lymphatic tributaries include the common, external, and internal iliac chains and inferior epigastric, circumflex iliac, and sacral vessels.

The retroaortic group of the para-aortic lymph nodes is located posterior to the aorta and has no discrete area of drainage other than possibly the posterior abdominal wall.

The paracaval group of lumbar lymphatics are located to the right of the vertebral bodies and up to 2 cm lateral to the vertebral body as seen on lymphangiogram. They are subdivided on the basis of their location to the inferior vena cava and include (1) precaval, (2) aortocaval, (3) retrocaval, and (4) lateral caval. Although the number of lymph nodes in the paracaval chain is greater than in the para-aortic chain, the number of paracaval lymph nodes seen on lymphangiogram is less. In about 70 per cent, the upper border of the paracaval chain is seen on lymphangiogram to be lower than the para-aortic chain; it is usually located at the L_3 level or below, although it may extend up to the L_2 in 20 per cent and L_1 in 10 per cent.

CISTERNA CHYLI AND THORACIC DUCT (Figs. 18–6 and 18–7)

The cisterna chyli is formed by the junction of the para-aortic and paracaval lymphatic trunks at about the T_{12} to L_2 level. It begins at the L_2 level in about 30 to 40 per cent, L_1 level in 40 to 50 per cent, and at T_{12} level in about 10 per cent. The cisterna chyli is about 5 to 7 cm in length and often has a beaded or ampullaceous configuration (Fig. 18–7*A*); its diameter is larger than that of the surrounding lymphatic vessels. It usually courses in the midline anterior to the spine and directly continues into the thoracic duct. It is seen on lymphangiography in up to 80 per cent. Rarely, the cisterna chyli may be absent and replaced by a network of small lumbar lymphatic trunks.

The thoracic duct begins at the upper end of the cisterna chyli at about the T_{12} level. It enters the thoracic cavity through the aortic hiatus of the diaphragm and courses anteriorly, slightly to the right of the thoracic spine in the posterior mediastinum to about the T_5 to T_6 level, where it crosses to the left. The thoracic duct is 38 to 45 cm in length. Its termination is variable, usually draining into the left internal jugular vein or junction of the left internal jugular and subclavian veins at about the C_7 level. Duplication of the thoracic duct occurs in about 10 per cent, with one duct coursing along each side of the aorta. Partial duplication is most frequent in the lower thoracic region. The thoracic duct can be divided into three parts—abdominal, thoracic, and cervical portions. The thoracic portion of the thoracic duct includes the segment from the aortic hiatus to the thoracic inlet. This portion of the thoracic duct connects with lymph nodes from the posterior mediastinum, thoracic wall, and heart. Occasionally, a hemithoracic duct is located to the left side of the main thoracic duct.

The cervical portion of the thoracic duct lies between the thoracic inlet and its termination in the venous system. The highest level the thoracic duct reaches is between C_6 and T_2. The cervical thoracic duct is a single vessel in 25 per cent of individuals, double in about 50 per cent, and between two and four vessels in the remainder. It drains into left-sided veins in 90 to 95 per cent, and in 1 to 5 per cent, it terminates into either right-sided or bilateral veins. On the left, it drains into the internal jugular vein in 60 per cent, subclavian vein in 15 per cent, between the external and internal jugular veins in 7 per cent, left innominate in 1.5 per cent, and between the external jugular and subclavian veins in less than 2.5 per cent. A valve is usually present at its venous insertion to prevent reflux of blood into the lymphatics. The sentinel lymph node at the terminal portion of the thoracic duct in the supraclavicular region is the Virchow-Troisier node (Fig. 18–7D). The cervical portion of the thoracic duct receives the left subclavian and left mediastinal lymphatic trunks draining the left arm, left hemithorax, left side of the head and neck, and occasionally the left bronchomediastinal trunk. A right-sided lymph vessel, which is about 1 cm in length, joins the junction of the right subclavian and internal jugular veins. This vessel receives the right-sided drainage from the head and neck, arm, hemithorax, heart, and superior portion of the liver bound by the coronary ligament.

LYMPHATICS OF UPPER EXTREMITIES, AXILLA, AND BREASTS (Figs. 18–8 and 18–9)

The superficial lymphatics in the upper extremities are greater in number than the deep; both deep and superficial lymphatics interconnect as in the lower extremities. In the forearm and arm, the superficial lymphatic vessels follow the superficial veins; the two main divisions are the ulnar (basilic or medial) group and the radial (cephalic or lateral) group. The ulnar group drains the third to fifth fingers and ulnar side of the hand and forearm. It then follows the basilic vein to the prefascial axillary lymph nodes; one or two lymphatics may join the deep subfascial lymphatics of the upper extremities. The radial group drains the first and second fingers and the radial side of the hand and forearm. It then follows the cephalic vein and enters the lateral group of axillary lymph nodes; a few lymphatics may enter the infraclavicular lymph nodes. The deep lymphatics of the arm follow the muscles, nerves, and deep vessels to terminate in the axillary lymph nodes.

The axillary lymph nodes are the first regional lymph nodes of the upper extremity and are divided into five groups: (1) lateral axillary, (2) anterior or pectoral, (3) posterior or subscapular, (4) central axillary, and (5) apical axillary groups. The lateral axillary group drains the majority of the arm except for that drained by the radial group. The anterior or pectoral group drains the skin and muscles of the anterolateral thoracic wall, part of abdominal wall, and most of the breasts. The posterior or subscapular group drains muscles and skin of the lower neck and posterior thorax. The apical axillary group drains lymphatics of the arm following the cephalic vein. Both central and apical axillary groups receive drainage from the other axillary lymphatic groups. Other axillary lymphatics drain into the subclavian, internal jugular, or deep cervical lymph nodes. In addition, the axillary lymph nodes receive about 75 per cent of the lymphatic drainage from the breasts. The remainder of the lymph from the medial and lateral portions of the breasts drains predominantly into the parasternal lymph nodes.

The thoracic viscera are drained by three major groups of lymphatics: the (1) brachiocephalic, (2) posterior mediastinal, and (3) tracheobronchial groups, which then join the thoracic duct. The brachiocephalic trunk drains the thymus (also drained by tracheobronchial and parasternal groups), thyroid, pericardium, and lateral diaphragmatic lymph nodes; it then joins the right and left bronchomediastinal trunk. The posterior mediastinal group drains the esophagus (also drained by deep cervical group), posterior pericardium, diaphragm, lateral and posterior diaphragmatic, and occasionally left hepatic lobe lymph nodes; it then joins the thoracic duct or occasionally the tracheobronchial lymph nodes. The tracheobronchial lymph nodes are some of the largest in the body and consist of five main groups: (1) paratracheal, (2) superior tracheobronchial, (3) inferior tracheobronchial, (4) bronchopulmonary (hilar), and (5) pulmonary lymph nodes. The lungs and pleura are drained by superficial and deep lymphatics; both then drain into hilar lymph nodes. The superficial group drains the borders of the lungs, visceral pleura, and fissures. The deep group follows the pulmonary arteries and bronchi. The parietal pleura drains into the parasternal and posterior mediastinal lymph nodes.

The heart is drained by three lymphatic plexuses, which include the (1) subcardial, (2) myocardial, and (3) subepicardial groups. In addition, the left side of the heart, including portions of both ventricles, drains into tracheobronchial lymph nodes. The right side of the heart, including the right atrium and right border of the right ventricle, drains into the brachiocephalic lymph nodes.

LYMPHATICS OF THE HEAD AND NECK (Fig. 18–10)

In the head and neck, most of the superficial tissues drain into local lymph node groups, which then enter the deep cervical lymph nodes. Major regional lymph node groups of the head include the occipital, retroauricular, parotid, and buccal groups. Regional lymph nodes of the neck include the submandibular, submental, anterior cervical, and superficial cervical groups. Much of the face is drained by the submandibular group. The mouth, teeth, tonsils, and tongue are drained by submandibular, deep cervical, retropharyngeal, and submental lymph nodes. The nasal cavity, nasopharynx, pharynx, and middle ear drain into submandibular, deep cervical, or retropharyngeal lymph node groups. The posterior portion of the nasal cavity may drain into parotid nodes. The pharynx and cervical esophagus drain into the cervical, retropharyngeal, or paratracheal groups. The larynx drains into deep cervical or occasionally pretracheal and prelaryngeal lymph nodes. The cervical trachea drains into pretracheal, paratracheal, or deep cervical nodes. The thyroid drains via the tracheal plexus into the prelaryngeal, pretracheal, and paratracheal and deep cervical nodes.

The deep cervical group of lymph nodes lies along the carotid sheath and drains the entire head and neck. The deep soft tissues of the head and neck usually drain into deep cervical nodes directly or indirectly via adjacent lymphatic groups, which include the retropharyngeal, pretracheal, lingual, infrahyoid, prelaryngeal, and pretracheal nodes. Efferent lymphatics from the deep cervical group form the jugular trunks bilaterally. The right jugular trunk drains into the junction of the right subclavian and internal jugular veins or right lymphatic duct. The left jugular trunk drains into the thoracic duct or occasionally into internal jugular or subclavian veins.

REFERENCES

1. Fischer HW, Zimmerman GR: Roentgenographic visualization of lymph nodes and lymphatic channels. AJR 81:517–534, 1959.
2. Fischer HW, Lawrence MS, Thornbury JR: Lymphography of the normal adult male: observations and their relation to the diagnosis of metastatic neoplasm. Radiology 78:399–406, 1962.
3. Greening RR, Wallace S: Further observations in lymphangiography. RCNA, 1:157–173, 1963.
4. Gregl VA, Heitmann D: Indikation zur Lymphographie in der Urologie unter besonderer Berucksichtigung des Peniskarzinoms. Fortschr Rontgenstr 126:339–344, 1977.
5. Herman PG, Benninghoff DL, Nelson JH, Mellins HZ: Roentgen anatomy of the ilio-pelvic-aortic lymphatic system. Radiology 80:182–193, 1963.
6. Larson DL, Lewis SR: Deep lymphatic system of the lower extremity. Am J Surg 113:217–220, 1967.
7. Lechner VG, Riedl P, Zechner O: Zum Mechanismus der Kontrastmitteldarstellung der Leber nach Lymphographie. Fortschr Rontgenstr 125:355–357, 1976.
8. Malek P, Kolc J, Belan A: Lymphography of the deep lymphatic system of the thigh. Acta Radiol 51:422–428, 1959.
9. Matoba N, Kikuchi T: Thyroidolymphography: A new technic for visualization of the thyroid and cervical lymph nodes. Radiology, 92:339–342, 1969.
10. Merrin C, Wajsman Z, Baumgartner G, Jennings E: The clinical value of lymphangiography: Are the nodes surrounding the obturator nerve visualized? J Urol 117:762–764, 1977.
11. Roth VS, Vielhauer E, Ludwig KG, Haberich H: Indirekte Lymphographie der retrosternalen Lymphbahnen und des Ductus thoracicus. Fortschr Rontgenstr 125:349–351, 1976.
12. Steckel RJ, Cameron TP: Changes in lymph node size induced by lymphangiography. Radiology 87:753–755, 1966.
13. Vitek J, Kaspar Z: The radiology of the deep lymphatic system of the leg. Brit J Rad 46:120–124, 1973.

Figures 18–1 through 18–10 on following pages.

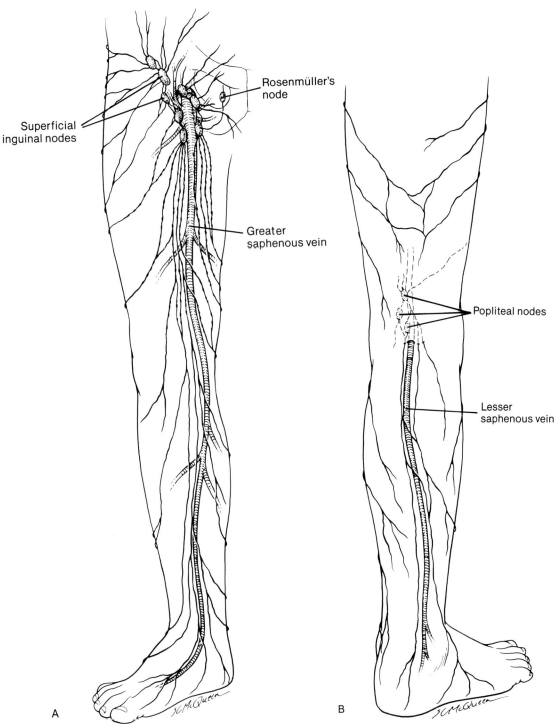

Figure 18–1. The lymph channels of the lower extremity. *A,* Medial superficial
lymphatics. *B,* Lateral superficial lymphatics.

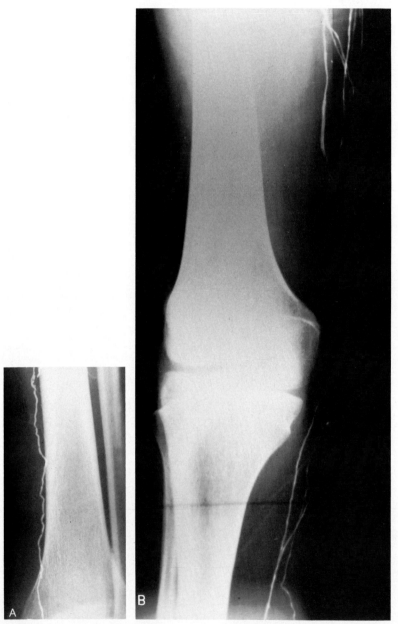

Figure 18–2. Radiographs illustrating normal lymph channels. *A* and *B,* Along lower leg. *C,* Along the upper thigh. Arrows point to extravasation of contrast medium.

Illustration continued on opposite page.

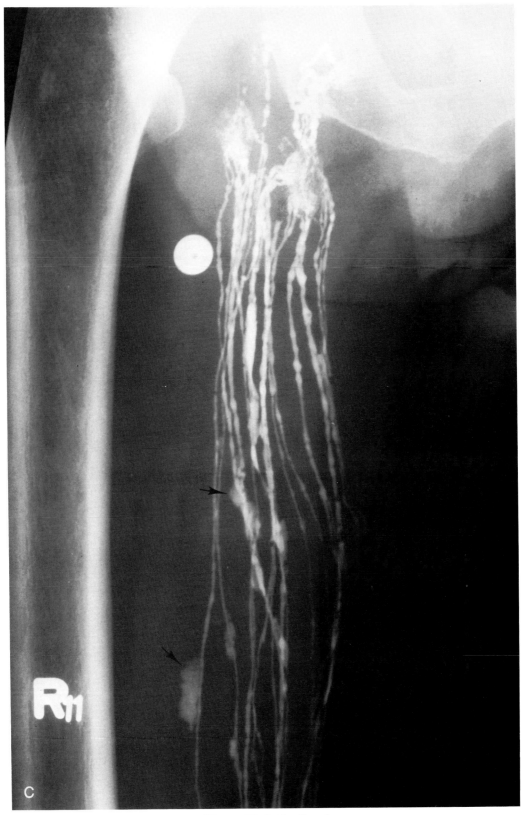

Figure 18–2. *Continued.*

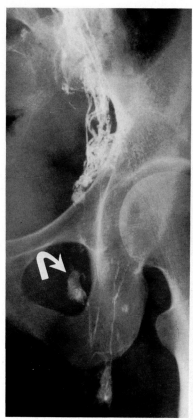

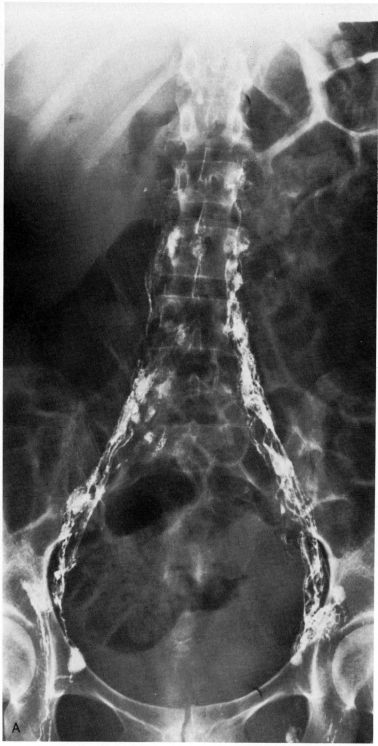

Figure 18–3. Node of Rosenmüller (*curved arrow*). (From Kadir S: Diagnostic Angiography. Philadelphia, WB Saunders Company, 1986.)

A

Figure 18–4. *Legend on opposite page.*

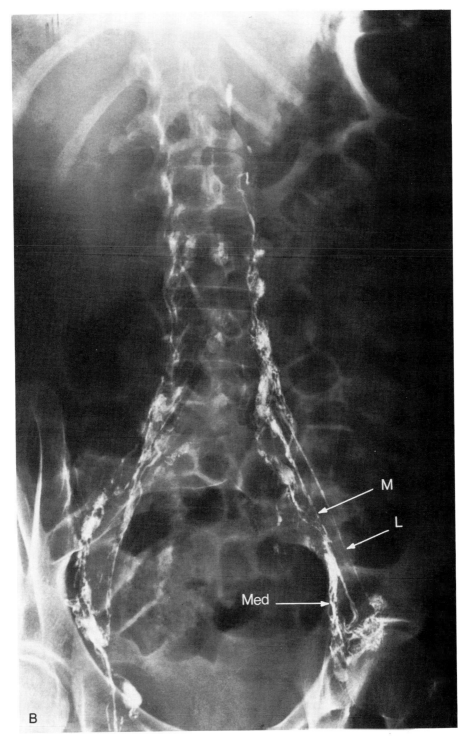

Figure 18–4. Channel phase of normal bipedal lymphangiogram. *A*, Anteroposterior view. *B*, Left posterior oblique view.

L   Lateral
M   Middle
Med Medial lymphatic channels

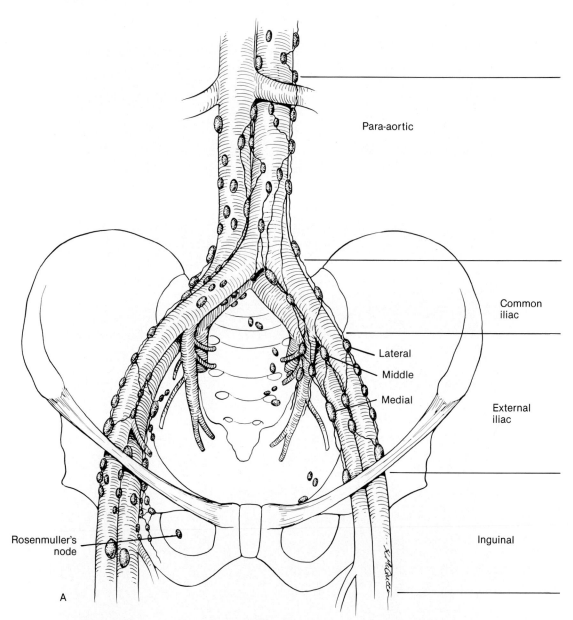

Figure 18–5. *A* and *B,* Diagrams illustrating the lymph nodes visualized on petal lymphangiography. *C* to *G,* AP, LPO, RPO, and lateral abdominal and pelvic radiographs showing the nodal phase.

Illustration continued on opposite page.

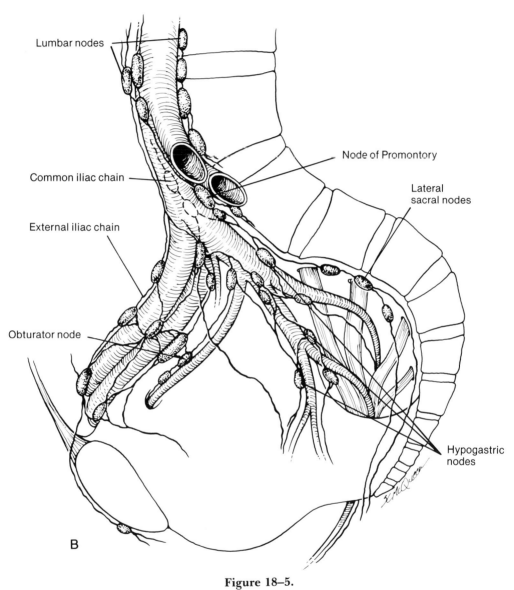

Lumbar nodes

Common iliac chain

External iliac chain

Obturator node

Node of Promontory

Lateral
sacral nodes

Hypogastric
nodes

B

Figure 18–5.

Illustration continued on following page.

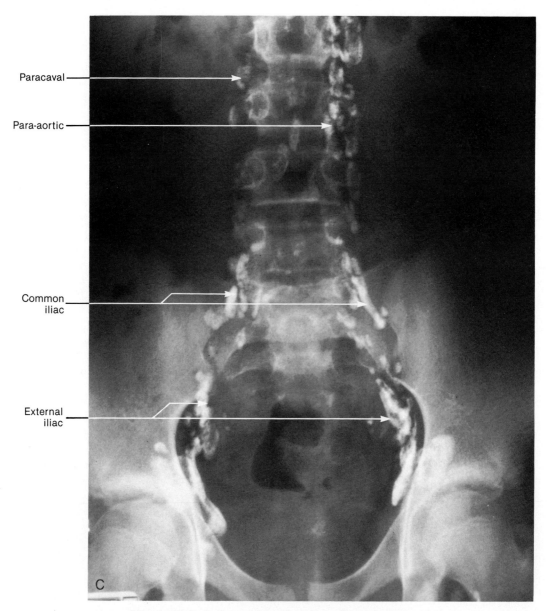

Paracaval

Para-aortic

Common
iliac

External
iliac

C

Figure 18–5. *C*, Anteroposterior view of nodal phase.

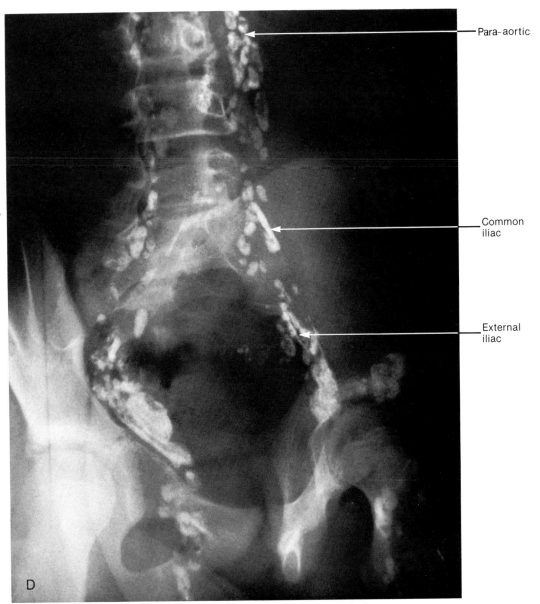

Para-aortic

Common
iliac

External
iliac

D

Figure 18–5. *D*, LPO view of nodal phase.

Illustration continued on following page.

Paracaval

Para–aortic

Common
iliac

External
iliac

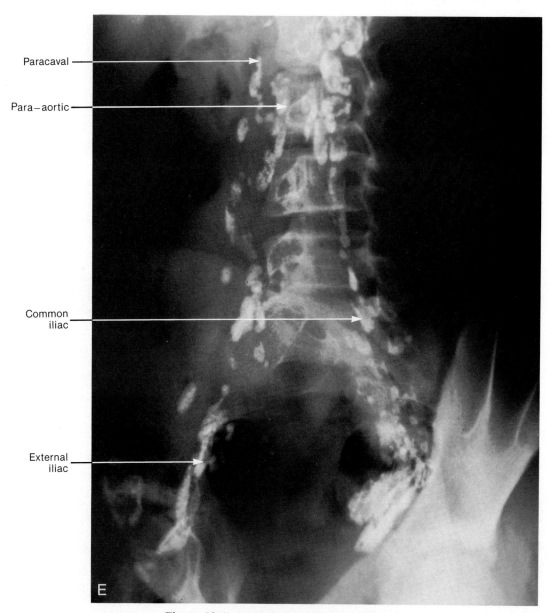

Figure 18–5. *E*, RPO view of nodal phase.

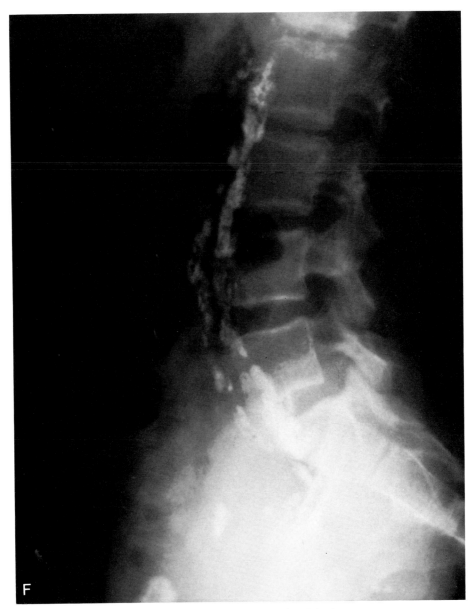

Figure 18–5. *F*, Lateral view of nodal phase.

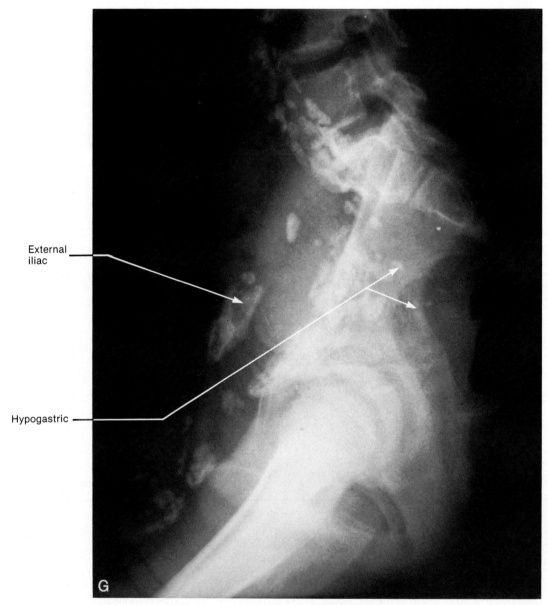

External
iliac

Hypogastric

Figure 18–5. *G,* Lateral view of pelvic nodes.

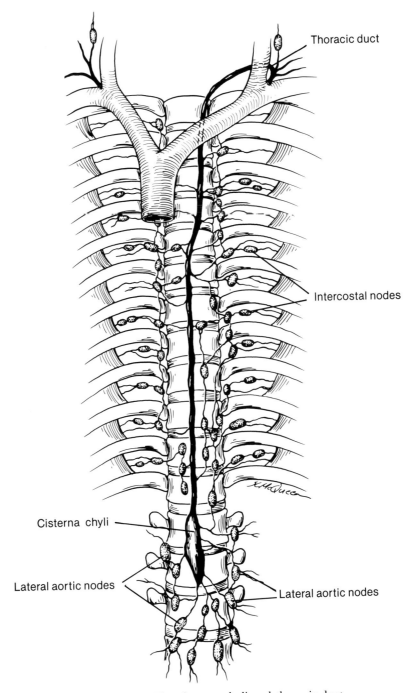

Figure 18–6. The cisterna chyli and thoracic duct.

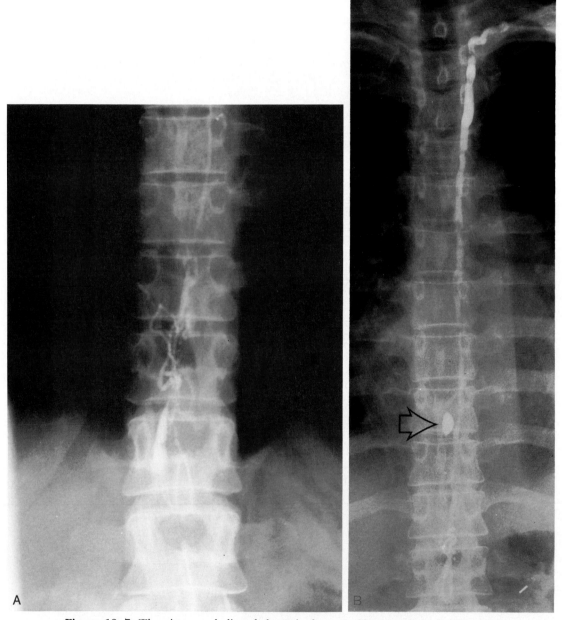

Figure 18–7. The cisterna chyli and thoracic duct. *A,* Cisterna chyli. *B,* Thoracic duct. *C,* Thoracic duct in another individual. *D,* Virchow's node *(arrows).*

Illustration continued on opposite page.

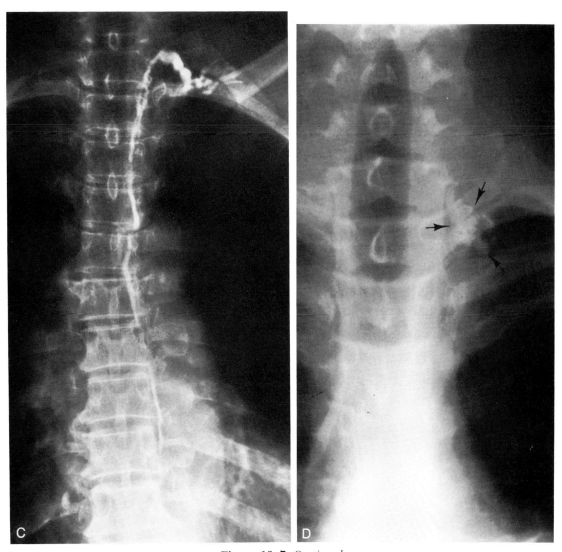

Figure 18–7. *Continued.*

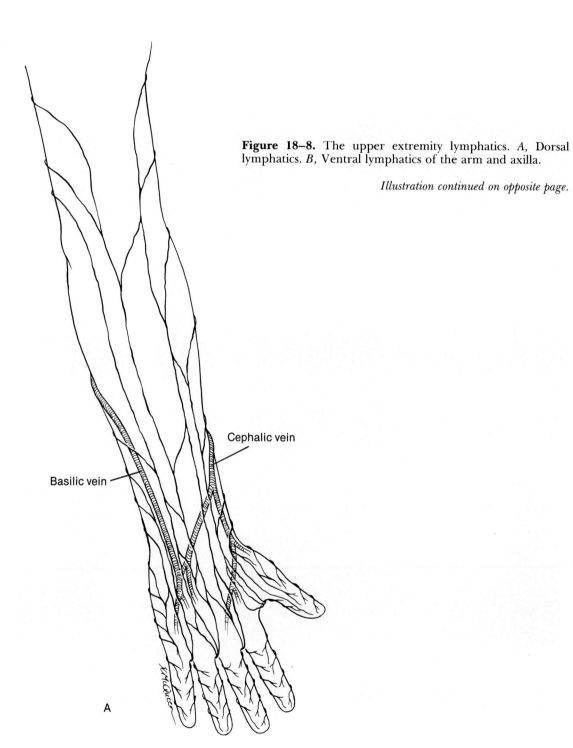

Figure 18–8. The upper extremity lymphatics. *A,* Dorsal lymphatics. *B,* Ventral lymphatics of the arm and axilla.

Illustration continued on opposite page.

Cephalic vein

Basilic vein

A

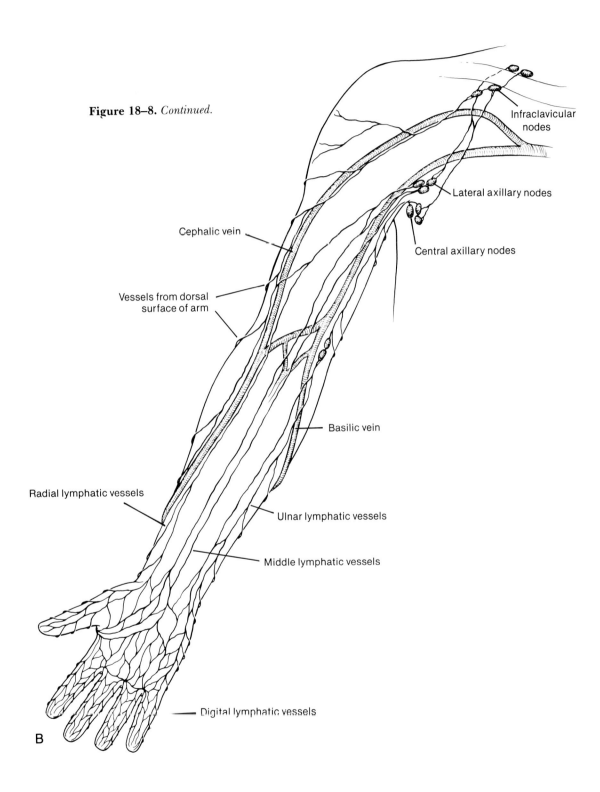

Figure 18–8. *Continued.*

Infraclavicular nodes

Lateral axillary nodes

Cephalic vein

Central axillary nodes

Vessels from dorsal surface of arm

Basilic vein

Radial lymphatic vessels

Ulnar lymphatic vessels

Middle lymphatic vessels

Digital lymphatic vessels

B

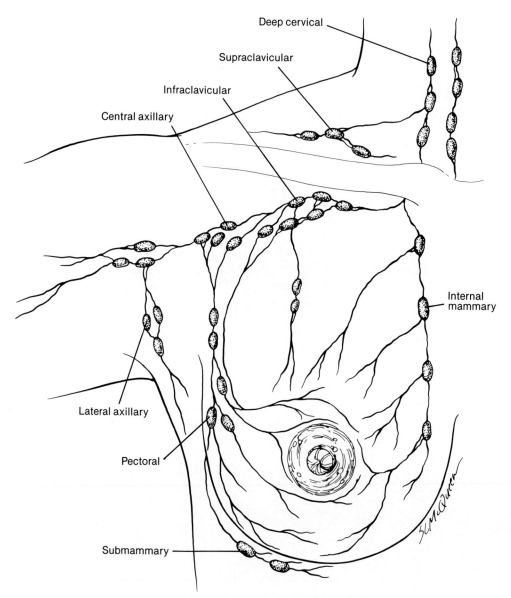

Figure 18–9. Lymph drainage of the female breast.

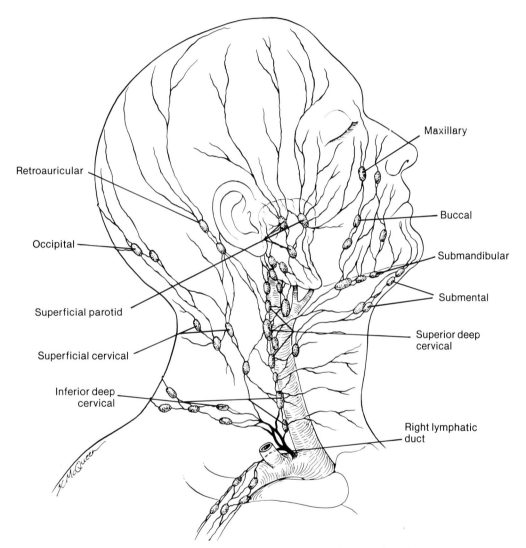

Figure 18–10. Lymphatic drainage of the head and neck.

INDEX

Note: Page numbers in *italics* refer to illustrations; page numbers followed by t refer to tables.